Clinical Decisions and Laboratory Use

Publications in the Health Sciences

Publication of this book was assisted
by a McKnight Foundation grant to the
University of Minnesota Press's program
in the health sciences.

Clinical Decisions and Laboratory Use

edited by *Donald P. Connelly,*
Ellis S. Benson, M. Desmond Burke,
and *Douglas Fenderson*

University of Minnesota
Continuing Medical Education
Volume I

University of Minnesota Press □ Minneapolis

Published by the University of Minnesota Press,
2037 University Avenue Southeast, Minneapolis, MN 55414
Printed in the United States of America.

Library of Congress Cataloging in Publication Data
Main entry under title:

Clinical decisions and laboratory use.

    (University of Minnesota continuing medical education;
v. 1) (Publications in the health sciences)
    Includes index.
    1. Medicine, Clinical—Decision making. 2. Medical
laboratories—Utilization. 3. Diagnosis, Laboratory.
I. Connelly, Donald P. II. Series. III. Series: Publications
in the health sciences. [DNLM: 1. Decision making. 2. Diagnosis,
Laboratory—Methods. 3. Laboratories—Utilization.
W1 UN944T v.1 / QY 4 C58]
RC48.C53   616   81-19825
ISBN 0-8166-1001-0   AACR2

Contents

Contributors

Adelin Albert, PhD
Department of Clinical Chemistry
University of Liège
Liège, Belgium

Charles H. Altshuler, MD
Department of Pathology
St. Joseph's Hospital
Medical College of Wisconsin
Milwaukee, Wisconsin

Barbara J. Andrew, PhD
National Board of Medical Examiners
Philadelphia, Pennsylvania

Ellis S. Benson, MD
Department of Laboratory Medicine
    and Pathology
University of Minnesota Medical School
Minneapolis, Minnesota

M. Desmond Burke, MD
Department of Pathology
Health Sciences Center School of
    Medicine
State University of New York
    at Stonybrook
Stonybrook, New York

Joyce A. Campbell, MD
Clinical Pathology Service
Veterans Administration Medical
    Center
Portland, Oregon

Jean-Paul Chapelle, PhD
Department of Clinical Chemistry
University of Liège
Liège, Belgium

Donald P. Connelly, MD, PhD
Department of Laboratory Medicine
    and Pathology
University of Minnesota Medical School
Minneapolis, Minnesota

John M. Eisenberg, MD, MBA
Section of General Medicine
Department of Medicine
University of Pennsylvania School
    of Medicine
Philadelphia, Pennsylvania

Arthur S. Elstein, PhD
Office of Medical Education Research
    and Development
Michigan State University College of
    Human Medicine
East Lansing, Michigan

Douglas A. Fenderson, PhD
Office of Continuing Medical Education
University of Minnesota Medical School
Minneapolis, Minnesota

Thomas F. Ferris, MD
Department of Medicine
University of Minnesota Medical School
Minneapolis, Minnesota

William R. Fifer, MD
Center for Health Services Research
University of Minnesota School of
  Public Health
Minneapolis, Minnesota

Stan N. Finkelstein, MD
Alfred P. Sloan School of Management
Massachusetts Institute of Technology
Cambridge, Massachusetts

Howard S. Frazier, MD
Center for the Analysis of Health
  Practices
Harvard School of Public Health and
  Harvard Medical School
Boston, Massachusetts

Robert S. Galen, MD, MPH
Department of Pathology
Overlook Hospital
The Columbia University College of
  Physicians and Surgeons
Summit, New Jersey

Werner A. Gliebe, MA
Health Systems Agency of Northeast
  Kansas
Topeka, Kansas

Stephen E. Goldfinger, MD
Department of Continuing Education
Harvard Medical School
Boston, Massachusetts

G. Anthony Gorry, PhD
Baylor College of Medicine
Houston, Texas

Paul F. Griner, MD
Department of Medicine
University of Rochester School of
  Medicine and Dentistry
Rochester, New York

Ilene B. Harris, PhD
Office of Curriculum Affairs
University of Minnesota Medical School
Minneapolis, Minnesota

Joseph Henny, PhD
Center of Preventive Medicine
Vandoeuvre-les-Nancy, France

Camille Heusghem, PhD
Department of Clinical Chemistry
University of Liège
Liège, Belgium

Margaret M. Holmes, PhD
Office of Medical Education Research
  and Development
Michigan State University College of
  Human Medicine
East Lansing, Michigan

Gerald B. Holtzman, MD
Office of Medical Education Research
  and Development and
  the Department of Obstetrics
  and Gynecology
Michigan State University College of
  Human Medicine
East Lansing, Michigan

Penny A. Jennett, MA
Office of Medical Education Research
  and Development
Michigan State University College of
  Human Medicine
East Lansing, Michigan

Eugene A. Johnson, PhD
Division of Biometry
University of Minnesota School of
  Public Health
Minneapolis, Minnesota

Paul E. Johnson, PhD
Department of Management Sciences
University of Minnesota School of
  Management
Minneapolis, Minnesota

Jerome P. Kassirer, MD
Department of Medicine
Tufts University School of Medicine
Boston, Massachusetts

Anthony L. Komaroff, MD
Laboratory for the Analysis of Medical
   Practices
Harvard Medical School and
   Harvard School of Public Health
Brigham and Women's Hospital
Boston, Massachusetts

John E. Kralewski, PhD
Center for Health Services Research
University of Minnesota School of
   Public Health
Minneapolis, Minnesota

Michael T. Makler, MD
Clinical Pathology Service
Veterans Administration Medical
   Center
Portland, Oregon

Barbara J. McNeil, MD, PhD
Division of Nuclear Medicine
Harvard Medical School Department
   of Radiology
Brigham and Women's Hospital
Boston, Massachusetts

Randolph A. Miller, MD
Department of Medicine
University of Pittsburgh School of
   Medicine
Pittsburgh, Pennsylvania

Robert E. Miller, MD
Department of Laboratory Medicine
The Johns Hopkins University School
   of Medicine
Baltimore, Maryland

John M. Murray, MD, D.Sc.
Department of Medicine
University of Minnesota Medical School
Minneapolis, Minnesota

Jack D. Myers, MD
Department of Medicine
University of Pittsburgh School of
   Medicine
Pittsburgh, Pennsylvania

Lynn E. Neitz, BS
Department of Laboratory Medicine
   and Pathology
University of Minnesota Medical School
Minneapolis, Minnesota

Theodore M. Pass, PhD
Laboratory for the Analysis of Medical
   Practices
Brigham and Women's Hospital
Boston, Massachusetts

Stephen G. Pauker, MD
Department of Medicine
Tufts University School of Medicine
Boston, Massachusetts

Harry E. Pople, Jr., PhD
University of Pittsburgh Graduate
   School of Business
Pittsburgh, Pennsylvania

Michael M. Ravitch, PhD
Office of Medical Education Research
   and Development
Michigan State University College of
   Human Medicine
East Lansing, Michigan

Stanley J. Reiser, MD, PhD
Program in the History of Medicine
Harvard Medical School
Boston, Massachusetts

David R. Rovner, MD
Office of Medical Education Research
   and Development and
   the Department of Medicine
Michigan State University College of
   Human Medicine
East Lansing, Michigan

Philip N. St. Louis, BS
Department of Laboratory Medicine
   and Pathology
University of Minnesota Medical School
Minneapolis, Minnesota

Herbert Sherman, DEE
Harvard School of Public Health

and Harvard Medical School
Brigham and Women's Hospital
Boston, Massachusetts

Gerard Siest, PhD
Center of Preventive Medicine
Vandoeuvre-les-Nancy, France,
and
Laboratory of Pharmacological
  Biochemistry
University of Nancy
Nancy, France

Harold C. Sox, Jr., MD
Department of Medicine
Stanford University School of
  Medicine
Palo Alto, California

Eugene A. Stead, Jr., MD
Department of Medicine
Duke University School of Medicine
Durham, North Carolina

Homer R. Warner, MD, PhD
Department of Biophysics and
  Bioengineering
University of Utah College of Medicine
LDS Hospital
Salt Lake City, Utah

Lawrence L. Weed, MD
Department of Medicine
University of Vermont College of
  Medicine
Burlington, Vermont

John H. Westerman, MHA
Hospital Administration
University of Minnesota Hospitals
  and Clinics
Minneapolis, Minnesota

Donald S. Young, MB, PhD
Department of Laboratory Medicine
Mayo Medical School
Rochester, Minnesota

Preface

Appropriate utilization of diagnostic services is one of the more complex problems facing medicine today. The escalating cost of health care and the public's desire to contain costs adds urgency to the need to examine the use of diagnostic services, including clinical laboratory services. In addition to the major effect of inflation, much of the increase in clinical laboratory expenditures has arisen from the expanding laboratory workload. Recurring concerns have been expressed that a significant fraction of the workload growth is inappropriate and not beneficial to the care of the patient. However, translating this concern into studies that will foster understanding and effective action is no easy task. During a period in which health care costs have skyrocketed and laboratory testing has proliferated, this relatively new field of research endeavor has grown in importance.

Drawn together by this concern, a small planning group was formed in the fall of 1978 to develop a conference that would focus on the many important issues of clinical use of the laboratory. The aim of the conference developers was to promote the exposition and synthesis of current knowledge by bringing together key researchers, medical educators, clinicians, laboratory directors and health systems planners. The efforts of the planning committee, the commitment, zeal, and cooperation of the scholars studying various aspects of clinical decision making, and a stimulating group of attendees brought into being the Conference on Clinical Decision Making and Laboratory Use held in Minneapolis, June 9-11, 1980, from which this book has been developed.

This book is divided into six major sections. The first section (Chapters 1-4) establishes perspective and a general basis for our concern for effective use of the clinical laboratory resource. This section sets the stage for the rest of the book, describing challenges as well as obstacles, answers and dilemmas, great potential but also surprising limitations.

Section II (Chapters 5-8) reflects the contention of the conference organizers that improved laboratory use will come through a better understanding of clinical decision processes. Strategies for improved test selection and laboratory use will be most acceptable if they can be integrated smoothly into established patterns of clinical practice. There are many extremely important reasons to study the process of medical decision making. In defining the process, if a unified definition can be formulated, medical educators should be able to help students develop clinical reasoning skills. It would be far easier to teach clinical decision-making skills to novices if the steps were clear and concrete. If the most effective principles and strategies of clinical reasoning can be discerned, then methods that enhance decision-making skills can be developed, enabling more efficient patient care. Finally, if the decision-making process were understood, decision-making aids might be incorporated more smoothly and effectively into the process.

Section III (Chapters 9-13) explores the role of the laboratory, the use of tests, and the effectiveness of such use in clinical decision making. Assessing the efficacy of clinical decision making, as it is related to the use of the clinical laboratory, presents major methodological challenges. Approaches used in health care quality assessment may prove helpful in developing methods for studying laboratory use. The identification of more nearly optimal strategies will require some means of assessing the effectiveness of laboratory use and the evaluation of alternative approaches.

Medical education appears to be a key determinant in effective laboratory utilization and is the focus of Section IV (Chapters 14-18). Physicians must be educated to promote the adoption of more rational approaches to the use of laboratory resources. The major educational burden must be borne by those teaching medical students and residents, for at this stage lifelong patterns of use are developed. Physician education at all career stages is important.

With the rapid changes in and increasing complexity of medical science, educational efforts cannot be the sole means of promoting more nearly optimal laboratory use. Prescriptive decision tools using decision theory, statistics, protocols, automated decision support systems, and artificial intelligence are now beginning to be applied to problems of laboratory use. A number of these tools are described in Section V (Chapters 19-26). Such tools must be proved clinically effective and be smoothly integrated into the decision-making process before wide acceptance and positive influence can be expected.

The last section (Chapters 27-32) discusses a number of recent projects related to the theme of this book. Research efforts identifying the causes of inappropriate laboratory use and evaluating means of effecting more appropriate use are growing in number. Further development of practical research methodologies is critically needed. Research findings related to laboratory use and clinical medicine must be rapidly disseminated; techniques that improve such use must be applied in other settings to benefit patient care and reduce costs.

It is our hope that this book will provide a useful synthesis of the ideas presented at the conference; we attempted to foster such a synthesis among the conference participants through the Nominal Group Process technique. This technique is designed to promote the generation of useful ideas within a group and allow a sort of consensus to be reached about important issues. The results of this process are presented in the final chapter of this book. Although these results were obtained with some controversy and concern about the approach used to gain consensus, we hope that the prudent reader will gain from a careful and critical reading of this chapter.

The discussion periods in any conference often focus on the most current and important concerns related to a general problem. In the appendix the discussion emanating from four panels are presented. For the convenience of the reader, the order of the discussion has been modified so that, for the most part, the questions and answers parallel the order of the chapters in this book.

The development and implementation of a conference and book like this one depends on the efforts of many individuals and groups. We thank especially those groups that helped sponsor the conference and publication of the proceedings. Among these groups are the Kaiser Family Foundation, the National Center for Health Services Research, the General Mills Foundation, and the Board of Governors of the University of Minnesota Hospitals. Though their generous support does not suggest endorsement of any one view, it is indicative of an important concern and commitment on their part that is deeply appreciated. For their contributions of ideas, hard work, and commitment, we recognize Drs. Paul Griner, G. Anthony Gorry, and John Kralewski who joined us in making up the conference planning group. We acknowledge our indebtedness to the conference participants and other attendees. The superb cooperation of our contributors has allowed the generation of this book.

Members of the support groups at the University of Minnesota, especially Darla Eckroth of the Continuing Medical Education Office and Richard Abel of the University of Minnesota Press, have provided outstanding advice, guidance, and service at every step. We are most grateful for the help that Dr. Eileen Harris of the Medical School Curriculum Office provided in implementing the nominal group process sessions.

This book is dedicated to the researchers, educators, clinicians, pathologists, and planners who choose to read it. Our sincere hope is that this publication is useful to you, the reader, in providing information and facilitating new directions of thought. If this book serves as a stepping stone to new knowledge, we have achieved our goals.

Section I. Medical Decisions, Technology, and Social Needs

CHAPTER ONE

Medical Technology and Public Policy

John E. Kralewski, PhD, and
John H. Westerman, MHA

One of the most important public policy issues in the health care field today centers on the appropriate use of state of the art technology. Since the National Institutes of Health were formally established in the 1930s, federal public policies favoring technological development have dominated the health field. In the mid 1960s, growing concern over the distribution of health services caused a slight but highly publicized shift in these policies as a number of governmental programs, such as the Regional Medical programs, were initiated to expedite the diffusion of technologies from research and teaching centers to the field of practice. These policies were assumed efficacious and concentrated on distribution of services and access to care. The major concern at that time was the growing dissatisfaction over perceived inequities in access to health services and the effective distribution of medical know-how from research centers to the field of practice.[1] Little attention was devoted to the costs associated with those technologies and the relative benefits derived from their use. More was considered better. Physicians largely trained in high technology medical centers welcomed this trend and encouraged hospitals to adopt these innovations indiscriminately. Hospitals noting the potential for economic growth and prestige were all too willing to comply and furnished the economic and organizational environment for what soon became a technology-driven system.

As a result, physicians became increasingly technology dependent, both through training and practice, and as health insurance coverage removed financial constraints, lucrative markets were created (and, according to some, exploited) by the so-called medical/industrial complex.[2] Physicians were consequently encouraged by patient expectations, financial incentives, and peer pressures to use—in many cases overuse—medical services in general, especially the high technologies. As is the case in any decision-making process, clinicians want to gain as much knowledge as possible about a patient and therefore tend to use every means of gathering information available to them. Their professional values further this process by committing clinicians to do everything possible for patients, regardless of the costs and potential benefits. As Dr. Relman aptly noted in a recent paper:[3]

> Physicians have the habit of wanting to know as much as possible about a patient and wanting to do something for him if there is any possible chance of benefit. The latter sentiment, if not the former, is certainly shared by patients.

This orientation, coupled with the fact that physicians are the consumers of medical resources in the economic sense and are, therefore, suppliers who determine, and in fact create, demand, has caused alarming increases in health care costs. The overuse and the misuse of these technologies also have disturbing quality-of-care implications, since often some risk is associated with their use. In this context and specifically relating to laboratory technology, one author recently noted that[4]

> The excessive and inappropriate use of laboratory facilities is a step toward domination by technology since the physician abandons his self-confidence, judgment and reasoning powers and unnecessarily exposes his patients to degrading, painful or dangerous diagnostic procedures.

The prospects of a national health insurance program that may further reduce financial constraints and the potential surplus of physicians, threatens to greatly exacerbate these quality and cost problems in the future.

The cost dimension is rapidly becoming the number one national issue. During this past decade the cost of personal health services has increased nearly threefold and is now estimated to be over $185 billion annually.[5] This represents an average of $822 per person, and this sum continues to grow at about 13 percent per year. Although inflation accounts for a great portion of this increase, changes in intensity largely reflecting technological development accounted for about 25 percent of the cost increases during the 12-month period ending September, 1979. According to Health Care Financing Administration data, cost increases due to changes in intensity since 1969 represent an estimated $30 billion in today's health care budget.[6] Clinical laboratory tests are growing by about 15 percent per year; diagnostic radiologic procedures now consume nearly $10 billion of today's personal health services budget; and the number of coronary bypass operations and total hip replacements are rapidly expanding—these are but a few examples of intensity changes underlying these cost increases.[7,8]

Although few people seriously propose to curtail technological development in the health field, considerable public concern has been expressed over this cost picture, and the realization is growing that for the first time in the United States, health services may soon be rationed by resource constraints. Other industrialized countries have, of course, rationed services for the past two decades with varying degreees of success, usually by limiting the supply of high-cost specialty services.[9]

Waiting lists have proved to be effective methods of allocating scarce resources; to some degree, they also increase the effective use of technologies as clinicians attempt to gain maximum benefit from their fixed resource. Clearly, however, major equity and quality questions are inherent in this approach, since its focus is rationing rather than the benefits of the technologies and procedures and the effective use of resources. Current cost containment policies in the United States appear to be ignoring these potential problems. Those favoring the market approach believe that restructuring the health care system to enhance competition through market forces will serve to allocate scarce resources in an effective and efficient manner. Much of this effort is focused on HMOs and other competitive health care programs and the development of health insurance plans designed to provide consumers incentives. These incentives take the form of consumer choice in the selection of the level of benefits and choice of vendor.[10] Others, less impressed with the free market performance in the human services fields, believe government control and regulations to be the answer with a national health insurance program being the main mechanism to that end.[11-13]

As is usually the case in public policy formation, the resultant health policy will likely be a mixture of these rather divergent approaches. The fundamental difficulty with these policies, however, is that they fail to address the real issue underlying cost containment and attempt to obtain optimal utilization of highly complex technologies and procedures through economic marketplace pressures and/or rationing through regulation. Both will likely reduce utilization but may do so at the expense of quality and equity in access to health care rather than selectively reducing ineffective services. Under the competitive systems, this solution could result in substantial inequities in the distribution of services, with the wealthy using a disproportionate share of the resources. It could also lead to two systems of care, reminiscent of the past, with underutilization of technology for low income groups and overutilization for the wealthy. It seems evident, therefore, that to protect the equity gains achieved in health services during the past two decades and improve quality of care under conditions of constrained resources, public policy must be focused on the cost and benefits of the clinical techniques, procedures, and technologies and on the clinical decision-making process. These judgments must derive from cost considerations coupled with clinical evidence of the benefits of the procedures and must therefore mix economic and clinical research. A program such as this, linked with provider incentives to improve the efficiency of the health care delivery system, will create a receptive environment for the effective utilization of technologies and will protect quality and access to appropriate services as it reduces costs. Public policy must, therefore, consider both the incentives for clinicians to practice cost-effective medicine and the development and provision of adequate cost/benefit information to facilitate their decision-making process.

At the national level, beginning efforts to formulate policies reflecting these values are evident. The formation of the National Center for Health Care Technology to initiate studies focused on technology assessment, the medical practice evaluation studies funded by the National Center for Health Services Research, and the cost/benefit research sponsored by NIH are some tangible examples of the efficacy dimensions of this policy initiative. The HMO legislation and Senator Durenberger's Health Incentive Reform Act, designed to provide consumers and providers incentives to reduce costs are collateral policy initiatives focused on theses issues.[14] These initiatives are serving to clarify the policy issues surrounding the general theme of clinical decision making and technology assessment. The first of these policy subsets focuses on cost containment, taking into account the use of services and the cost of those services. The second deals with the appropriate use of existing high cost technologies that have been proved effective. Who will be authorized to use these technologies, under what circumstances should they be used, what guidelines should be developed to control the use, who should develop those guidelines, and how should those who use these technologies be reimbursed for their services are some of the policy questions being considered. A third set of policy questions focuses on the character and style of medical practice. Should medical practice be changed to reduce dependency on even the low cost technologies? Is it realistic or desirable to expect practitioners to bring the element of cost into the clinical decision-making process and if so, how?—through incentives, education, regulation, or all of these, and perhaps other means as well? A fourth set of policy concerns centers on control of newly developed technologies. These policies deal with the need to assure the efficacy of new technology in the future, before it is introduced into the field, and its equitable distribution once approved. Who should control this process and the dissemination of the proven technology, determine its location in the field (physician offices, hospital HMO, etc.), control its use, and establish reimbursement rates are issues relevant to this policy area.

In view of this range of issues, some policy analysts believe these federal initiatives to be far too limited to meet the challenge of the 1980s. Kane,[15] for example, noting the inability of the field to limit utilization, suggests a national policy wherein third party payers at both the federal and local levels would not reimburse for services that use new technology until that technology was proved effective by controlled clinical trials. He further suggests selected institutions be designated to conduct those studies for the health care system. Although these suggestions appear radical in today's social, economic, and political environment, they probably portend future policy unless the field of practice exercises its presently available options and captures the initiative in the medical practice assessment arena. And yet the general theme of most health solutions is to avoid government intervention and rely on nongovernmental approaches to problem solving. Clearly, the decade of the '80s will focus much of the policymakers' attention and effort on these issues. Many policy analysts foresee the converging forces of (1) a rapidly expanding population in the over 60 age group (who use three to four times the health care resources as those under 60), (2) increased expansion of health insurance coverage through continued union and management support for nontaxable worker benefits, and (3) the highest ratio of physicians to population since the Flexner studies; all of these forces occur during an era of continued technological expansion, constituting one of the most serious threats yet encountered to the survival of private sector medicine. A major effort must be initiated nationwide by the private sector to meet this challenge and help shape the policies guiding the allocation of medical care resources in the future. Two important considerations must be underscored in this regard. First, the nature of public policy dictates that policy decisions *will* be made in this, as in other arenas, regardless of the availability of information on which to base those decisions or assure their success. Policy is made with or without good policy analysis and information. Second, without these data, policies tend to be made by default and to reflect a much higher degree of political influence.

Health science centers and academic teaching hospitals within those centers provide one of the most promising environments for these research and development activities. First of all, major gains in the effectiveness of resource allocation by clinicians will be accomplished only by integrating those skills and values in their medical education program. University hospitals provide the basic laboratory for this process and therefore have an excellent opportunity to work with medical schools to influence future clinicians' orientation toward the practice of cost-effective medicine. Second, few institutions have the capacity and capabilities of the university hospitals to mount a technology assessment program. These hospitals have proven research track records, are dedicated to scientific discovery, and have financial support to further research and teaching efforts. More important, these hospitals are sufficiently removed from the day to day economics and politics of health care to be able to pursue what inevitably will be some unpopular lines of inquiry without fear of reprisal.

Unlike the expansionist era of the past, today, conflicting economic and political forces can be expected to be a major consideration in any medical practice or technology assessment program that might be developed in the future and the influence of these factors should not be underestimated. Physicians' incomes will be affected and in some of the subspecialties, incomes will be greatly reduced. Powerful private sector medical/industrial complexes will be challenged, and some community hospitals highly dependent on technology derived revenue will not survive. Local community groups, planning agencies, lobbying groups, and local and national politicians can be expected to take up the cause in one way or another as professional and consumer prerogatives and "rights" are challenged. Given these circumstances, only prestigious institutions protected from these political forces and at least partially removed from economic dependence on service income will be able to develop and sustain a creditable technology assessment effort.

In many ways, health science centers and academic hospitals have been reluctant to assume a leadership role in this arena. Although highly committed to quality of care and medical research, their efforts in this regard have largely focused on the development of structure and process standards rather than cost and efficacy or outcome considerations. In the laboratory medicine area, this emphasis has generated performance standards that have influenced accreditation standards, architectural designs, and training programs. It has not, however, furnished the decision-making infrastructure, information systems, and economic incentives to consider the efficacy costs and outcomes of medical practices.

Some academic centers are unable to assume this role because they are vulnerable to the economic and political forces previously outlined. Academic teaching hospitals lacking a separate Board of Trustees and those totally dependent on patient revenue for operating funds will find it difficult, if not impossible, to withstand the economic effects of these studies and the pressures from the professional and political community. If a successful private sector effort is to be mounted, however, it will largely depend on the initiative of the leading academic teaching hospitals to at least facilitate such a program if not play the lead role in its development.

The need for this degree of involvement and commitment at the institutional level largely stems from the organizational imperatives demanded by this type of research effort. Many clinical faculty members in the academic medical community are willing and committed to engage in studies focused on clinical decision making and technology assessment. The nature of the inquiry, however, often necessitates involvement of a number of clinical disciplines, cutting across several organizational units in the medical school and the teaching hospital. It also requires the involvement of people in disciplines outside the medical arena, such as economists and health services researchers. Without the organizational support of a medical center and especially the support of the academic teaching hospital, it will be extremely difficult for a clinical faculty, however committed, to establish these interorganizational linkages and mount a sustained effort of the magnitude required to influence and shape national policies. Laboratory medicine is a good example. Laboratory functions tend to be conceptualized as diagnostic support services. Use patterns are seldom subject to rigorous review or assessment, and introduction of new technology is more often negotiated than planned. Reconceptualization of this role into a medical practice partnership is an essential first step for a successful technology assessment program. This will require the joint efforts of faculty in laboratory medicine, the major clinical departments, health services researchers, and the administration of the academic hospital. The academic hospital then needs to accommodate and institutionalize this change through organizational structure and process.

Second, and of equal importance, a number of organizational subsystems must be available to facilitate this effort. A management information system, linking resource utilization to diagnostic categories delineated according to intensity measures, and a data system that allows long-term evaluation of outcomes on a large scale are essential to this process. To facilitate information transfer and capture data from sufficiently large population groups, these data systems will need to be linked to other medical centers engaged in similar work. Financial subsystems must also be reorganized to facilitate this effort. In some cases, institutional budgets will need to be restructured to remove a dependency on technology-derived income and to furnish financial incentives for clinicians to engage in activities that will eventually result in the loss of personal and institutional income.

Third, an organizational mechanism must be developed to assure rapid translation of the results of this research and development effort into policies guiding the field of practice. Formalized linkages with policymakers at the national and local levels, professional organizations influencing medical practices, and educational programs preparing clinicians for the field are essential. In essence, these institutions then become the research and development arm for policymakers dealing with appropriate resource utilization in the health care sector.

For these reasons, an institutional commitment is essential to a clinical decision-making and technology assessment research effort great enough and durable enough to influence policies regulating the use of resources; in addition, it must provide physicians sufficient information and guidelines to enable them to practice quality medicine within those resource constraints. This is not to say that important contributions will not be made by individual clinicians working alone or in small groups to further this effort. Rather, it reflects the magnitude of the problem and the importance of sustained large-scale studies designed to increase the effectiveness of medical practices during a time of economic retrenchment. We believe that selected health science centers and especially academic teaching hospitals within those centers should take the initiative in this regard and formally establish this role as part of their mission.

In summary, cost escalations resulting from converging forces of a provider-driven health care economy, rapidly expanding technologies, and shifts in financial responsibilities toward health insurance are serving to refocus health care policies from development and distribution to cost containment and retrenchment. These policy options range from highly regulated systems limiting supply, to competitive systems allocating resources according to market economies. Both approaches and their derivatives center on limiting costs rather than the effective use of scarce medical resources to achieve high quality cost/effective care. Consequently, important quality and access (equity) issues are at stake; an erosion of the modest gains made in these areas during the past decade could occur unless policies are refocused. Although a beginning effort is occurring at the national level to address clinical decision-making and medical technology assessment issues, it is far too limited to have a significant effect on the field. Since health science centers and especially medical school/academic teaching hospital alliances have contributed centrally toward the growth and development of the medical care field and the expansion of technologies underpinning the field, they should appropriately now address their organizational and financial capacity to policy-relevant studies linking resource utilization to these technologies and should develop closer alliances with policymakers and practitioners to translate the research findings into practice.

This effort will require an institutional commitment that in some ways will redefine the mission of these organizations and, in the case of the academic teaching hospitals, may in fact provide the major set of characteristics differentiating them from technology intense community hospitals that are now rapidly encroaching on their roles. Now may be an opportune time for academic teaching hospitals to assume these new responsibilities and reorient their organizations toward these policy concerns.

References

1. Battistella RM. The course of regional health planning: Review and assessment of recent federal legislation. Med Care 1967;5:153-61.
2. Waitzkin H. A Marxian interpretation of the growth and development of coronary care technology. Am J Public Health, 1979;69:1260-68.
3. Relman S. The allocation of medical resources by physicians. N Engl J Med 1980 55: 99-104.
4. Ford HC. Use and abuse of clinical laboratories. NZ Med J 1978;88:16-18.
5. Health Care Financing Administration, Office of Research, Demonstrations, and Statistics. Health Care Financing Review, Summer 1979, Vol. 1, No. 1. (DHEW publication no. (HCFA) 03002-8/79); Health Care Financing Administration, Office of Research, Demonstrations, and Statistics. Health Care Financing Review, Winter 1980, Vol. 1, No. 3 (DHEW publication no. (HCFA) 03027-3/80); Health Care Financing Administration, Office of Research, Demonstrations, and Statistics, Health Care Financing Trends, Winter 1980, Vol. 1, No. 2 (DHEW publication no. (HCFA) 03028-3/80).
6. Health Care Financing Administration, Office of Research, Demonstrations, and Statistics. loc. cit.
7. Bailey RM. Clinical laboratories and the practice of medicine. Berkeley, California: McCutcheon Publishing Corp., 1979.
8. Health Care Financing Administration, Office of Research, Demonstrations, and Statistics. loc. cit.
9. Blanpain J, Delesie L, Nys H. The policies. In: National health insurance & health resources: the European experience. Cambridge: Harvard University Press, 1978:209-52.
10. Havighurst CC, Hackbarth GM. Private cost containment. N Engl J Med, 1979;300: 1298-1305.
11. Luft H. HMOs and the medical care market. Socioeconomic issues of health, 1980. American Medical Association, July, 1980.
12. Navarro V. Under capitalism. New York: Prodist, 1976.
13. Reinhardt E. The future of medical enterprise: Perspectives on resource allocation in socialized markets. J Med Educ 1980;55:311-32.
14. Health Incentive Reform Act of 1979, Senate Bill 1968.
15. Kane RL. Strengthening health services research programs (Editorial). Community Health 1977;3:1-2.

CHAPTER TWO

Decision Making and the Evolution of Modern Medicine

Stanley Joel Reiser, MD, PhD

The physician's search for evidence to provide clues to sources of the patient's complaints has always occupied a preeminent place in the hierarchy of medical tasks. Discussion of how this process evolved is often cast as a succession of techniques, the better techniques thought, generally, to replace the inferior. Yet the change from one order of diagnostic procedure to another involves far more than a change of technique: it involves, basically, a transformation of the criteria we use to decide what to direct our attention to from the universe of possible observations that can be made on the person who is sick. It is the alteration of these fundamental norms of selection that, when speaking of diagnosis, demarcates one historical period from another.

It is difficult to understand the norms of selection influencing the modern period without understanding something about those dominating the era preceding it, which spanned virtually the entire nineteenth century. This was the heyday of physical diagnosis. It began in 1819 when the French doctor René Laënnec gave convincing evidence in a newly published treatise, *De l'Auscultation Médiate*, that the diagnoses of chest disease could be made far more accurate if physicians learned the significance of the sounds produced by the organs within that cavity, using an instrument Laënnec had invented that he called the stethoscope. His procedure of proof involved linking the acoustic signs with lesions uncovered at autopsy; it was one of the early testaments to the power of the clinicopathological correlation. But the proposal involved far more than urging doctors to learn a new set of diagnostic signs. It was a call to reevaluate the sort of evidence doctors should seek and value. The era in which Laënnec had learned medicine as a student placed a great emphasis on the patient's story: the experiences, sensations, and interpretations about the illness that it revealed. Laënnec urged a turning away from such evidence, and replacing it with data doctors gained through their own senses. The arguments for the change were powerful. Physicians should place more credence in what they heard, or saw, or felt than in what others (patients) heard, or saw, or felt—an appeal to the doctor's ego and desire for authority. Physical evidence linked to anatomical change was superior to functional evidence without such explicit causal associations—an appeal to the view of medicine as science.

Case histories of illness reflected this changed idea of what constituted the most crucial data. They focused less on the patient's view of the symptoms and more on the doctor's view. A clinical report written by Laënnec illustrates this perspective:

> A woman, aged 40, had been long subject to much cough, and dyspnoea, varied by temporary aggravations, especially by certain states of the weather. These symptoms, which she called asthma, had not incapacitated her for labour, until the last fifteen days, at the end of which time she came into hospital. At this time she could not at all lie down,—the respiration was very short and difficult, the lips violet, and there was anasarca of the lower limbs. The chest yielded, on percussion, a pretty good sound throughout, though, perhaps, somewhat less than natural. Immediately below the clavicle on each side, the cylinder [stethoscope] discovered a well-marked *rattle*. The thoracic parietes were much and forcibly elevated at each inspiration. The cough was very frequent, and followed by expectoration of opaque yellow sputa. Pectoriloquism was not discoverable. The pulse was frequent, small, and regular; the external jugulars were swelled and distinctly pulsative; the pulsations of the heart [examined by the stethoscope] were deep, regular, little sonorous, and without impulse to the ear. From this examination I thought myself justified in considering the heart as sound, notwithstanding the contrary indication afforded by the general symptoms; and accordingly gave my diagnostic—*Phthisis without disease of the heart*. A few days after, the contraction of the ventricles gave some impulse, a symptom which, taken along with the pulsation of the jugulars, gave reason to suspect slight hypertrophia of the right ventricle. The symptoms, especially the anasarca, got gradually worse; and she died on the 19th of February. The day before her death evident pectoriloquism was discovered in the anterior third of the fourth intercostal space, on the right side, a point which had not been examined before.[1]

The portrait of illness revealed in this case is dominated by the anatomical dimensions of illness, and largely drawn from the testimony of the doctor's senses. We learn little about what the patient thought or experienced.

Laënnec directed doctors doubly inward—in urging that the basic communication in medicine proceed from the interior of the patient to the interior of the doctor. The doctor's "aim" was to penetrate the skin and bypass the experiences of the patient. The doctor's senses became the main agents of diagnosis.

In the twentieth century, the gaze of medicine shifted away from the visible physical characteristics of patients, and from using the doctors' senses as the principal media of diagnosis. The human senses increasingly became replaced by instruments and machines, which used mechanical and chemical probes to evaluate the innermost features of biological existence. The evidence these machines produced were characteristically expressed as graphs or numbers, which became the dominant forms of modern medical evidence. More precise-seeming, able to be viewed and evaluated by groups of clinicians, the product of a science-generated technology, such evidence appeared superior to that gained by the mere human senses. Physicians turned from themselves as gatherers of diagnostic evidence and toward technicians and machines.

The use of the diagnostic laboratory has been a key aspect of this evolution. Spurred by advances in chemistry and microscopy during the nineteenth century, the ward laboratory became part of many major hospitals as the twentieth century dawned. Representing a leading avenue of the application of science to clinical medicine, laboratory evaluation became increasingly essential to physicians, and began to turn them away from clinical evidence, often intemperately. Noted one medical observer of that time: "No urine-caster in his wildest dreams thought that the attempt would ever be made to do what is done now every day by the least expert, when he finds sugar or albumin in the urine, and tells the accompanying symptoms or the consequences."[2]

By the mid-twentieth century, the spell of laboratory findings bound most graduates of medical schools. A revealing dialog between Groucho Marx and a medical intern epitomized the problem:

Groucho: If I were found unconscious on the sidewalk, what would you do?

Intern: I would work up the patient.

Groucho: How would you start?

Intern: Well, I would do the laboratory work first. I would do a red count and hemoglobin and then a total white and differential count.[3]

In the 1950s in the United States the number of laboratory tests ordered was doubling every five years; by the 1970s the cost of ordering laboratory tests and X rays was nearly ten percent of total medical expenditures. Automated analyzers now became a common feature of hospital laboratories, giving 6, 12, 18, 24 tests literally for the price of one produced manually. Indeed it is difficult now for doctors to request just one or two tests from the laboratory, although that is all they may want. The argument that more tests for the price is better ignores the problem of extra procedures generating more false positive and false negative results. Although doctors of today are attracted to the comforting presence of machines, a sense of uneasiness about their distant effects prevails, even among laboratory experts, as one scenario of the future warns:

Dr. H. A. Zbin peered mournfully through the carefully polished eyepieces of his obsolete light microscope. His was in an obscure cubicle in a dark basement corner of the great Metrocolossal University Hospital laboratory.

He fumbled through old collections of faded slides, dating back to 1964. No one sent Dr. Zbin current material for microscopical study. In the new, brightly lighted portions of the tremendous multistory laboratory the automated gizmos burbled, bubbled, rotated and transmitted test results (to the sixth decimal place) to the battery of computers . . . . A meager pension awaited him. For decades he had been without assistants or residents. He would not be replaced. His position was being abolished.[4]

Indeed of all the machines introduced into medicine in modern times the computer, with its capacity not merely to sense but to *interpret* evidence, has created more excitement and uneasiness than any other.

There is no such thing as a neutral technique or technology. The so-called wisdom offered in clichés such as "It's not the gun but the person using it" is flawed. Techniques and machines, such as those used in medicine to diagnose illness, play active roles in shaping our perceptions and actions, irrespective of the users. They direct our attention to certain aspects of illness and divert our attention from others; they provide us with a certain power to manipulate our environment and thus tempt us to use them. Many of the contemporary dilemmas of the diagnostic aspect of medical practice stem directly from the view of illness that modern diagnostic media projects, from the self-image they instill in the healer, and the form of the medical relationship they help impose.

The most dependable portraits of patients in an era in which the most valued evidence is quantitative and graphic are, not surprisingly, flow charts and printouts. Although adequate, even valuable, for an aspect of illness, such evidence is necessarily a partial statement of the problems of a patient. The often disproportionate role it assumes in evaluation stems not only from modern views of its inherent value, but from a related decline in modern ability to gather or evaluate forms of diagnostic evidence gained through the doctor's senses or the patient's experiences. The more we value machine-gathered data, the less medical schools teach and physicians seek nontechnological evidence. One feature of illness assumes even greater prominence, seems more accurate than it really is, and gradually begins to stand for the whole. Naturally, physicians depending increasingly on evidence gathered by technicians and machines become more dependent on them, and thus feel out of place in environments of practice where such data are not readily at hand. This accounts, in part, for the concentration of physicians in urban medical centers. It follows too that when graphic and numerical data dominate, chart rounds become as important as bedside rounds, records seem adequate stand-ins for people, and problems in the medical relationship develop.[5]

None of these problems is insoluble. We can begin to remedy them now by giving explicit attention in the process of medical education to the effects of diagnostic techniques on physicians and patients. In specific terms we might, for example, seek to stem the relative decline in our desire and ability to gather, evaluate, and use those forms of evidence that appear subjective, and that link the experiences of the patient to the problems of the illness. We might cultivate modern knowledge of the interview process that has been developed in the behavioral and social sciences, and in the medical humanities, that would allow us to go far beyond our predecessors in making the medical interview a highly accurate tool of diagnostic fact-finding, and a significant medium to establish bonds of trust and rapport between doctor and patient essential in a therapeutic alliance. We might lift the veil of secrecy concerning observer variation and error in medicine. A literature does exist on the subject, but to my knowledge, no American medical school systematically explores with students the discrepancies between observers viewing the same evidence—both technological and nontechnological—nor helps them to learn their own strengths and weaknesses in perceiving different kinds of medical evidence. There also is more to do from the viewpoint of teaching students to understand and influence public policy to rationalize and ration the use of technology. Although in this paper I have not touched subjects such as reimbursement schemes, legal imperatives, and efforts to evaluate the effectiveness of medical technology, clearly they all have a strong bearing on these problems. Yet at the heart of the matter are the views of the age about what sort of evidence counts, and the imperatives taught and transmitted in medical schools to seek and value technologic more than other evidence. Unless and until these matters are forthrightly addressed by educators, our dilemmas over the technology of diagnosis will remain.

References

1. Laënnec RTH. A treatise on the diseases of the chest, trans. John Forbes. New York: Hafner Publishing Co., 1962:395-96.
2. Da Costa JM. Modern medicine. Philadelphia: J.B. Lippincott, 1872:16.
3. Maes U. The lost art of clinical diagnosis. Am J Surg 1951;82:107.
4. Foraker G. The end of an era. N Engl J Med 1965;272:37.
5. These themes are more fully developed in Reiser SJ. Medicine and the reign of technology. New York: Cambridge University Press, 1978.

CHAPTER THREE

Medical Decisions and Society

Howard S. Frazier, MD

INTRODUCTION

As autonomous practitioners, we share the belief that we have choices. We assume that, in the course of our professional activities, we make decisions that, if prudently arrived at, will not affect the care of patients adversely, and may significantly reduce the resources used in their care. We believe that we can do good (or at least as well) by using fewer resources and save some money.

I subscribe to the first assumption; it has the ring of motherhood and the flag, and circularity as well. The validity and implications of the second assumption, that we can do as well for less, are the subjects of this discussion. I will first briefly examine some of the determinants of resource allocation in the health sector and the magnitude of those resource components. Next, I will attempt an estimation of the improvements in cost efficiency that might be achieved by influencing decisions made by autonomous practitioners on behalf of their patients. We will be principally concerned with decisions involving personal health care. Finally, given prudent medical decisions, what problems will remain? I suggest that elimination of the inefficiencies resulting from our present habits of medical decision making is important, but mainly because it will clear the air for a discussion of a more fundamental issue. We must demonstrate convincingly our efficient use of resources, in order to focus public attention on the much more difficult issue of resource allocation to the health sector when available resources become truly rate-limiting. Elimination of waste is not a solution to the problems of equity and entitlement that soon will confront us. Elimination of inefficiency is, however, a necessary condition for productive public discussion of the deeper issue.

Supported in part by a grant from the Robert Wood Johnson Foundation to the Center for the Analysis of Health Practices.

RESOURCE ALLOCATION IN THE HEALTH SECTOR

We are concerned here with medical decisions made by individual practitioners on behalf of individual patients. These decisions affect society in two related but distinguishable ways. First, they affect the outcomes of singular encounters between patient and practitioner. Second, in the aggregate, they also affect the patterns of productivity, but more important, those of social investment. The magnitude and characteristics of this investment are designed to anticipate the needs or cultivated expectations of the patient, on the one hand, and to provide the practitioner with a wide range of possible responses on the other. "Designed," implying a single architect and a coherent plan, is precisely the wrong word.

For the year ending in September of 1979, expenditures for personal health care in the United States totaled $184 billion, of which some $83 billion represents charges for hospital care.[1] I cannot find equally well-documented figures for the charges for laboratory studies during the same period, but a reasonable estimate based on prior experience would be approximately $16 billion. Of this amount, roughly $4 billion can be attributed to charges for the information provided by clinical laboratory tests.[2-6] There is some degree of overlap between hospital charges and those for laboratory studies, but approximations will suffice for the points that follow.

The capacity to produce this aggregate volume of services exists and operates not on the basis of any single assessment of needs, but as the result of the efforts of a variety of principal actors responding to different sets of incentives. These include, but are not limited to, patients, who perceive consumption of health services as the route to health and whose market signals have been attenuated; autonomous practitioners, who have been trained to allocate all those resources that may be of potential benefit to individual patients; and an industrial infrastructure sensitive both to demand for services and to possibilities for profit.

Is $184 billion, 8% of our gross national product (GNP), too much or too little to devote to the package of services called personal health care? At one extreme are those who argue that the very size of the enterprise and its need for workers of all levels of skill make it an exemplary public work. At the opposite pole are those who see it as an infinite sink for resources, the social return on which is at best very much less than that available from alternative forms of investment. In the middle are the rest of us, groaning at the fiscal burden of our appetite for services while ordering up more of the same.

Prospects for an early consensus on how much is enough, and how it should be divided, seem dim indeed. The pluralism of interests involved, the absence of a widely accepted yardstick of medical need, and our lack of familiarity with possible tools for comparing expected benefits and costs across the whole spectrum of public investment all conspire against it. I would like to emphasize my belief that our lack of agreement about means and ends is *not* primarily a manifestation of wrongheadedness, greed, or indifference to others. No enterprise of this size can be viewed in its entirety from a single vantage point. And the alternative perspectives we adopt lead to very different approaches to the allocation of our public resources.

The economist, for example, has both methodology for and experience in establishing the costs of the inputs to the health care industry. Assignments of value to the outputs is a different matter. With respect to the caring function of personal health services, abundant anecdotal evidence testifies to the value it has in the minds of consumers, but I am not aware of any systematic studies of its inputs and differential outcomes in economic terms. The component of personal health services made up of technical interventions can, in principle, be treated on the input side by the economist. The outcomes of such interventions are multi-attributed, however, and the task of scaling them before their aggregation will at best suppress individual values and, at worst, ignore the strongly held preferences of sizable groups in the population.

If an inspired economist can successfully resolve the problems of scaling and aggregation, personal health services would be described by the cost of obtaining one more unit of valued outcome, that is, by their marginal utility. By the economist's approach, our pattern of public investment within the health sector and across all sectors of public interest would be determined either by a hierarchy of marginal utility, or by the finding that a given allocation would provide an outcome greater in value than the costs of the inputs.

From an ethical perspective, resource costs are not a primary concern and, on the output side, technical efficacy of an intervention in the usual medical sense is perhaps of less importance than the value attached to a particular outcome by the recipient, and to its consequences for those involved with the recipient. The discussion would focus on whether or not an individual had a right or entitlement to consume personal health services, expressed as first call on resources, as compared with those who simply had an interest in their consumption. Issues of cost and benefit would be examined from the standpoint of the equity of their distribution rather than their magnitude.[7]

Our perspective as practitioners leads us to still another set of behaviors in our role as autonomous decision makers, allocating resources in the public domain. For most of us, resource needs in the health arena are not considered to be in competition with the requirements of other sectors. Personal health services clearly are unique, exercising a preemptive position with respect to alternative forms of social investment. Our implicit contract to act as agent and advocate for our patients, taken one at a time, virtually removes from consideration issues of cost effectiveness; the important question is whether a given decision regarding a single individual is more likely to be of benefit or harm. Patients unseen are not party to a contract, and society's major role is to act as a producer of services from among which the patient and physician may choose those deemed relevant to the problem at hand.

EXPECTATIONS FOR IMPROVING EFFICIENCY
IN RESOURCE USE

Under the circumstances, it seems most productive to focus our attention on the most familiar set of actors, ourselves, and to ask what might be the impact on allocation of resources of changing our present behavior within the limits of current ethical imperatives. How much might we save on personal health care without compromising that care? For a variety of reasons, not least of which is the paucity of data on the relation of service inputs to health outcomes, detailed estimates are not available. For the purposes of this argument, however, reasonable upper bounds will suffice.

The largest single component of personal health care is the $83 billion hospital bill. Health maintenance organizations report rates of hospital utilization among their patients approximately 75% of the national average, without apparent decline in health outcome.[8] Since a substantial fraction of this lower utilization is attributed to the provision of a wider range of services to ambulatory patients, the full 25% of $83 billion is not realizable as savings. Let us assume that the net is 15%, or about 12 billion, still a considerable sum.

Our prior estimates of the concurrent bill for laboratory studies, $16 billion, is, as was noted previously, not cleanly separable from total hospital costs. Let us make the favorable assumption that savings resulting from the decision not to hospitalize are over and above those resulting from changes in laboratory utilization. How much of the latter might realistically be affected by altered patterns of decision making by practitioners? With respect to tests offered by clinical laboratories, evidence is accumulating that overutilization is substantial and pervasive, ranging, for specific tests, from more than 50 to 95%.[9,10] Fewer estimates are available for other types of tests. Personal experience suggests overutilization is not quite so flagrant, perhaps because of barriers such as queuing and the effort required of the decision-maker. In the aggregate, reduction to 50% of present levels, or $8 billion, would be a reasonable guess as to savings short of risk to the quality of patient care.

Similar arguments could be advanced with respect to the $16 billion spent for drugs and related items.[1] The only other large discretionary component of the bill for personal health care is physicians' services at $38.7 billion. In the interests of personal survival, I shall leave to the experience and conscience of my colleagues an estimate of potential savings to be achieved in this item.

Excluding potential savings to be achieved by reducing the costs of physicians' services, we arrive at a rough estimate of the maximum annual savings achievable by changing the patterns of decision making of individual practitioners of some $28 billion. The purview of this conference, of course, covers a much narrower range of medical decisions, and the potential savings to be achieved by improving the rationality of our test ordering and reducing the force of perverse incentives is substantially less.

At this point, it is worth putting these figures into their economic surroundings. Over the three-year period ending in September of 1979, the costs of personal health care increased at an average rate of $19 billion per year.[1] The savings for which we have developed rough estimates are a one-time event; in terms of absolute rates of expenditure, we would be back to our current position only 18 months after having achieved the greatest increase in efficiency in personal health care that we believe is possible. In addition, the costs of personal health care are rising faster than the value of the GNP, by about 0.1% of the GNP per year over the past three years. This amounts to the allocation of more than $2 billion extra to personal health care in the last year, beyond the amount provided by a constant proportion of an expanding GNP. This increment includes nondiscretionary items, such as a change in the age structure of the population. New services, or the more intense application of existing ones, constitute discretionary components to the extent that they can be shown to confer negligible benefit.

The health care enterprise is huge, and the most optimistic estimates of change in the efficiency with which we allocate resources are relatively small. Is the effort to achieve change worthwhile? We turn to this issue in the final part of the discussion.

THE FUTURE OF THE RESOURCE-EFFICIENT
SYSTEM OF HEALTH CARE

As I have tried to make clear, I believe the economic impact of improving the quality of our medical decisions, particularly with respect to the use of the laboratory, will be modest. That result does not reduce my enthusiasm for the work of this conference. The reasons are two.

My own experience, my observations of physicians in training, and what understanding I have of the process of clinical decision making all suggest that the process itself and the teaching of it are ripe for reexploration. Significant improvements are possible, and their achievement surely will improve the quality of the outcomes we seek on behalf of our patients. In addition, I think it likely that this improvement in health outcomes can occur despite a reduction in the resources utilized, a reduction brought about by a more pointed and appropriate selection of the information to be sought in the clinical encounter and the interventions undertaken. Less will indeed yield more. In these terms, this conference is simply a continuation of a long line of efforts to improve the prospects we can offer our patients.

There is another, less cheerful, but more important reason to push forward. I believe that, given the present structure and incentives in our system of personal health care, even the elimination of waste and inefficiency will fail to bring the increases in spending below the rate of rise of the GNP per capita. However efficiently applied, resources simply will not be available to do everything that might be done for everyone who might want it to be done. The form and timing of the message are uncertain, but our fellow citizens soon will indicate their unwillingness to shrink other forms of social investment continually to expand the resources available for health care.

At that point, we will begin the unpleasant job of choosing among valued outcomes. It is true that the elimination of waste and inefficiency will delay the arrival of painful resource constraints, but it cannot, in my opinion, prevent it.

Nevertheless, rigorous efforts to improve the efficiency of personal health care will have another beneficial effect. As resource limitations have begun to pinch our system of welfare support services, for example, we have grasped at all sorts of simple but empty explanations, such as welfare fraud, to avoid confronting the difficult and deeply moral task of deciding whether and how we want to help each other. The same danger will exist when the time comes to consider how we shall go about rationing that amount of personal health care we elect to produce. In order to focus the public discussion on the real issues of allocating constrained resources, we shall first have to make a credible showing that we have made the most efficient use of the resources we have. To that enhanced efficiency, the subject of this conference can make a powerful contribution.

References

1. Health Care Financing Trends/Winter 1980. Table A-1: National health expenditures, by type of expenditure. DHEW, Washington, DC.
2. Smithson LH Jr. The clinical laboratory report. Prepared for the Long Range Planning Service, Stanford Research Institute, 1975.
3. Kosowsky DI. New opportunities in the clinical laboratory industry. Arthur D Little Inc. Executive Forum on Healthcare under the Carter Administration, 1977.
4. Zucker B, ed. National survey of hospital clinical laboratories. Laboratory Management 1976;14:17-39 (May).
5. Zucker B, ed. National survey of non-hospital clinical laboratories. Laboratory Management 1976;14:17-36 (Nov).
6. Fineberg HV. Clinical chemistries: the high cost of low-cost diagnostic tests. In: Altman SH, Blendon R, eds. Medical technology: the culprit behind health care costs?. Proceedings of the 1977 Sun Valley Forum on National Health. (DHEW publication no. (PHS) 79-3216).
7. One point of entry into this expanding literature is provided by the following review article: Callahan D. Shattuck Lecture—Contemporary biomedical ethics. N Engl J Med 1980;302:1228-33.
8. Klarman HE. Cited, p. 52, by Hughes EFX, Baron DP, Dittman DA, et al. Hospital cost containment programs: a policy analysis. Cambridge: Ballinger, 1978.
9. Sandler G. Costs of unnecessary tests. Br Med J 1979;2:21-4.
10. Dixon RH, Laszlo J. Utilization of clinical chemistry services by medical house staff. Arch Intern Med 1974;134:1064-7.

CHAPTER FOUR

Use of Computers in a Clinical Library

Eugene A. Stead, Jr., MD

Clinical practitioners of medicine are artists, with some training in methods of the more exact sciences. Patients are people who wish to stay well or who have diseases. In only a few of the diseases that are more or less completely understood can treatment be controlled by the scientific method. Doctors so far have little to offer adults in the way of disease prevention; they are at their best when caring for patients with acute illness. They are at a great disadvantage in caring for patients who have chronic illness because the methods of collecting data over time have not been perfected. The doctor who treats acute illness can link current states to known outcomes. In chronic illness, however, current states cannot be linked to known outcomes.

The interested practitioner can easily become expert in the care of the patient with acute illness. Because the process is acute, the illness will terminate before time-dependent processes occur in organs other than those involved in the current acute process. The doctor can anticipate a stable situation, except for the current acute process. As information is entered into the doctor's brain from the history, physical examination, and laboratory procedures, it is checked off against patterns previously laid down. If the information fits a known pattern, it can be carried with no effort expended in memorizing a great many details. If it does not fit, the doctor has no trouble remembering the nonfitting information, because the situation has to be reexamined to see if the correct pattern was selected. The physician selects a course of action, and with quick feedback is allowed to continue if the course is favorable or to change it if it is unfavorable. Economic, social, and cultural influences have minimal influence, because acute processes by definition terminate quickly. If doctors practice in a place like the Duke Medical Center, they will learn about the care of acute problems not only from their own patients but from those of their colleagues.

The problem in acute medicine is to decide how much information a physician needs to care for the acute problem and how many dangerous drugs and procedures should be used. The average internist frequently confuses patient care and diagnosis. Acute patient care requires doctors to collect that amount of information which assures them that the patient is not immediately threatened by treatable illness. This amount of information may be insufficient to establish a definitive diagnosis. A diagnosis is not essential when the patient has a self-limited illness and dangerous, treatable illnesses have been excluded or when none of the possible diagnoses leads to change in the treatment of the patient.

Having collected the minimal essential data, what should the doctor do? When there is a specific treatment substantiated by scientific inquiry, everyone agrees on the action. Pneumococcal pneumonia is always treated with antimicrobial agents, pernicious anemia with B_{12}, myxedema with the appropriate thyroid hormone replacement. When the disease is self-limited or when no treatment can restore the patient to his or her usual health state, the doctor may or may not initiate treatment. Here the art dominates over the science and the range of acceptable physician behavior is very wide.

In the course of caring for the acute problem, doctors collect some data that may characterize patients in whom the same or different acute problems are likely to occur. The presence of diabetes or agammaglobulinemia predisposes to infections. The feet of persons with impaired circulation are very susceptible to trauma. The asymptomatic person with elevated serum calcium and depressed serum phosphorus is at risk from mental symptoms and from renal calcification and stones. The finding of hypertension identifies persons more likely to have strokes. No general agreement exists on the amount of data that should be collected beyond that needed for the care of the immediate problem. The internist collects a great deal and the general practitioner relatively little. Because of three unsolved problems, there is no general agreement that forces doctors to act in the same way:

First, the cost of identifying an instance of an easily treatable disease—say, carcinoma of the sigmoid colon—in an asymptomatic population is very high. When you add the risk of the travel to the doctor's office, the risk of x-ray exposure, and the risk of perforation of a normal bowel by the sigmoidoscope, repeated examinations to detect carcinoma of the sigmoid colon in its early stages may not be as sensible as we are taught. If you are killed by some process not prevented by these repeated examinations, all the examinations might better have been omitted. The second problem is that we have no method of preventing the progress of many diseases that our tests reveal. Third, if the disease process cannot be removed, the doctor must care for the patient over months or years. The method of practice so successful for acute medicine does not work in the care of the patient with chronic illness. The doctor has no pattern for behavior of the disease over time to relate to the care of a new patient. The doctor cannot remember the initial states of the patients, doesn't know what treatment they have had during the duration of the chronic process, and doesn't know what happened to them. Physicians are at an even greater disadvantage in learning from the patients of their colleagues. In short, the multiple pattern systems with known outcomes that stabilize the practice of acute medicine have not been developed for the care of patients with chronic illness.

Medical science has made considerable progress in identifying the presence or absence of disease in organs. We have made less progress in determining the cause, prevention, and treatment of such common disease processes as cancer and atherosclerosis. By defining the amount of organ disease present in a broad group of persons by appropriate subgrouping of these patients and by following the persons until they die, we can predict with some accuracy the outcome of organ disease in a new patient seen today. This prediction uses the methods developed by the science of biostatistics. Since the integrated behavior of the person arises from many inputs into the nervous system besides just that from the diseased organ, it is to be expected that behavior of the patient will have little relationship to the amount of disease in the organ until very late in the process, when the organ is nearly completely destroyed. Thus persons with minimal organ disease may be completely incapacitated and persons with severe organ disease may live nearly normal lives.

At present the science of medicine concerns itself primarily with organ disease and not integrated human behavior. In time we will be able to relate the behavior of well and ill persons to the structure of the brain. Understanding of these relationships is in its infancy. The present situation is analogous to the understanding or lack of understanding about protein structure and immunity when I took immunology in 1930. We knew that immunity had to have a structural basis but we had no idea what it would be.

The Duke group, spurred by Rosati, Starmer, and Wallace, has started the development of a computerized library to allow doctors caring for patients with chronic illness to quickly determine what has happened to patients who have the characteristics of his current patient. The library is structured to contain information about patients who have those diseases for which the patient and the doctor are willing to spend time and money to accurately characterize the initial state of the patient. No attempt is being made to include data on patients with conditions that do not require descriptions in depth or that do not require the continuing services of doctors. The library bears the cost of processing the data and making them easily available to the practicing physician but bears none of the costs of producing the data. Patients with many chronic illnesses remain under the care of their doctor, and therefore data over time are usually charged to the cost of continuing patient care. When outcomes cannot be determined from medical records, much information can be made available by telephone calls to the patient. These telephone costs are borne by the computerized library.

We have information in depth on all patients over an 8-year period who were judged to have enough of a problem with chest pain or previous myocardial infarction to warrant cardiac catheterization (6,403 patients). We have up-to-date information on death or current status on 99+% of those patients. The information in the system is machine searchable. Once a doctor has defined the characteristics of a new patient, a search can be made on-line for patients who have descriptors like those of the current patient. Similarities and differences between the current patient and those in the subgroup are noted. Doctors can use their own judgment on which descriptors they will drop to make the match of the remaining characteristics more exact or they can ask our biostatisticians to weight the data so that the match excludes those descriptors that they know have the least weight in determining outcomes. This information, called a prognostigram, is available to any physician who wishes to use it at a cost of slightly under $50. The data kept in the bank are carefully screened for quality and no one except the Duke staff can add to this database, but any doctor can use it. How worthwhile doctors will find it will depend on their judgment in collecting the descriptors of the patient and their compulsiveness in determining the exactness of the descriptors. In the past we have divided diseases into those that were common and those that were rare. We have appreciated that special methods had to be used to collect data on rare diseases. In our new library we recognize that the combination of a person with a chronic disease process produces a unique product and that in fact each person represents a rare disease. With the data stored on-line in the computer, each person with a disease can be treated as a rare situation. A complete search of the entire Duke experience can produce data related to that patient and not to the entire gamut of the patients in the category of coronary arterial disease.

This method of collection, storing and using data created in practice to determine to what extent the care by a doctor modifies the long-term outcomes in patients with chronic illness is the first step in creating a new library for use by the practicing doctor. It requires the development of a new library system supported by clinical epidemiologists, biostatisticians, computer scientists, and bioengineers, and by institutional dollars. A system that starts and then stops is worthless.

We envision that 10 libraries located in different parts of the country will eventually be developed for processing and using data for care of patients with chronic illness. These institutions will eventually become branches of the National Library of Medicine.

A library of this type supplies the raw data that are essential for technologic evaluation of a variety of medical procedures. For example, we can already select with noninvasive techniques a sample of 100 men with angina pectoris, 95% of whom will be alive five years later. If all 100 are submitted to cardiac catheterization, five men will be identified who might have their life prolonged by coronary artery bypass. It is doubtful if more than two would achieve this. Physicians will unequivocally opt to catheterize the entire 100. Society has the data to consider whether this is a wise choice.

Section II. The Process of Clinical Decision Making

CHAPTER FIVE

The Clinical Decision-Making Process

Jerome P. Kassirer, MD

INTRODUCTION

It is probably not merely an accident that the clinical decision-making process is the target of research efforts in so many institutions. The new interest in this area of research can be attributed in part to the development of new methods, but increased public awareness of medicine undoubtedly has contributed importantly. Decisions, particularly those involving the use of expensive diagnostic equipment, have come under public scrutiny largely as the result of the highly visible national expenditures for medical care and the widespread concern that these expenses are uncontrolled and possibly uncontrollable. Investigators are motivated by the desire to develop a richer understanding of the clinical decision-making process: the motivation stems in part from dissatisfactions with the way that physicians make decisions. By and large physicians make good decisions, but presumably some make better decisions than others, some make good decisions only some of the time, and presumably some make poor decisions much of the time. We often make glib comments about good decisions and bad decisions, when in fact standards of decision making are sorely deficient.[1] Substituting for such standards are tangential measurements including assessments of the number and kind of tests carried out in given clinical disorders and checks of the completeness of the medical record. Indeed, we are able to assess the outcome of medical care on large populations of patients; but a reproducible, objective methodology to evaluate individual complex life-and-death decisions made by physicians each day is yet to emerge.

Most of the current dogma on the decision-making process is derived from the opinion of experts reflecting on their own problem-solving methodologies.[2-13]

This publication was supported in part by National Institutes of Health, Grants 1 P04LM 03374 and LM 07027 from the National Library of Medicine.

These introspective descriptions have served us well over the years, allowing us to take care of patients and to pass on our practices to others. Drawing on recent research in problem solving, investigators now believe that there are cogent reasons to suspect that the introspective method is at best incomplete. Individuals who try to explain how they solve problems often do an inadequate job.[14] Moreover, if one inspects textbooks designed to teach medical students and house officers the dynamics of the problem-solving process, most of these texts emphasize elements that, albeit important, do not focus on how to approach a diagnostic problem or how to make complex decisions. That is, they do not explain how to interpret data of variable validity, how to assess the potential value of the benefits and risks of various tests and treatments, or how and when to act under conditions of diagnostic uncertainty.

A deeper understanding of the clinical decision-making process may provide better methods for getting these complex clinical ideas across. It also may provide a basis for avoiding some of the innate limitations of normal individuals. Recent investigations by cognitive psychologists have shown that some of the tasks most important to clinical decision-making are those which normal intelligent people handle suboptimally. Such studies show that people tend to be insensitive to rates of disease prevalence and that they distort probabilities when the outcome is potentially serious.[15-17] People also have a strong tendency to utilize irrelevant data to support their hypotheses, and they resist giving up hypotheses even when there is convincing opposing evidence.[16-19] People find it easier to recall events that are most recent or those that occur more often than those of the past or those that are less frequent.[17, 19-21] People are distractable and not always reliable, and they are subject to physical and emotional stresses that may distort their problem-solving practices. Given the goals of improving the quality of medical care and of medical teaching, and the promise that standards of care might emerge from research efforts directed at the clinical decision-making process, the critical question is how to approach the problem.

SOME ELEMENTS OF THE CLINICAL DECISION-MAKING PROCESS

The diagnostic process has always been characterized by some mystique. Physicians in academic medical centers often are amused by the apocryphal story of a medical student who, when presenting the history of an elderly man with pain in the back, opined that the patient must have pancreatic cancer. Later this diagnosis was proven accurate, and the student, when asked how he alone had arrived at the correct diagnosis replied, "What else causes back pain?" Part of the amusement in this tale derives from the widespread acknowledgement in medicine that the diagnostic process is not simple, that diseases come packaged in many misleading forms, and that a given constellation of nearly identical clinical findings may be the manifestation of one disease process in one patient and a different disease process in another.

Physicians must integrate a great mass of data during the clinical decision-making process. They must have a concept of the prevalence of various diseases and a thorough knowledge about the clinical and laboratory manifestations of a large number of disease processes. They also must deal with a large number of findings specific to the patient and must be able to make a link between their patients' findings and the known manifestations of various disease entities. They must be aware of the possibility that on occasion they may unknowingly treat a patient for a disease that is not present and may occasionally unknowingly fail to treat a patient who has a treatable disease. The physician must have a wide-ranging knowledge about diagnostic tests, particularly their risks, their values, and their pitfalls and must be able to integrate the results of these tests into a diagnostic framework. Simplistic views of the testing process such as "Sutton's Law" provide little insight into the diagnostic decision-making process. The concept that in diagnostic testing one should order the test that will go to the core of the problem just as the thief robs banks because "that's where the money is," fails to recognize that even the most rational planning of the sequence of diagnostic tests will not always provide the most direct solution to a complex diagnostic problem. Exploring the abdomen of a febrile patient with left upper quadrant abdominal pain and guarding may be the appropriate approach according to "Sutton's Law" when the tentative diagnosis is subphrenic abscess, but it is both a futile and hazardous plan if the clinical manifestations are in reality those of incipient acute pericarditis.

The large quantity and variety of data are molded by the physician into a diagnostic and therapeutic plan, but most physicians carry out this integration in an implicit, inchoate fashion. The mechanisms physicians use have escaped explicit analysis until recently.

THE EXPLICIT DESCRIPTION OF THE CLINICAL DECISION-MAKING PROCESS

Two of the principal directions of studies of the clinical decision-making process have been labeled *prescriptive* and *descriptive.* Prescriptive strategies are explicit problem-solving and decision-making methodologies; most were developed in other disciplines and have been applied in medicine recently. Such strategies include flow charts, the problem oriented medical record, quantitative decision making using statistical probability theory and decision analysis, and artificial intelligence techniques. Descriptive studies are based on observations of physicians during the process of problem solving and decision making. The basis for these studies is the concept that it is possible to identify tactics and strategies that physicians use by observing physicians engaged in the actual task of problem solving.

The Prescriptive Approach

Flow charts have become popular methods of describing the clinical decision-making process, and many algorithms have been developed for use by medical personnel with varying levels of expertise: from the physician's assistant and nurse practitioner to the surgical resident and practicing physician.[22,23] Because the decisions described by such algorithms must be shown in a branched logic structure, the complex decision making that goes into the development of this structure is implicit. In other words, the reasoning process is built into the flow chart rather than being explicitly described by it. This method cannot handle complex clinical problems or multiple simultaneous clinical problems and is thus rather inflexible. In addition, flow charts are rigidly fixed in a sequential mode and this sequence becomes redundant on repeated use. This method is not likely to be the most fruitful approach to the explication of clinical decision making.

Quantitative decision-making methods that employ Bayesian analysis and decision analysis, however, are major advances that show considerable promise.[24-37] These quantitative methods describe decisions explicitly. They require that a clinical problem be described clearly and precisely and that probabilities and utilities of outcomes be identified as numerical values. The method clarifies the relation between the quality of the decision and the quality of the outcome; it demands that possible outcomes of tests and treatments be identified in advance; it enables the clear interpretation of the relations between the result of a test and the population from which the patient is derived.

The critics of these quantitative techniques argue that the probability and utility data required for use in decision analysis are "soft"; that the method is cumbersome, and that there is a need to compare the results of this technique with some other standard of performance. Some of these criticisms have been answered by the development of methods to test the effect of "soft data." In particular, the concepts of *sensitivity analysis* and *threshold analysis* make it possible to assess the effect of the softness of the data on the ultimate decision. Sensitivity analysis is a method of testing the effect on the decision of changes in one or more variables. The threshold concept is based on the familiar notion that when two courses of action are perceived as having equal potential value, the decision maker should be indifferent to selecting one choice or the other.[24,36,37] A threshold, once derived, serves as a reference point for decision making: after assessing probabilities and utilities in a given patient and finding that values lie above a given threshold, one action is the optimal choice. If values fall below the threshold, however, the alternate action is the optimal choice. A threshold between two decisions can be formulated in terms of a probability of an outcome, a probability of disease, or even of a given utility (i.e., a value of an outcome). Two types of threshold analysis that can be applied to a variety of clinical problems are described elsewhere.[24,36] Proponents of decision analysis point out that even if the probability and utility are not firmly established, it is better to use the best available estimates of these data rather than make the decision without reference to such data.

Artificial intelligence techniques have been applied recently to problem solving in medicine. The advances in computer technology that make it possible to apply these techniques in medicine include the capacity of computers to store large bodies of facts and to use programs that are "goal directed," that is, programs that use knowledge only when it is required.[38] Several successful models have been developed, one for the diagnosis and treatment of glaucoma,[39] one for the diagnosis and treatment of edema-forming states,[38] one for the treatment of infectious diseases,[40] and one large program that encompasses all of internal medicine.[41] Nevertheless, artificial intelligence-oriented computer programs also are based principally on a subjective data base. They have neither been extensively compared with some standard of performance, nor tested on large enough populations of patients; thus their validity remains unproven.

The Descriptive Approach

Recently some efforts have been made toward studying the clinical decision-making process by observing the behavior of physicians engaged in the process. The most extensive study is that carried out by Elstein, Shulman, and Sprafka.[18] The approach in this study was patterned on investigations carried out by Newell and Simon on problem solving in nonmedical domains such as crypt-arithmetic, logic, and chess.[14] In this kind of study the experimental protocol involves observing an individual who is solving a problem, having the individual explain how he is approaching the problem solving (usually during the time that the problem is being solved), recording the remarks of the problem solver, converting these remarks into a transcript, and subsequently analyzing the transcript. Our recent description of physician behavior is an example of this approach.[42] In our study the findings of a real patient were simulated by a physician totally familiar with all of the patient's clinical data. The patient had analgesic nephropathy complicated by acute pyelonephritis, renal insufficiency, and metabolic acidosis. The experimental subject was given minimal data and was required to elicit the rest. In this experiment, immediate introspection was requested. The subject was asked why he had asked a question and how he interpreted the answer. No lists of possible answers were provided. There was no retrospective review of the protocol by the subject, only a terminal summary. Figure 1 shows an example of how hypotheses appeared and disappeared and how levels of diagnostic confidence were attained during a typical problem-solving session.

On the basis of such studies, we and others have concluded that physicians use a hypothetico-deductive method of clinical problem solving, that they do not simply gather data until a solution becomes obvious.[18,42,43] These studies show that physicians form hypotheses early in a clinical encounter and that they cannot be convinced to do otherwise. The early diagnostic hypotheses may be very general (such as infection) or very specific (such as acute pyelonephritis). The number of active hypotheses at any given time is small (approximately five to seven),[18,42] consistent with the finding of Miller that short-term memory has the capacity for only a small number of items.[44] It seems virtually certain that

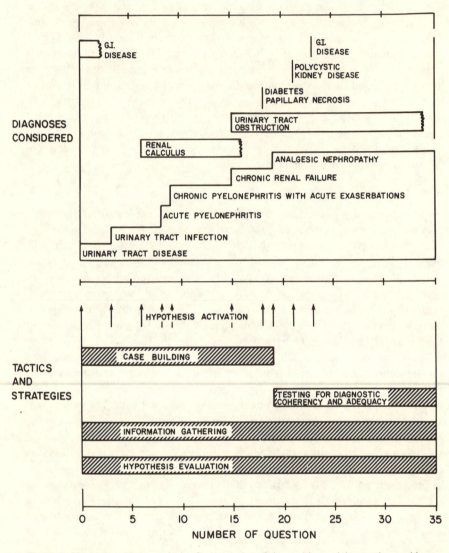

Figure 1. Illustration of the analysis of a transcript of the problem solving tactics used by a physician in diagnosing a patient with analgesic nephropathy. "Building a case" toward the final diagnosis is illustrated at the top. Despite relative confidence in the diagnosis, other alternative diagnoses and possible complications are sought late in the session (after question 20). The irregular ends of several bars represent the analyst's uncertainty regarding whether a given diagnostic hypothesis had been dropped from consideration. Explanation of the various tactics and strategies is given elsewhere.[42]

hypotheses are used as a context for further information gathering. In fact, most questioning seems to be hypothesis driven. Some "routine" questioning is also used, first to give the physician time to think, and second, to provide clues to alternative hypotheses not previously considered. [18,42,43] Our study of the problem-solving process also suggested that experts can be identified, but that expert behavior is probably not a function of a special problem-solving capacity; more likely, it is related to the greater body of factual material held by the expert.

These new descriptive experimental methods have many pitfalls. Factors that may distort results include the experimental design; in particular distortion is likely to occur if information is gathered from the experimental subjects in retrospect, i.e., after the outcome is already known.[45] Misleading results also may derive from interpretation of the transcript; though the data in transcripts are often unambiguous, differing interpretations are possible and the methods of transcript analysis are not precise. With the refining of these experimental methods, it should be possible to avoid many of these pitfalls. Such experiments hold promise for developing further information about the clinical decision-making process, particularly how physicians deal with the complex balancing of risks and benefits of tests and treatments.

DIRECTIONS FOR FUTURE RESEARCH

Considerable further development of decision analysis is warranted: no technical obstacles stand in the way of gathering more precisely the data required for this technique. The necessary probabilities can be obtained by careful data collection, as long as the application of the data is kept in mind. The same is true of the data required on the reliability of diagnostic tests. It should be pointed out, however, that there is considerable resistance on the part of many individuals to describe their data in a probabilistic format. This is not a readily soluble problem. The methodologies for assessing utilities, particularly multidimensional utilities, will require considerable attention. These utility assessments will eventually require methods for placing on the same scale such divergent characteristics as death, disability, discomfort, mental anguish, and financial cost. It will also be necessary to devise methods for factoring into these utility assessments the values held by individuals, the families, and society. A more extensive application of decision analysis to generic clinical problems should also prove highly useful because it is these explicit analyses of general clinical problems that can be measured against current performance. Methods must be developed, however, to expedite the clinical use of decision analysis, specifically to simplify the complex calculations required for sensitivity and threshold analyses.

Further developments in artificial intelligence are also needed. The particular problem that requires further work involves the way in which medical knowledge is structured in the computer. It is not yet clear whether medical data are best represented by probabilistic associations, deterministic associations, physiological linkages, lists of attributes, or some combination of these and other as yet undescribed techniques.

More promising is the possible interrelationship of the descriptive and prescriptive techniques. It is possible that the prescriptive techniques can serve as hypotheses to explain medical problem solving and that descriptive studies can be developed to determine whether or not expert physicians solve problems using such techniques.

One interaction of investigative methods that offers considerable potential in advancing this effort is a marriage of the techniques of artificial intelligence and cognitive psychology. The concept of using the computer as a laboratory to simulate intelligent behavior originated with the studies of Newell and Simon in the simple problem-solving areas referred to earlier.[14] The technologies of artificial intelligence have made it possible over the past few years to represent in the computer both a considerable body of knowledge and the methods with which to manipulate this knowledge. Simultaneously, concepts of language, reasoning, and learning have moved forward. These advances make it possible to explore the use of computer programs as models of the clinical cognitive process. To obtain the data for such programs, it may be possible to turn to the transcripts of the protocols of physicians solving clinical problems. Although the explanations physicians give of their problem-solving activities during a session may be incomplete or even somewhat inaccurate, the protocol nonetheless is likely to be a luxuriant source of clues regarding the thought processes that physicians use to solve problems. From the analysis of these protocols it should be possible, using the methods of Newell and Simon, to develop hypotheses concerning clinical cognitive processes that can be stated precisely as a computer program. This unambiguous statement (i.e., the computer program) can be tested by simulating clinical events, tracing the sequence the program selects to solve problems, and assessing both the method used and the outcome of the procedure. The prospect of applying these new methods to research in clinical cognition is exciting and promising, but we are only at the beginning of this endeavor.

References

1. Burnum JF. The "scientific" value of personal care. Ann Intern Med 1979;4:643-5.
2. Feinstein AR. An analysis of diagnostic reasoning. I. The domains and disorders of clinical macrobiology. Yale J Biol Med 1973;46:212-32.
3. Morgan WL Jr., Engel GL. The clinical approach to the patient. Philadelphia: WB Saunders Co, 1969.
4. MacLeod JG, ed. Clinical examination. New York: Churchill Livingstone, 1976.
5. Feinstein AR: Clinical judgment. New York: RE Krieger Publishing Co, 1967.
6. Bouchier AID, Morris JS, eds. Clinical skills. London: WB Saunders 1976.
7. Stevenson I: The diagnostic interview. 2nd ed. New York: Harper & Row, Publishers, 1971.
8. Wulff HR: Rational diagnosis and treatment. Oxford: Blackwell Scientific Publications, 1976.

9. DeGowin EL, DeGowin RL: Bedside diagnostic examination. 3rd ed. New York: Macmillan Publishing Co, Inc, 1976.
10. Enelow AJ, Swisher SN: Interviewing and patient care. New York: Oxford University Press, 1972.
11. Judge RD, Zuidema GD, eds. Methods of clinical examination: a physiologic approach. 3rd ed. Boston: Little, Brown and Co, 1974.
12. Price RB, Vlahcevic ZR. Logical principles in differential diagnosis. Ann Intern Med 1971;75:89-95.
13. Levinson D. Teaching the diagnostic process. J Med Educ 1968;43:961-8.
14. Newell A, Simon HA. Human problem solving. Englewood Cliffs, NJ: Prentice Hall Inc, 1972.
15. Casscells W, Schoenberger A, Graboys TB. Interpretation by physicians of clinical laboratory results. N Engl J Med 1978;299:999-1001.
16. Slovic P, Fishhoff B, Lichtenstein S. Behavioral decision theory. Ann Rev Psychol 1977; 28:1-39.
17. Tversky A, Kahneman D. Judgment under uncertainty. Heuristics and biases. In: Wendt D, Vlek C, eds. Utility, probability, and human decision making. Boston: D. Reidel Publishing Co, 1975:141-62.
18. Elstein AS, Shulman LS, Sprafka SA. Medical problem solving: an analysis of clinical reasoning. Cambridge, MA: Harvard University Press, 1978.
19. Kahneman D, Tversky A. On the psychology of prediction. Psychol Rev 1973;80:237-51.
20. Tversky A, Kahneman D. Judgment under uncertainty: Heuristics and biases. Science 1974;185:1124.
21. Tversky A, Kahneman D. Availability: a heuristic for judging frequency and probability. Cognitive Psychology 1973;5:207-32.
22. Feinstein AR. An analysis of diagnostic reasoning. III. Construction of clinical algorithms. Yale J Biol Med 1974;27:5-32.
23. Eiseman B, Wotkyns RS. Surgical decision making. Philadelphia, Pa: WB Saunders, 1978.
24. Pauker SG, Kassirer JP. Therapeutic decision making: a cost-benefit analysis. N Engl J Med 1975;293:229-34.
25. Raiffa H. Decision analysis: Introductory lectures on choices under uncertainty. Reading, MA: Addison-Wesley, 1968.
26. Ginsberg AS. Decision analysis in the clinical patient management with an application to the pleural-effusion syndrome. Rand Corp R-751-RC/NLM Santa Monica 1971.
27. Schwartz WB, Gorry GA, Kassirer JP, Essig A. Decision analysis and clinical judgment. Am J Med 1973;55:459-72.
28. Emerson PA, Teather D, Handley AJ. The application of decision theory to the prevention of deep venous thrombosis following myocardial infarction. Q J Med 1974;43: 380-98.
29. Schoenbaum SG, McNeil BJ, Kavet J. The swine influenza decision. N Engl J Med 1976; 295:759-65.
30. Sisson JC, Schoomaker EB, Ross JC. Clinical decision analysis: the hazard of using additional data. JAMA 1976;236:1259-63.
31. McNeil BJ, Hessel SJ, Branch WT, Bjork L, Adelstein SJ. Measures of clinical efficacy: III. The value of the lung scan in the evaluation of young patients with pleuritic chest pain. J Nucl Med 1976;17:163-9.
32. Kassirer JP. The principles of clinical decision making: an introduction to decision analysis. Yale J Biol Med 1976;49:149-64.
33. Pauker SG. Coronary artery surgery: the use of decision analysis. Ann Intern Med 1976; 85:8-18.
34. Pauker SP, Pauker SG. Prenatal diagnosis: a directive approach to genetic counseling using decision analysis. Yale J Biol Med 1977;50:275-89.

35. Safran C, Desforges JG, Tsichlis PN, Bluming AZ. Decision analysis to evaluate lymphangiography in the management of patients with Hodgkin's disease. N Engl J Med 1977; 296:1088-92.
36. Pauker SG, Kassirer JP. The threshold approach to clinical decision making. N Engl J Med 1980;302:1109-17.
37. Pauker SG, Kassirer JP. Clinical application of decision analysis: a detailed illustration. Semin Nucl Med 1978;8:324-35.
38. Pauker SG, Gorry GA, Kassirer JP, Schwartz WB. Toward the simulation of clinical cognition. Taking a present illness by computer. Am J Med 1976;60:981-96.
39. Kulikowski CA, Weiss S, Safir A. Glaucoma diagnosis and therapy by computer. Proceedings of Annual Meeting of Association for Research in Vision and Ophthalmology: Sarasota, Florida, May 1973.
40. Shortliffe EH, Axline SG, Buchanan BG, Merigan TC, Cohen SN. An artificial intelligence program to advise physicians regarding antimicrobial therapy. Comput Biomed Res 1973;6:544.
41. Pople HE, Jr. The formation of composite hypotheses in diagnostic problem solving: an exercise in synthetic reasoning. Proceedings 5th International Joint Conference on Artificial Intelligence. Available from Carnegie Mellon Univ, Pittsburgh, 1977.
42. Kassirer JP, Gorry GA. Clinical problem solving: a behavioral analysis. Ann Intern Med 1978;89:245-55.
43. Barrows HS, Bennett K. The diagnostic (problem solving) skill of the neurologist. Experimental studies and their implications for neurological training. Arch Neurol 1972;26: 273-7.
44. Miller GA. The magical number seven, plus or minus two: some limits on our capacity for processing information. Psychol Rev 1956;63:81-97.
45. Wood G. The knew-it-all-along effect. J Exp Psychol [Hum Percept] 1978;4:345-53.

CHAPTER SIX

Cognitive Models of Medical Problem Solvers

Paul E. Johnson, PhD

For years those who studied the problem-solving process hoped that individuals at different levels of training and experience would differ in characteristic, predictable ways. However, beginning with the classic work of DeGroot[1] and Chase and Simon[2] in chess, and continuing to present day work in a number of areas including medicine,[3-5] the dominant message seems to be that similarities outweigh differences in comparisons between individual problem solvers.

In medicine as well as other areas, problem solving consists of an application of hypothetico-deductive reasoning in which the basic units are questions, cues, and diagnostic hypotheses. Clinical problem solving typically begins with the elicitation of a small number of cues obtained through questions (usually through the taking of a patient history) that suggest a limited number of diagnostic hypotheses. Additional cues are interpreted with respect to the diagnostic hypotheses, suggesting new, revised hypotheses. Eventually, hypotheses are evaluated with respect to their relative ability to account for cues. Clinicians seem to generate hypotheses in similar quantities, use those hypotheses to guide collection and interpretation of additional patient data, and evaluate the relative ability of the hypotheses to account for that data. Differences between experts and novices (and among members of each group) are found at a more detailed, qualitative level in the content of physician knowledge and the features of a case.[6]

This work was supported by grants from the Dwan Fund of the University of Minnesota Medical School, the University of Minnesota Graduate School, and The Center for Research in Human Learning through grants from the National Institute for Child Health and Human Development and the National Science Foundation.

Numerous colleagues as well as former and current students have contributed to the work reported here. I am particularly grateful to Paul Feltovich for the analysis and discussion of data on the SubAS case reported here (see Feltovich, 1981; Feltovich et al., 1980, for a more detailed description of this case and others).

There is usually large variation in problem-solving behavior, both within the same physician and among physicians. This variation appears to be due to problem-specific differences in cases and individual differences in physician knowledge. Varying the domain from which a case originates results in changes in the degree of skill a clinical problem solver displays. As a function of their knowledge of an area, individual clinicians have profiles of competence that vary across case domains and across similar cases that differ at a detailed level. Little can be predicted, at a detailed level, about the problem-solving behavior of a specific physician on a specific case without extensive knowledge of the characteristics of the case and of the way those characteristics interact with the physician's knowledge of the medical domain from which the case is drawn.

To advance our current understanding of problem solving in medicine it will be necessary to represent the formal knowledge individual physicians have of the domain in which cases occur as well as the experiential knowledge they have from their past encounters with such cases. In addition, it will be useful to represent the cognitive skills physicians have developed for applying this knowledge to the task of diagnostic thinking.

This paper presents a model of physician knowledge for what patients with particular diseases or conditions should "look like." The model, which has also been partially formalized as a computer program,[7] is used to interpret behavior in tasks in which physicians are asked to diagnose particular patient cases.[8] The model allows for the interpretation of success as well as error in diagnostic thinking.

A COGNITIVE MODEL OF DIAGNOSTIC REASONING

The proposed model embodies a memory store of disease models each of which specifies, for a particular disease, the set of clinical manifestations that a patient with the disease should present clinically (see also Rubin's disease "templates"[9] and Pople's "disease entities."[10] In the theory of the expert, this set of disease models is extensive[1,2] and hierarchically organized.[10,11] At upper (more general) levels of the hierarchy are disease categories consisting of sets of diseases that present similarly because of physiological similarity. Particular diseases occupy middle ranks of the hierarchy and these, in turn, are differentiated at the lowest hierarchical levels into numerous variants of each disease, each of which presents slightly differently in the clinic for reasons of underlying anatomy, severity, or patient's age at time of presentation.

In novices, prototype knowledge is developed around "classical" cases. Initial training materials,[12] as well as the probability distribution of diseases presenting in the hospital, emphasize the most common versions of diseases, which then constitute "anchorage points" for subsequent elaboration of the store of diseases.[13] In the novice, disease knowledge also lacks extensive cross-referencing and connection among disease models in memory.[14,15] It is with experience that the starting-point store of diseases is augmented, and both generalized into categorical clusters, as similarities among diseases are discovered, and discriminated into finer distinct entities, as differentiation points among diseases are discovered.[16,17]

For a model of memory to function in a diagnostic task two types of process or skill must be defined: generation of hypotheses and evaluation of hypotheses with respect to the available data.

Hypothesis Generation

The generation of hypotheses in a specific problem-solving encounter is accomplished through direct links between patient data and one or more disease models in memory (we shall call these data-driven heuristics). Figure 1 gives a model for illustrating the relationships between patient data and schema for disease knowledge in memory. According to the model, a given piece of data (age 60 months) triggers three schema in memory, atrial septal defect (ASD), functional murmur, and mild heart disease. Each of these represents a separate entity with expectations for what individuals with the presumed abnormality should look like. Once generated the three hypotheses are placed in working memory to be considered in light of eventual data.

In addition to hypotheses generated because of direct links to patient data, there are also hypotheses generated because they are linked to other hypotheses (hypotheses-driven heuristics). In this case when a given disease has been triggered, additional schema are generated as elaborations of further specifications of the given hypothesis and perhaps as variants of it. According to the model shown in Figure 1, the original datum, (patient age 60 months) activates the classic ASD heuristic, which in turn triggers the variant, severe ASD. As before, the hypothesis is placed in working memory to be evaluated with respect to additional data.

Hypothesis Evaluation

The evaluation of hypotheses that have been triggered in the manner specified above takes two forms. The first is based on the use of micro-decision rules and is termed exact reasoning. The second is based on the use of more global or macro-decision rules and is termed inexact reasoning.

Exact Reasoning: The data collected from a patient form a context in which certain evidence (e.g., pathognomonic findings) indicate nearly invariant conclusions to be drawn, either to accept a specific hypothesis or to unconditionally reject a specific hypothesis (e.g., if a difference is observed in blood pressure reading taken by the flush method between the arm and the leg, then conclude coarcation of the aorta). These micro-rules are embedded in both data-driven and hypothesis-driven heuristics. Embedding such rules in the context of heuristics allows many hypotheses to be eliminated by the time the final piece of evidence has been gathered. If, however, the micro-rules for exact reasoning are not sufficient to isolate a single hypothesis, then the macro-rules of inexact reasoning must be invoked.

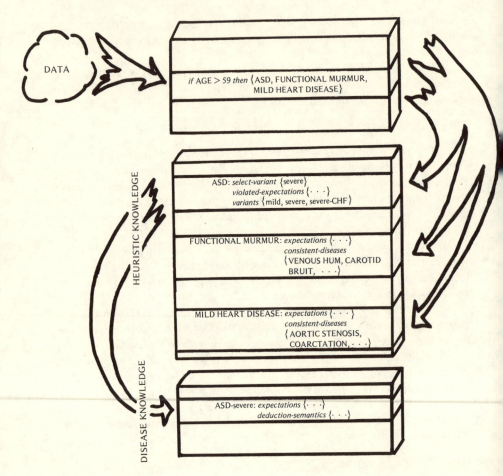

Figure 1. Illustration of model process of triggering disease knowledge from patient data.

Inexact Reasoning: If the evaluation of hypotheses during the course of diagnostic thinking does not converge to a single conclusion, then more contextually independent procedures must be used. Typical schemes of inexact reasoning are represented by models in which expert knowledge is augmented with statistical data and Bayesian procedures. Arguments against this approach are based primarily on (a) the assumption of conditional independence of symptoms,[18] (b) the stability of the conditional probabilities,[19] and (c) the reliability of complex stochastic modeling over simple methods.[20]

The model described here uses relatively simple macro-decision rules to perform a differential diagnosis based on the final set of disease candidates. Differential diagnosis involves a comparative evaluation among hypotheses; specifically, hypotheses are rated according to their relative ability to account for patient findings. These ratings are used to rank the hypotheses, with the hypothesis receiving the highest ranking at the end of a case being the final diagnosis. Macro-decision rules have been used in several studies of medical problem solving[3,4] based on "how well" the obtained patient data fit the hypotheses in question.

In the model, patient data are classified into four groups according to their relevance to the expected findings identified in the disease schema triggered from the knowledge base. Patient data, when evaluated in the context of a specific disease hypothesis, may be judged as (a) not relevant (they are filtered out by data heuristics), (b) confirmed expectations (an abnormal finding was expected and obtained or a normal finding was expected and obtained), (c) unobtained abnormals (an abnormal finding was expected but a normal finding was obtained), or (d) unexplained abnormals (a normal finding was expected but an abnormal was obtained).

When all of the available patient data have been received, and all of the active disease hypotheses have been considered with respect to that data, the macro-decision rule used to order diseases for differential diagnosis simply counts confirmed expectations, unobtained abnormals, and unexplained abnormals for each candidate disease hypothesis and combines them in one of several alternative ways (see Swanson,[7] for a more complete discussion). Each alternative rule yields a value, which can be used to form a preference ordering of hypotheses.

EVIDENCE FROM THE DIAGNOSIS OF
CONGENITAL HEART DISEASE

Let us now turn to a consideration of some data recently collected in our laboratory by Paul Feltovich, as part of his Ph.D. thesis research.[21,22] One of Feltovich's cases, subaortic stenosis, was selected from the files of the University Heart Hospital because it is described in introductory texts on congenital heart disease but is often confused with other cardiac anomalies that present similarly, and hence form a set of competing alternatives leading to a possible misdiagnosis of a given instance of the disease.

The competing alternatives for the case presented here are all variations of aortic stenosis: valvular aortic stenosis (ValAS), subvalvular aortic stenosis (SubAS), and supravalvular aortic stenosis (SupAS). All of these disease variants involve obstruction to left ventricular outflow with different variants defined by slight differences in the locus of obstruction: ValAS is an obstruction at the aortic valve itself; SubAS is an obstruction slightly "upstream" from the valve; SupAS is obstruction slightly "downstream" from the valve. Because these disease variants are only subtly different anatomically and physiologically, they differ only slightly in clinical presentation. ValAS is the most common of the three and receives the greatest amount of exposition in introductory training materials of pediatric cardiology (for example, Moller[12]). Hence it might be expected that subjects' knowledge for ValAS will develop more rapidly than for others. The question addressed in Feltovich's experiment was the extent to which subjects at differing levels of training and experience would confuse these three alternative conditions and misdiagnose a given case of SubAS.

Data for the case were drawn from the case files of the University of Minnesota Hospital. The patients' data were summarized in 23 verbal statements, each presenting a particular aspect of the medical history, physical examination, or laboratory data. These statements were constructed with the help of a consulting cardiologist and were placed into standard patient data groupings of history, physical examination, x-ray findings, and electrocardiographic readings.

Subjects and Method

Four experts (board-certified staff in pediatric cardiology and fifth and sixth year specialty fellows), four trainees (first and second year specialty fellows and residents), and four medical students who had completed a 6-week elective in pediatric cardiology served as subjects. All were volunteers. Each of the 23 statements was read to the subject in turn in the order in which the data appeared in the patient chart (history, physical examination, x-ray, ECG). After each statement, subjects were asked to describe their thoughts; upon completion of all 23 statements, subjects were asked to make a final diagnosis. The complete problem-solving session for each subject was tape-recorded and transcribed. The simulation model was also given the data.

Results

The case of subaortic stenosis was correctly diagnosed by four subjects (two experts and two trainees). The simulation model also correctly diagnosed the case as SubAS. All subjects generated the basic disease hypothesis, valvular aortic stenosis, six subjects generated the variant supra-aortic stenosis, and six subjects generated the operative disease subaortic stenosis. The simulation generated each of the three alternatives.

To evaluate the performance of subjects and the simulation model on the SubAS case more precisely, an analysis was performed on just those hypotheses that were from the competitor set (ValAS, SubAS, SupraAS). The patient data responsible for eliciting each of these hypotheses in subjects as well as the simulation model are shown in Table 1.

Table 1. Evaluations of Target Data Items with Respect to Members of the Competitor Set

	Target Data Items																	
	(10) Normal Facies			(17) Thrill			(18) No Click			(19) Murmur			(20) Aortic Insufficiency			(22) Prominent Aorta		
Subjects	ValAS	SubAS	SupAS*	ValAS	SubAS	SupAS	ValAS	SubAS	SupAS	ValAS	SubAS	SupAS	ValAS	SubAS	SupAS	ValAS	SubAS	SupAS
S_1			−				−			+						+		
S_2	o		−		+		+			+			+			+		
S_3					+		+			+			+					
S_4					+					+						+		
T_1					+		−			+		+			+	+	+	
T_2										+						+	+	
T_3					+	+	−		o	+			+		+	−	+	
T_4					+	+	−			+						+		
E_1					o	+	−			+	o		+	+		+	−	−
E_2						+	−	+		+	+	+	+		+	+	+	+
E_3			−		+	+	−	+	+	+	+	+	+		+	+	+	+
E_4					+		−	+		+	+	+	+		+	+		
Simulation					+		−			+	+	+				+	−	−

*ValAS = Valvular Aortic Stenosis; SubAS = Subvalvular Aortic Stenosis; SupAS = Supravalvular Aortic Stenosis.

Table 1 shows all evaluations for the competing hypotheses with respect to the set of data items that are central to successful solution of the case. A mark (+, –, o) under a disease variant and data item in this table indicates that the data item was judged to be positive, negative, or neutral evidence for the disease variant as a hypothesis. For example, a negative evaluation of "no click" with respect to ValAS would be: "The lack of a systolic ejection click is against valvular aortic stenosis." Table 1 shows a general increase, from students to experts, in the active evaluation of data items as evidence for or against the variants of aortic stenosis. The evaluation of any particular data item in relation to all three variants is one indication that a subject is actively attempting to weigh the variants against each other to determine which is the best explanation for the case. No students,, two trainees (T_1, T_3), three experts (E_1, E_3, E_4), and the simulation model meet this criterion. A second criterion of expertness is the extent to which all three variants were evaluated in relation to more than one data item. No students, no trainees, three experts (E_1, E_3, E_4), and the simulation model meet this criterion.

The analysis thus far suggests that the more expert subjects and the simulation model consider and actively evaluate a set of good alternative hypotheses. Examination of the two most experienced subjects, E_3 and E_4, yields some clues as to the knowledge structure that supports this performance. Figure 2 shows the protocols of these subjects at two data points: 17, which is the first strong evidence for valvular aortic stenosis and other variants, and 18, which is the strongest evidence against ValAS. E_3 raises all three variants together (in the same "breath" so to speak) at the time of the first strong evidence. These hypotheses are then available to be evaluated comparatively against subsequent data, in particular, data item 18. This same form characterizes subject E_1. Subject E_4, however, aggressively focuses on the "classic" member of the competitor set at 17, but immediately expands to the full set on receiving negative evidence at 18. This form is shared by subject T_3 and less clearly, subject T_1.

One explanation for these patterns is that in the expert, a disease and the set of alternatives most likely to be confused with it during a diagnostic encounter constitute a memory unit or category, so that when one of the members is triggered, the others are also activated. The expert can then choose to consider category members in two modes. In the first mode, he tests all members simultaneously. This first mode might be termed "precautionary" since if any hypothesis encounters disconfirmatory evidence, alternative explanations for which the same evidence might be compatible are already under consideration. In the second mode, the expert tests only the most likely member (in his current judgment). This mode of reasoning might be termed one of "extraction" because its general success depends heavily on "rejection" of the target disease when appropriate, which, in turn, depends heavily on the precision in the diagnostician's model for the disease. Once the target disease is rejected, other category members provide a ready "back-up" set of alternative hypotheses.

A final analysis of the results of this case involves an attempt to discern

(17) There is a systolic thrill felt below the right clavicle, along the mid-left sternal border, and in the suprasternal notch.

E_3:   This thrill is most consistent with a diagnosis of bicuspid aortic valve or aortic valvular stenosis. It would also be consistent with supravalvular stenosis and discrete subaortic stenosis.

E_4:   Until proved otherwise, now, he must have valvular aortic stenosis.

(18) The first heart sound is normal and there is no systolic ejection click.

E_3:   The absence of a systolic ejection click in the presence of what I would consider to be an aortic outflow thrill makes aortic valvular stenosis and bicuspid aortic valve less likely. Aortic valvular stenosis of a very severe degree might be associated without a click. On the other hand, uh, it makes us think more seriously of discrete membranous subaortic stenosis.

E_4:   Absence of the click is against valvular aortic stenosis. Then perhaps instead he has subvalvular or supravalvular aortic stenosis.

Figure 2. Protocols from experts E_3 and E_4 at data points 17 and 18.

the causes for subjects' errors in final diagnosis. Six subjects (S_1, S_3, S_4, T_2, T_4, E_2) never considered subvalvular aortic stenosis at all, although all generated valvular aortic stenosis. At least three explanations could apply to this lack of activation. First, and most basically, it could be that subjects do not know about SubAS. However, postexperimental interviews with all these subjects confirmed that they had some knowledge of this disease and could describe it. A second possible explanation is that these subjects have not built up strong "bottom-up" associations in memory between any data item of the case and the subvalvular disease. Even lacking such a "trigger" for SubAS itself, it would have been possible for subjects to generate SubAS as a side effect of their activation of ValAS, if these two diseases were related in a memory unit, through a process of "spreading activation"[23] or "top-down" activation.[24,25] This suggests that for these subjects, their knowledge representations for the variants of aortic stenosis exist more in isolation than they do in the more experienced subjects.

For those subjects who generated ValAS as a hypothesis but failed to abandon it in the face of strong negative evidence, examination of their handling of this disconfirmatory evidence yields insight into the nature and precision of their disease models for ValAS. Discussion will focus on data item 18, the strongest evidence against ValAS.

Two subjects (S_2, S_3), evaluated 18, "no click," as confirmatory for ValAS. This appears to reflect, simply, an error in important factual knowledge about this disease. Two subjects (S_4, T_2) did not evaluate 18 at all with respect to ValAS. Significantly, they also did not generate any variant of aortic stenosis until after data item 18. This suggests that the memory store of bottom-up associations between data items and aortic stenosis variants for these subjects is not as extensive as for other subjects and, in particular, that data item 18 is not recognized as a strong cue for aortic stenosis type diseases. A further implication is that the physical examination finding of a "systolic ejection click" and its import in ValAS are not represented in the ValAS disease models of these subjects since, if they were, the model itself should have led the subjects to reexamine this finding.

Finally, four subjects (S_1, T_4, E_1, E_2) who, although they evaluated 18 as negative for ValAS, maintained ValAS as a final diagnosis. The protocols of subjects S_1 and T_4 yield some insight into an explanation for these subjects. Figure 3 shows the protocols for these two subjects at data points 18 and 22, the latter consisting primarily of the finding of a "prominent aorta" on x-ray. Both subjects question ValAS at 18, but are much more satisfied with this diagnosis at 22 and thereafter.

There is a causal relationship between a "tight" or stenotic aortic valve and an enlarged or prominent aorta. To open a tight valve, the left ventricle of the heart must generate abnormally high pressure. Blood expelled under this high pressure forces against the aortic wall and expands it. For the two subjects under discussion, it appears that their causal knowledge attributes the "systolic ejection click" in ValAS to the enlarged aorta itself; that is, the click is caused by the large chamber into which the valve is opening, perhaps some kind of resonance phenomenon. For these subjects, the causal chain from the valve to the "click" is as follows.

tight valve → big aorta → click

Hence, for these subjects, the "big aorta" itself is predominant over the "click" as evidence for ValAS, with the click just additional evidence for a big aorta. Once they receive their best evidence for a "big aorta," 22, they are no longer worried about the lack of a "click."

The true state of affairs appears to be that a tight valve causes both the "click" and the enlarged aorta at the same level of cause.[26] The systolic ejection click is associated with the opening of the right valve itself as shown below.

tight valve → click → big aorta

Hence, both of these effects must be proved. Why might a number of subjects have misconstrued this relationship? One need look no further than the introductory textbook these subjects use,[12] where the erroneous causal relationship is stated, or at least strongly implied.

Discussion

Analysis of the pattern of hypotheses generated during the problem-solving process showed that the set of alternatives identified in the medical literature as competitors to the correct diagnosis was generated by both the simulation and subjects in response to the data of the case. Of the diseases in this set, valvular aortic stenosis was generated by all subjects and concluded (incorrectly) as the final diagnosis by eight subjects. Supra-aortic stenosis was generated by six subjects but was not concluded as the final diagnosis by any subject. Subaortic

(18) The first heart sound is normal and there is no systolic ejection click.

S_1:   Ah, well, this, the fact that there is no systolic ejection click present tells us that there is probably not a poststenotic dilatation of the aorta, which one would expect with the presence of aortic stenosis and some aortic insufficiency. However, this does not necessarily rule it out.

T_4:   Love it. Um, well, okay. I wonder if there is . . . , no click, that's funny. I would expect it if he has AS. I wish they had said whether the murmur went up into his neck. Okay.

X-RAY

(22) The chest x-ray shows normal cardiac size and contour and normal vascularity, but prominence of the ascending aorta.

S_1:   Ah, well this is what one would expect with a ah, aortic stenosis with secondary aortic insufficiency. One would expect that the aorta, ascending aorta distal to the ah, to the stenosis, would be dilatated due to the changes in the wall tension across the gradients. Therefore, ah, the fact that ah, a click was not heard on physical exam, may have been a subjective finding of the person examining. But, the x-ray does indeed suggest that there is some poststenotic dilatation.

T_4:   Ha ha! AS-AI.

Figure 3. Protocols from subjects S_1 and T_4 at data points 18 and 22.

stenosis was generated by six subjects and concluded (correctly) as the final diagnosis by four subjects. Of the twelve possible final diagnoses offered by subjects, the set of alternatives identified in the medical literature and also generated by the simulation accounted for all of them.

The errors responsible for a faulty diagnosis can be related to similar processes of hypothesis generation and evaluation in the simulation model (as described earlier): (a) errors of hypothesis generation —not all subjects generated the correct hypothesis as one of the responses to the data of the case; having failed to generate the correct hypothesis it could, of course, not be considered as one of the contenders for the final diagnosis (one expert, two trainees, and three students made this type of error), and (b) errors of hypothesis evaluation—although the correct disease was generated at some point, the fit between the expectations of the prototype for this disease and the data of the case was not judged sufficient to warrant its selection as the final diagnosis (one expert and one student made this type of error).

The data on subject errors also raise two important issues. First, they demonstrate how "small" knowledge errors can have major repercussions for the handling of a case, which in turn gives some insight into the case-specific nature of a clinician's diagnostic performance also found elsewhere.[3] Second, they suggest a sensitivity in less experienced clinicians to specific training experiences, e.g., training materials, particular patient cases, etc. As experience increases, so does the sample of "inputs" and the effects of particular experience might be expected to lessen accordingly.

Although the data presented here are based on a single task and a small sample of subjects, it was possible to represent the kind of detailed medical knowledge that is necessary for successful task performance. That such a representation can be embodied in a simulation model and tested against the behavior of human subjects supports the argument that development and evaluation of such representations may lead to a better understanding of the problem-solving process as well as possible improvement in the practice of problem solving itself, through improved education and decision support.[27,28]

References

1. DeGroot AD. Thought and choice in chess. New York: Basic Books, Inc., 1965.
2. Chase WG, Simon HA. Perception in chess. Cognitive Psychology, 1973;4:55-81.
3. Elstein AS, Shulman LS, Sprafka SA. Medical problem solving. Cambridge, Mass.: Harvard University Press, 1978.
4. Barrows HS, Feightner JW, Neufeld VR, Norman GR. Analysis of the clinical methods of medical students and physicians. Final report, Ontario Department of Health Grants ODH-PR-273 and ODM-DM-226, Hamilton, Ontario, Canada: McMaster University, March 1978.
5. McGuire C, Bashook P. A conceptual framework for measuring clinical problem solving. Paper presented at the meeting of the American Educational Research Association, 1978.
6. Connelly D, Johnson PE. The medical problem solving process. Hum Pathol 1980;11:412-19.
7. Swanson DB. Computer simulation of expert problem solving in medical diagnosis. Ph.D. thesis, University of Minnesota, 1978.
8. Johnson PE, Barreto A, Hassebrock F, Moller J, Feltovich P, Swanson D. Expertise and error in diagnostic reasoning. Cognitive science 1981,5, 235-55.
9. Rubin AD. Hypothesis formation and evaluation in medical diagnosis (MIT-AI Tech. Report 316). Cambridge, MA: MIT, 1975.
10. Pople HE. The formation of composite hypotheses in diagnostic problem solving: An exercise in synthetic reasoning. Paper presented at the International Joint Conference on Artificial Intelligence, 1977.
11. Wortman PM. Medical diagnosis: An information processing approach. Comput Biomed Res 1972;5:315-28.
12. Moller JH. Essentials of pediatric cardiology. Philadelphia: F. A. Davis Company, 1978.
13. Rosch E, Mervis CG, Gray W, Johnson D, Boyes-Braem P. Basic objects in natural categories. Cognitive Psychology 1976;8:383-440.
14. Elstein AS, Loupe MJ, Erdmann, JG. An experimental study of medical diagnostic thinking. Journal of Structural Learning 1971;2:45-53.
15. Shavelson RJ. Some aspects of the correspondence between content structure and cognitive structure in physics instruction. J Educ Psych 1972;63:225-34.
16. Reed SK. Category vs. item learning: Implications for categorization models. Memory and Cognition 1978;6:612-21.
17. Wortman PM, Greenberg LD. Coding, recoding, and decoding of hierarchical information in long-term memory. Journal of Verbal Learning and Verbal Behavior 1971;10:234-43.
18. Norusis M, Jacques J. Diagnosis. I. Symptom nonindependence in mathematical models for diagnosis. Comput Biomed Research 1975;8.
19. Shortliffe EH, Buchanan BG, Feigenbaum EA. Knowledge engineering for medical decision making: A review of computer-based clinical decision aids. Proc IEEE 1979;67 (No. 9):1207-24.

20. Dawes RM. The robust beauty of improper linear models in decision making. Am Psychol 1979;34(No. 7):571-82.
21. Feltovich PJ. Knowledge based components of expertise in medical diagnosis. Ph.D. thesis, University of Minnesota, 1981.
22. Feltovich PJ, Johnson PE, Moller JH, Swanson DB. The role and development of medical knowledge in diagnostic reasoning. Paper presented at the meeting of the American Educational Research Association, Boston, 1980.
23. Anderson JR. Language, memory and thought. Hillsdale, N.J,: Lawrence Erlbaum Associates, 1976.
24. Rummelhart DE, Ortony A. The representation of knowledge in memory. In: Anderson RC, Spiro RJ, Montague WE, eds. Schooling and the acquisition of knowledge. Hillsdale NJ: Lawrence Erlbaum Associates, 1977.
25. Bobrow DG, Norman DA. Some principles of memory schemata. In: Bobrow DG, Collins A, eds. Representation and understanding: Studies in cognitive science. New York: Academic Press, 1975.
26. Moss AJ, Adams FH, Emmanouilidies GC. Heart disease in infants, children and adolescents. Baltimore: Williams and Wilkins, Company, 1977:180.
27. Johnson PE, Severance DG, Feltovich PJ. Design of decision support systems in medicine: Rationale and principles from the analysis of physician expertise. Proceedings of the Twelfth Hawaii International Conference on System Sciences, Wester Periodicals Co., 1979;3:105-18.
28. Swanson DB, Feltovich PJ, Johnson PE. Analysis of expertise: Implications for the design of decision support systems. In: Shires DB, Wolf H, eds. Medinfo 77. Amsterdam: North-Holland Publishing Co., 1977:161-4.

CHAPTER SEVEN

Decision Making in Primary Care: The Case of Obesity

Michael M. Ravitch, PhD, David R. Rovner, MD, Penny A. Jennett, MA, Margaret M. Holmes, PhD, Gerald B. Holzman, MD, and Arthur S. Elstein, PhD

INTRODUCTION

Most studies of clinical decision making fall into one of two classes. Retrospective reviews use chart audit techniques to assess the performance of physicians in the light of predetermined criteria.[1] The criteria may deal with the steps to be performed in the work-up of a target condition, as in Payne's process index. Alternatively, evaluation may be concerned with frequency or rate of achieving desired outcomes of care, regardless of the process employed, as in the Performance Evaluation Program of the Joint Commission on Accreditation of Hospitals.[2] In either case, the record is evaluated retrospectively, in the light of some external standard.

Another major approach to research on clinical decision making uses decision analysis,[3,4] a frankly normative approach to determining the optimal strategy for a variety of difficult clinical decisions: weighing risks and benefits of an invasive diagnostic procedure,[5] or choosing a treatment where the safer treatment is also less effective, or determining an optimal subset from a battery of tests that are correlated to some extent.[6] The normative model in these situations is intended to guide future practice, though it can also be applied to retrospective evaluation.

Now it can be argued that these two approaches to studying clinical decision making focus so heavily on conformity to or departure from externally developed norms that the decisions of physicians, who may well be trying to achieve aims other than those implied by the norms, will almost inevitably

This research was supported in part by a grant from the National Library of Medicine, LM-03396. We wish to acknowledge the contributions of Marilyn L. Rothert, PhD, Paulette Valliere, and Rita Huang to the planning and execution of this investigation.

appear to be irrational or suboptimal.[7] But is such a conclusion warranted? It is easier to raise this question than to answer it, but at least it does point to the need for careful study of physician behavior and for efforts to understand this behavior as an attempt to cope with complexity, not as a perverse refusal to conform to rational guidelines. For by understanding why physicians behave as they do, we may be able to change behavior in ways that do not seem arbitrary, capricious, reductionistic, or imposed from without. We may even be able to persuade physicians to behave normatively!

This line of reasoning opens the door to a third paradigm for the study of clinical decision making. It postpones the question of normative appraisal and asks instead, What is this behavior and what are its determinants? The approach is thus descriptive and analytic, rather than evaluative, at least in its initial phases. It aims not so much to critique physician performance in the light of a model of perfect rationality—though such criticism may well emerge from these studies—as to understand how experienced clinicians make decisions when they are not guided by the explicit criteria of a normative chart audit or by the rigorous structuring of decision analysis.

The analysis of clinical decision making proposed here is essentially psychological. It views the clinician as an information processor of limited rational capacity[8,9] trying to cope with an exceedingly complex probabilistic environment. The psychological representation of this environment will almost surely be simpler than the environment itself. Thus, one aspect of the investigation can focus on what is included and what is omitted in the representation of the task. Certain characteristics of clinical reasoning are understood as consequences of a serial processing strategy and the limited rationality of the human information processing system.[10]

A number of research methods are subsumed within this general paradigm. The process-tracing or information-processing analysis of clinical reasoning is one of these methods. Earlier work concentrated on a detailed analysis of a limited number of physicians solving an even smaller number of diagnostic problems. It relied heavily on analysis of clinicians thinking aloud as they solved clinical problems. The assets and liabilities of this approach have been the subject of much discussion[9,11,12] and need not be repeated here. Suffice it to say that in embarking on new investigations, an approach was sought that would survey physicians' decisions more extensively than was possible with process-tracing and thinking aloud. One way to accomplish this goal is to study the decisions recorded in charts, without evaluating them according to external criteria, and using multiple regression or discriminant function analysis to identify consistencies in the handling of clinical information or making decisions. These consistencies are conceptualized as a clinical policy for dealing with cases in a particular category, and studies of this type are therefore called policy capturing.[13] This method is currently being applied to the decision making of primary care physicians in regard to obese patients.

BACKGROUND

The investigation of the decision making of primary care physicians concerning obese patients began with the impression of the endocrinologist in our group (DRR) that most of the obese patients referred to his clinic do not have significant endocrine disease related to their obesity. Many, if not most, of these patients were in this sense inappropriate referrals. Hypothyroidism and Cushing's Syndrome could both be ruled out by history and physical examination alone in many cases, thus eliminating the need for an expensive endocrine work-up. He felt that if referring physicians properly weighted available cues, then diagnostic accuracy would increase. As a consequence, patients referred would be fewer and more likely to be obese because of conditions that an endocrinologist can treat. Indeed, many medical subspecialists feel that much of their referral practice is made up of "poor" or inappropriate referrals and that primary care physicians ought to be able to diagnose more accurately and not refer these patients to specialists needlessly. On the other hand, primary care physicians are also criticized for not referring appropriate patients early enough. Clearly, these decisions constitute an arena of problems.

Of course, specialists can see only the cases referred and have at best an imperfect understanding of how selective the referral process is. Given that hypothyroidism and Cushing's syndrome have very low rates of occurrence even in obese patients, it becomes clear that primary care physicians might be referring only a small fraction of their obese patients to specialists and that the vast majority of those referred could still have no significant endocrine disease (i.e., the false-positive rate is necessarily high). Under these conditions, the referral cohort that the endocrinologist construes as inappropriate is highly selected from the viewpoint of the referring physicians, the result of judgments and decisions that are, in the nature of medical practice, unknown to the physicians to whom cases are referred. Rather than being "inappropriate," the referrals may be the best that can be done in trying to detect a set of conditions with low base rates.

This analysis implies that the referral policies of primary care physicians are unknown to the specialists to whom they refer, since the specialists cannot readily know the reasoning used in deciding *not* to refer a patient; thus they form their impressions of primary care policies from a smaller subset of the entire range of decisions. One phase of our research will use policy capturing to identify consistent patterns in primary care decision making that cannot be clear to the specialists to whom referrals are sent.

METHOD

This line of reasoning suggests a series of questions revolving around two themes, one quantitative and the other qualitative. The quantitative questions have to do with the rate of referral and the incidence of suspected endocrine problems among those referred. The qualitative questions have to do with the clinical reasoning involved in the decision to refer a patient or not.

1. Suppose a cohort of patients is identified, all of whom are at least 15% above normal body weight, as determined from standard reference tables. Presumably not all of these patients will be identified as obese by their physicians nor will all of them be referred for endocrine work-ups. What are the determinants of the diagnostic judgment that a patient is obese? Is it weight alone or in combination with other factors? What are the other factors and how are they weighted? What is the relation between the judgment that a patient is obese and the decision to refer? How closely associated are they? Perhaps all or nearly all patients referred are obese but not all obese patients are referred. Why not? What other considerations can be identified as bearing on the referral decision?

2. What is the rate of referral of obese patients to an endocrine clinic? From a cohort of obese patients, how many will be referred and how many not? How many obese patients referred to the endocrine clinic do not have significant endocrine disease?

3. What are the reasons for referral as set forth in the referral letters? Why do primary care physicians seek endocrine consultations?

4. What are the medical and social variables associated with the decision to refer an obese patient to an endocrinologist? Put another way, is a high index of suspicion for endocrine disease needed to refer a patient to an endocrinologist? What other factors are involved in this decision? Is the degree of obesity a significant determinant of this decision? Or is it the presence of other problems whose management is made more difficult by obesity? Or is it the duration of the problem? How important is the social class of the patient and the ability to pay for endocrine work-up?

These questions may be summarized by asking, What guidelines and policies appear to be operating in these decisions? Can a statistical model of the policy be constructed by analysis of decisions involving a large series of patients? To what degree can such a model adequately represent the thought processes that produced the data used to construct the model?

These research questions are intended to be descriptive and analytic. We are trying to understand how physicians make these decisions by identifying the variables that singly or in combination distinguish between patients judged obese or not and patients who are referred to an endocrinologist or not. These variables and the weights assigned to them define a policy. We are not yet proposing guidelines for how these decisions ought to be made.

To study these questions, the charts of approximately 110 obese patients referred to the Endocrine Clinic at Michigan State University and approximately 300 obese patients randomly drawn from the entire clinic population are being reviewed according to a specially developed coding frame. Two criteria were used for including patients in the random sample: body weight 15% above normal and age greater than 15 years. A small number of obese patients in the random group will have been referred for endocrine work-ups; these will be deleted from the random sample. The major comparisons will be between referred and nonreferred groups. The retrospective review provides the data base needed to develop a statistical model of the cues and their weights that will predict the referral decisions of the primary-care physicians whose patients are the sample.

The quantitative questions—rates of referral and incidence of suspected endocrine problems—can be answered fairly easily. The more difficult problem is the analysis of the determinants of the decision to refer. Policy capturing addresses this difficulty by using multivariate statistical analysis to develop a model of the features in the patient's charts that will predict referral decisions. The model must identify the cues and assign weights to them. When the model has been constructed, it will be possible to determine how well it can capture the decisions of a large group of primary-care physicians. This approach to clinical decision making analyzes a large number of decisions and tries to find a formula that reproduces them.

COMMENTS ON THE RESEARCH DESIGN

In the early stages of planning, direct observation of care was considered. This method was rejected as too expensive, time-consuming, and too reactive. The costs of obtaining data on several hundred cases were simply too high. Observers would have to spend much time in physicians' offices awaiting the visits of obese patients. One could question whether physicians who would permit observation were representative of those who would not and whether the presence of an observer would affect to unknown degrees the care provided and the decisions made. These concerns led to the choice of retrospective chart review, which permits analysis of a large number of decisions made in actual clinical circumstances on real patients without the method of data collection affecting the decisions studied.

Since chart review is a naturalistic, not an experimental method, it has certain design flaws: (1) It is unlikely that each physician in the series will be represented by an equal number of patients, so that the range of physicians' decisions will be unevenly sampled. (2) Since each patient is seen by a different primary physician and each physician has a different panel of patients, differences in referral policy cannot be systematically attributed to patients or physicians. In most chart review studies, these differences are confounded or investigators must set aside the search for differences in policy between physicians. In this study, the chart review will be used to develop an overall referral policy for the panel of primary physicians studied, but reliable, stable policies for each physician will not be developed. It will not be possible to determine if there are systematic differences between physicians when patient variation is eliminated. This question will be approached in another phase of our study, which will use hypothetical case vignettes so that each physician will be presented with a standardized series of cases. Systematic differences in physicians' decisions can then be attributed more confidently to physician characteristics.

In the course of reviewing charts, one other serious problem has become apparent: How adequate is chart review for evaluating social factors in medical decision making? There is surely reason to believe that the socioeconomic status of the patient is an important determinant of medical decisions,[14,15] especially when the condition of concern is not immediately life-threatening, such as obesity, and/or when the decision concerns an elective procedure, for instance a diagnostic endocrine work-up. The patient's ability to pay may affect the physician's willingness to order an expensive, and possibly useless, diagnostic work-up. The social and personal significance of obesity may differ by social class and ethnicity, affecting the degree of the patient's insistence on care. Yet our preliminary impression is that the information needed for an accurate categorization of the patient's social class is missing in a significant fraction of the charts reviewed. Missing data may seriously impair the effectiveness of chart review as a tool for the analysis of social determinants of clinical policies and practices and may significantly limit the applicability of multivariate techniques like discriminant function analysis. It will be possible to be more precise about the extent of these problems as data analysis proceeds.

CONCLUSION

The referral of obese patients to endocrinologists is an illustration of a broader problem in the health care system—expectations regarding the use of laboratory tests in consultation. By understanding the determinants of referral decisions, we will be in a better position to develop guidelines for more rational, cost-effective laboratory use in these circumstances.

This study is designed to explore and model the reasoning of a large group of physicians on a common clinical problem by identifying and weighing cues, mainly from medical history and physical examinations, that are the determinants of the decision to refer. Policy capturing might be thought of as a variant of input-output analysis. The research strategy is intended to complement process-tracing studies,[9,16] which can explore the reasoning process in depth but which are necessarily limited in sampling both of physicians and cases. Policy-capturing research can sample cases and physicians more broadly, favoring generalizability. The price paid is that important determinants of certain types of decisions may not be entered in charts and their contributions cannot be analyzed. Multiple approaches are thus needed to study clinical reasoning. The policy-capturing strategy is applied here to obesity, but it need not be limited to that problem, for the tactics outlined have broader generality.

References

1. Payne BC and Study Staff. The quality of medical care: evaluation and improvement. Chicago: Hospital Research and Educational Trust, 1976.
2. Studnick J, Saywell R. Comparing medical audits: Correlation scaling, and sensitivity. J Med Educ 1978;53:480-6.
3. Kassirer JP. The principles of clinical decision making: an introduction to decision analysis. Yale J Biol Med 1976;49:149-64.
4. Pauker SG. Coronary artery surgery: the use of decision analysis. Ann Intern Med 1975; 85:8-18.

5. Weinstein MC, Fineberg HV, Elstein AS, et al. Clinical decision analysis. Philadelphia: WB Saunders, 1980.
6. McNeil BJ, Varady PD, Burrows BA, Adelstein SJ. Measure of clinical efficacy: I. Cost-effective calculations in the diagnosis and treatment of renovascular disease. N Engl J Med 1975;293:216-21.
7. Einhorn HJ, Hogarth RM. Behavioral decision theory: Processes of judgment and choice. Annu Rev Psychol 1981;32 (in press).
8. Newell A, Simon HA. Human problem solving. Englewood Cliffs: Prentice Hall, 1972.
9. Elstein AS, Shulman LS, Sprafka SA, et al. Medical problem solving: an analysis of clinical reasoning. Cambridge: Harvard University Press, 1978.
10. Elstein AS. Human factors in clinical judgment: discussion of Scriven's 'clinical Judgment.' In: Engelhardt HT Jr, Spicker SF, Towers B, eds. Clinical judgment: a critical appraisal. Boston: Reidel, 1979.
11. Elstein AS, Sprafka SA, Shulman LS. The information processing approach to clinical reasoning: reflections on the research method. Presented at the 1978 Annual Meeting of the American Educational Research Association.
12. Elstein AS, Bordage G. The psychology of clinical reasoning: current research approaches. In: Stone G, Cohen F, Adler N, eds. Health psychology. San Francisco: Jossey-Bass, 1979.
13. Slovic P, Lichtenstein S. Comparison of Bayesian and regression approaches to the study of information processing in judgment. Organizational Behavior and Human Performance 1971;6:649-744.
14. Barr DM. Factors influencing clinical decision making by physicians: a conceptual framework and literature review. Presented at the Eighth World Congress of Family Medicine, 1978.
15. Eisenberg JM. Sociologic influences on decision-making by clinicians. Ann Intern Med 1979;90:957-64.
16. Johnson PE. Cognitive models of medical problem solvers. Presented at the Conference on Clinical Decision Making and Laboratory Use, Chapter 6 this volume.

CHAPTER EIGHT

Evaluating Skills in Clinical Decision Making

Barbara J. Andrew, PhD

We know that problem solving is a process that involves several interrelated stages, and that experienced problem solvers store, organize, and retrieve knowledge in a somewhat different fashion than do inexperienced problem solvers. Problem solving is certainly not the sole component of clinical competence, although it is, I believe, the principal one. Humanism and effective communication and psychomotor skills can enhance the quality and effectiveness of health care, but they cannot compensate for a failure to reach a quick, accurate diagnosis or for an ineffective or inappropriate treatment plan.

My task here is to discuss methods being used to assess skills in decision making. I will comment briefly on some current methods and will describe two new evaluation methods that should enhance our capacity to assess decision-making skills. To avoid confusion over terminology, let me clarify my use of "decision making." In my view, it is not an activity separate from problem solving, but rather is an integral component, an activity that underlies or is embedded in every facet of problem solving. Decisions are made regarding the diagnostic hypotheses that should be considered, regarding the specific types of history, physical examination, and laboratory data needed, and regarding the meaning of the data once they have been gathered. In weighing the elements of an entire data set, decisions must be made about the overall significance of the data set and whether there are conflicting elements in it that require further investigation or that will have an effect on the approach to management and treatment.

That problem-solving skills have a bearing on competence of physicians is certainly not a novel or recent concept. In the early 1960s, the National Board of Medical Examiners commissioned a critical incidents study of clinical competence by the American Institutes for Research.[1] The purpose of this study was to identify incidents in the behavior of interns and residents that in the judgment of faculty observers had a significant positive or negative impact on health outcome. Over 3,000 such critical incidents were reported and analyzed, and these were subsequently classified into nine dimensions of clinical competence. Of particular relevance to our discussion of problem solving is the dimension of competence which was labeled "Diagnostic Acumen." The following behaviors were generalized from the critical incidents and used to describe this component of competence:

- identifies initial pertinent hypotheses;
- tests all pertinent hypotheses;
- reevaluates hypotheses in the light of new findings;
- recognizes when sufficient data have been obtained and does not jump to conclusions;
- integrates data into one or more meaningful conclusions; and
- selects appropriate management and treatment plans.

From this critical incidents study emerged several evaluation methods: the patient management problem, the motion picture film examination, and the multiple-choice question based on comprehensive clinical vignettes.

Through extensive use of and experimentation with these evaluation methods, their limitations have become known, and these limitations have suggested directions for further research and developmental work.[2] Misunderstandings about these evaluation methods have also arisen, as have unrealistic expectations for evaluation methods in general. Most observers have come to accept that no single evaluation method can effectively assess all facets of clinical problem solving. Thus the challenge is not to find the omnibus evaluation method, but to design multiple methods, each with specific objectives, and to determine the most valid mix of assessment techniques.

Perhaps the most pervasive misunderstanding about multiple-choice questions is the belief that they can only assess knowledge. Of course, we recognize that problem solving in medicine or in any field cannot take place in the absence of a body of knowledge and understanding. Yet we have also come to recognize that though knowledge and understanding are necessary to problem solving they are not sufficient to guarantee that physicians will be successful in reaching correct diagnoses or in selecting appropriate management and treatment plans. Nonetheless, multiple-choice questions *can* be written and indeed *are* written to test various elements of the problem-solving process. Some questions are designed to assess whether the examinee can reevaluate diagnostic hypotheses when additional clinical data are presented; others are designed to assess whether the examinee can evaluate the overall meaning of a set of clinical data and synthesize those data into one or more appropriate conclusions. Multiple-choice questions are also designed to assess whether the examinee can select appropriate management and treatment plans given a summary of relevant clinical data.

The obvious limitation of multiple-choice questions is that they tend to provide single snapshots of clinical decision making when what we are trying to assess is a logical thought process that has a beginning, a middle, and an end.

The receipt of these books is acknowledged, and this listing must be regarded as sufficient return for the courtesy of the sender. Books that appear to be of particular interest will be reviewed as space permits.

The Journal solicits reviews of new books from its readers. Books for review would ordinarily, but not necessarily, be selected from the Books Received lists. In any event the book is to be obtained independently by the reviewer.

If you wish to submit a review, before proceeding please send a letter of intent, identifying the book in question (title, author, and publisher), to Dr. Francis D. Moore, Book Reviews, New England Journal of Medicine, 10 Shattuck St., Boston, MA 02115. Instructions will then be sent to you.

If the book to be reviewed is not listed in the Journal, we may require that you send it to us with your review, but it will of course be returned. The Journal reserves the right of final decision on publication.

designed to provide extensive bibliographies.

Rheumatology in General Practice, on the other hand, is new. It is a 266-page paperbound handbook designed to provide primary-care physicians in Great Britain with a concise description of practical and clinical approaches to patients presenting with a variety of musculoskeletal symptoms. The section on principles of management includes recommendations for drugs available in Britain. Both books contain sections on self-assessment. I am particularly impressed with the problem-oriented approach in *Rheumatology in General Practice*. It is helpful for a primary physician to be able to refresh his memory quickly when he is confronted with a patient with pain in a lower limb. If only a few patients present with limb pain, the differential diagnosis does not come quickly to mind. In summary, both contributions have value, but the book by Rogers and Williams has greater emphasis on general practice. The relatively low cost of both books certainly adds to their attractiveness.

EUGENE V. BARNETT, M.D.
University of California, Los Angeles
Medical Center

Los Angeles, CA 90024

CLINICAL DECISIONS AND LABORATORY USE

(University of Minnesota Continuing Medical Education, Vol. 1.) Edited by Donald P. Connelly, Ellis S. Benson, M. Desmond Burke, and Douglas Fenderson. 355 pp. Minneapolis, University of Minnesota Press, 1982. $29.50.

According to Garrison's *History of Medicine*, medical diagnosis in the 19th century was "snap" diagnosis. Like sleight-of-hand surgery, it was the fashion. Hebra and Joseph Bell could detect the occupations as well as the diseases of their patients, and some of the greatest diagnosticians never admitted that a diagnosis was wrong. Perhaps future historians will characterize the last quarter of the 20th century as a time when medical theoreticians began to analyze the diagnostic process and to apply mathematical methods to quantitate the uncertainty that inevitably accompanies any process of clinical reasoning.

Most proceedings of medical or scientific conferences make rather dull reading for someone who has attended, and it was a pleasant surprise to find this book an exception. The material has been reorganized and edited extensively, and the participants have written ten chapters that could stand on their own merits.

The book is divided into six sections. The first addresses such societal concerns as the economic impact of technology on medicine, the necessity for developing better methods of allocating medical resources, and the reshaping of health-care policies from an emphasis on development and expansion toward one on cost containment and retrenchment. There are extensive analyses of the clinical decision-making process and of the ways in which the clinical laboratory is used or misused. There is a section directed toward improving the effectiveness of the process through education of students, house staff, and physicians.

The most interesting section deals with "tools" for supporting the decision making process. The tool kit contains algorithms, graphs (depicting false positive/true positive ratios), equations (for timing the resection of aortic aneurysms, for example), and computers and physicians.

The title of the final section, "Research Initiatives," is somewhat misleading, since it implies that previous sections dealt with state-of-the-art decision-making and that this section will describe the future. Actually, it does contain some new additions to the tool kit. This book will be useful to physicians who are interested in process, current approaches to the analysis of medical diagnosis, and effectiveness of patient care.

REX B. CONN, M.D.
Emory University
School of Medicine

Atlanta, GA 30322

BIOMEDICAL SCIENCE

Atlas of Surgical and Sectional Anatomy. By Bok Y. Lee. 322 pp., illustrated. Norwalk, Conn., Appleton-Century-Crofts, 1982. $35.

Bacterial Infections of Humans: Epidemiology and control. Edited by Alfred S. Evans and Harry A. Feldman. 702 pp. New York, Plenum Press, 1982. $59.50.

Child Nurturance. Vol. 3. **Studies of Development in Nonhuman Primates.** Edited by Hiram E. Fitzgerald, John A. Mullins, and Patricia Gage. 274 pp. New York, Plenum Press, 1982. $29.50.

Free Radicals and Cancer. Edited by Robert A. Floyd. 541 pp. New York, Marcel Dekker, 1982. $69.75.

Genetic Analysis of the X Chromosome: Studies of Duchenne muscular dystrophy and related disorders. (Advances in Experimental Medicine and Biology. Vol. 154.) Edited by Henry F. Epstein and Stewart Wolf. 203 pp., illustrated. New York, Plenum Press, 1982. $37.50.

New Researches in Biology and Genetics: Problems of science and ethics. Edited by Hakim Mohammed Said. 384 pp. Karachi, Hamdard Academy, 1980.

The Physician's Guide to Desktop Computers. By Mark Harrison Spohr. 222 pp., illustrated. Reston, Va., Reston Publishing, 1983. $21.95.

Recent Advances in Mucosal Immunity. Edited by Warren Strober, Lars A. Hanson, and Kenneth W. Sell. 435 pp., illustrated. New York, Raven Press, 1982. $80.

Reviews of Physiology, Biochemistry and Pharmacology 94. Edited by R. H. Adrian, H. zur Hausen, E. Helmreich, et al. 207 pp. New York, Springer-Verlag. 1982. $44.

Vitamins and Hormones: Advances in research and applications. Vol. 39. Edited by Paul L. Munson, Egon Diczfalusy, John Glover, and Robert E. Olson. 431 pp. New York, Academic Press, 1982. $56.

EDUCATION, HISTORY, AND BIOGRAPHY

Cancer Care: A personal guide. Revised edition. By Harold Glucksberg and Jack W. Singer. 435 pp. New York, Charles Scribner, 1982. $12.95.

The Diseases of Children and Their Remedies. (A Nutrition Foundation Reprint of the 1776 English edition.) By Nicholas Rosen von Rosenstein. 364 pp. New York, Johnson Reprint, 1977. (Distributed by Academic Press, New York.)

Leo Eloesser, M.D.: Eulogy for a free spirit. By Harris B. Shumacker, Jr. 483 pp. New York, Philosophical Library, 1982. $29.95.

The Social Transformation of American Medicine. By Paul Starr. 514 pp. New York, Basic Books, 1982. $24.95.

Women Scientists in America: Struggles and strategies to 1940. By Margaret W. Rossiter. 439 pp., illustrated. Baltimore, Johns Hopkins University Press, 1982. $27.50.

Work, Marriage, and Motherhood: The career persistence of female physicians. By Dorothy Rosenthal Mandelbaum. 303 pp. New York, Praeger, 1981. $29.95.

Writing a Scientific Paper and Speaking at Scientific Meetings. Fifth edition. By Vernon Booth. 47 pp. Colchester, England, Biochemical Society, 1981. $6.

HEALTH SERVICES

Alternatives to Traditional Family Living. (Marriage and Family Review. Vol. 5. No. 2.) Edited by Harriet Gross and Marvin B. Sussman. 128 pp. New York, Haworth Press, 1982. $20 (cloth); $9.95 (paper).

Beliefs and Self-Help: Cross-cultural perspectives and approaches. Edited by George H. Weber and Lucy M. Cohen. 359 pp. New York, Human Sciences Press, 1982. $29.95.

Blood — Gift or Merchandise: Towards an international blood policy. By Piet J. Hagen. 231 pp. New York, Alan R. Liss, 1982. $29.50.

Clinical Laboratory Management: A guide for clinical laboratory scientists. Edited by Karen R. Karni, Karen R. Viskochil, and Patricia A. Amos. 579 pp. Boston, Little, Brown, 1982. $24.95.

The D.O.'s: Osteopathic medicine in America. By Norman Gevitz. 183 pp. Baltimore, Johns Hopkins University Press, 1982. $18.50.

Health and the Law: A handbook for health professionals. By Tom Christoffel. 450 pp. New York, Free Press, 1982. $29.95.

Hospital Statistics in Europe. Edited by P. M. Lambert and F. H. Roger. 200 pp. New York, Elsevier/North-Holland, 1982. $37.25.

The Role of the University Teaching Hospital: An international perspective. Edited by Elizabeth F. Purcell. 258 pp. New York, Josiah Macy, Jr. Foundation, 1982. $10. (Distributed by Independent Publishers Group, Port Washington, N.Y.)

MEDICINE

Adult Leukemias I. (Cancer Treatment and Research 5.) Edited by Clara D. Bloomfield. 415 pp. The Hague, Martinus Nijhoff, 1982. $69.50. (Distributed in the U.S. by Kluwer Boston, Hingham, Mass.)

Archives of Family Practice. Vol. 3. Edited by John P. Geyman. 349 pp. Norwalk, Conn., Appleton-Century-Crofts, 1982. $38.50.

BOOKS RECEIVED

lished in French, German, and Spanish provides further testimony of the excellence of a valuable but brief handbook — one that the

Contrast Echocardiography. (Developments in Cardiovascular Medicine. Vol. 15.) Edited by Richard S. Meltzer and Jos Roelandt. 334 pp., illustrated. The Hague, Martinus Nijhoff, 1982, $69.50. (Distributed in the U.S. by Kluwer Boston, Hingham, Mass.)

Critical Care Gastroenterology. Edited by H. Juergen Nord and Patrick G. Brady. 364 pp., illustrated. New York, Churchill Livingstone, 1982. $36.

Debates in Nephrology. (Contributions to Nephrology. Vol. 34.) Edited by L. Minetti, G. Barbiano di Belgiojoso, and G. Civati. 131 pp. New York, S. Karger, 1982. $53.50.

Diabetes Mellitus and Obesity. Edited by Bernard N. Brodoff and Sheldon J. Bleicher. 816 pp., illustrated. Baltimore, Williams and Wilkins, 1982. $60.

Diseases of the Esophagus. (Contemporary Issues in Gastroenterology. Vol. 1.) Edited by Sidney Cohen and Roger D. Soloway. 305 pp., illustrated. New York, Churchill Livingstone, 1982. $43.

Diseases of the Gastrointestinal Tract and Liver. By David J. C. Shearman and Niall D. C. Finlayson. 974 pp., illustrated. New York, Churchill Livingstone, 1982. $79.

Endocrinology: New directions in therapy. (Second edition.) By Robert E. Bolinger. 503 pp. New Hyde Park, N.Y., Medical Examination Publishing, 1982. $39.50.

Handbook: Interactions of selected drugs and nutrients in patients. Third edition. By Daphne A. Roe. 142 pp. Chicago, American Dietetic Association, 1982. $17.50.

The Lymphocytes. (Clinics in Haematology. Vol. 11. No. 3.) Edited by G. Janossy. 776 pp., illustrated. Philadelphia, W.B. Saunders, 1982. $24.

Manual of Hemostasis and Thrombosis. Third edition. By Arthur R. Thompson and Laurence A. Harker. 219 pp. Philadelphia, F.A. Davis, 1982. $8.95.

The Modern Management of Congestive Heart Failure. By John Hamer. 168 pp. London, Lloyd-Luke, 1982.

Nephrology. (Continuing Education Review.) By David A. Ogden and Stanley M. Lee. 369 pp. New Hyde Park, N.Y., Medical Examination Publishing, 1982. $29.50.

Neurology for Non-Neurologists. Edited by Wigbert C. Wiederholt. 411 pp., illustrated. New York, Academic Press, 1982. $37.50.

Oral Leukoplakia. (Developments in Oncology. Vol. 8.) By Jolán Bánóczy. 231 pp., illustrated. The Hague, Martinus Nijhoff, 1982. $42. (Distributed in the U.S. by Kluwer Boston, Hingham, Mass.)

Prevention of Kidney Disease and Long-Term Survival. Edited by M. M. Avram. 324 pp. New York, Plenum Press, 1982. $35.

Reviews of Clinical Infectious Diseases. 298 pp. Academic Press, 1982. $24.95.

The Transformation-Associated Cellular p53 Protein. (Advances in Viral Oncology. Vol. 2.) Edited by George Klein. 180 pp., illustrated. New York, Raven Press, 1982. $32.

PATHOLOGY

Advances in Pathology (Anatomic and Clinical). (Laboratory Medicine.) Vol. 2. Anatomic Pathology, Cytopathology, and Forensic Pathology and Toxicology. Edited by Emmanuel Levy. 572 pp., illustrated. New York, Pergamon Press, 1982. $135.

General Pathology. (Medical Outline Series.) By Ivan Damjanov. 393 pp., illustrated. New Hyde Park, N.Y., Medical Examination Publishing, 1982. $23.50.

TNM Classification of Breast Cancer. Edited by M. H. Harmer. 17 pp. Geneva, International Union Against Cancer (UICC), 1982.

TNM Classification of Malignant Tumours. Third edition. Edited by M. H. Harmer. 169 pp. Geneva, International Union Against Cancer, 1982.

TNM Classification of Paediatric Tumours. By M. H. Harmer. 28 pp. Geneva, International Union Against Cancer, 1982.

PEDIATRICS

Advances in Pediatrics. Vol. 29. Edited by Lewis A. Barness, Alfred M. Bongiovanni, Grant Morrow, Frank Oski, and Abraham M. Rudolph. 568 pp. Chicago, Year Book, 1982. $49.50.

The Child with Multiple Birth Defects. By M. Michael Cohen, Jr. 189 pp., illustrated. New York, Raven Press, 1982. $32.

Management of the Physically and Emotionally Abused: Emergency assessment, intervention, and counseling. Edited by Carmen Germaine Warner and G. Richard Braen. 329 pp., illustrated. Norwalk, Conn., Appleton-Century-Crofts, 1982. $28.95.

Pediatric Otolaryngology: New directions in therapy. Edited by David D. Caldarelli. 277 pp. illustrated. New Hyde Park, N.Y., Medical Examination Publishing, 1982. $32.50.

The Psychoanalytic Study of the Child. Vol. 37. Edited by Albert J. Solnit, Ruth S. Eissler, Anna Freud, and Peter B. Neubauer. 588 pp. New Haven, Conn., Yale University Press, 1982. $37.50.

Tumours of the Central Nervous System in Infancy and Childhood. Edited by D. Voth, P. Gutjahr, and C. Langmaid. 438 pp., illustrated. New York, Springer-Verlag, 1982. $44.

PHARMACOLOGY AND SUBSTANCE ABUSE

Basic and Clinical Pharmacology. Edited by Bertram G. Katzung, 815 pp. Los Altos, Calif., Lange, 1982. $23.50.

Lithium and Animal Behavior. Vol. 2. (Lithium Research Review Series.) By Donald F. Smith. 134 pp. New York, Human Sciences Press, 1982. $16.95.

Critical Problems in Psychiatry. Edited by Jesse O. Cavenar, Jr., and H. Keith Brodie. 498 pp. Philadelphia, J.B. Lippincott, 1982. $29.50.

Family Therapy: Complementary frameworks of theory and practice. Edited by Arnon Bentovim, Gill Gorell Barnes, and Alan Cooklin. 543 pp. in two volumes. New York, Grune and Stratton for the Institute of Family Therapy, 1982 $22.50 per volume.

Mechanism and Management of Headache. Fourth edition. By James W. Lance. 260 pp., illustrated. Boston, Butterworths, 1982. $39.95.

The Neurology Handbook. Second edition. By Labe C. Scheinberg, Barbara S. Giesser, and Herbert H. Schaumburg. 184 pp., illustrated. New Hyde Park, N.Y., Medical Examination Publishing, 1982. $11.95.

The Parietal Cortex of Monkey and Man. (Studies of Brain Function. Vol. 8.) By Juhani Hyvärinen. 202 pp., illustrated. New York, Springer-Verlag, 1982. $39.50.

Phobic and Obsessive-Compulsive Disorders: Theory, research, and practice. By Paul M. G. Emmelkamp. 357 pp. New York, Plenum Press, 1982. $27.50.

Phospholipids in the Nervous System. Vol. 1. Metabolism. Edited by Lloyd A. Horrocks, G. Brian Ansell, and Giuseppe Porcellati. 378 pp. New York, Raven Press, 1982. $44.

Psychological Approaches to the Management of Pain. Edited by Joseph Barber and Cheri Adrian. 211 pp. New York, Brunner/Mazel, 1982. $20.

Questions and Answers in the Practice of Family Therapy. Vol. 2. Edited by Alan S. Gurman. 317 pp. New York, Brunner/Mazel, 1982. $27.50.

Terminology of Communication Disorders: Speech, language, hearing. Second edition. By Lucille Nicolosi, Elizabeth Harryman, and Janet Kresheck. 319 pp., illustrated. Baltimore, Williams and Wilkins, 1982. $18.50.

RADIOLOGY

Administration and Supervision in Laboratory Medicine. Edited by John R. Snyder and Arthur L. Larsen. 564 pp. Philadelphia, Harper and Row, 1982. $35.

Advanced Interpretation of Clinical Laboratory Data. (Clinical and Biochemical Analysis. Vol. 13.) Edited by Camille Heusghem, Adelin Albert, and Ellis S. Benson. 420 pp. New York, Marcel Dekker, 1982. $55.

Atlas of Radionuclide Hepatobiliary Imaging. By Christopher C. Kuni and William C. Klingensmith. 222 pp., illustrated. Boston, G.K. Hall, 1982. $39.95.

Essentials of Chest Radiology. By John V. Forrest and David S. Feigin. 152 pp., illustrated. Philadelphia, W.B. Saunders, 1982. $12.95.

Neuroradiology: A neuropathological approach. By R. Kautzky, K. J. Zülch, S. Wende, and A. Tanzer. 324 pp. illustrated. New York, Springer-Verlag, 1982. $98. (Translated by W. M. Boehm and V. B. Kellett from Neuroradiologie auf Neuropathologischer Grundlage [second edition, Heidelberg, 1976] with minor revisions.)

Radiology of the Pancreas. By Patrick C. Freeny and Thomas L. Lawson. 624 pp., illustrated. New York, Springer-Verlag, 1982 $125.

Treatment Planning and Dose Calculation in Radiation Oncology. Third edition. By Gunilla C. Bentel, Charles E. Nelson, and K. Thomas Noell. 262 pp., illustrated. New York, Pergamon Press, 1982. $35 (cloth); $12.95 (paper).

REPRODUCTIVE BIOLOGY, OBSTETRICS AND GYNECOLOGY

Advances in Psychosomatic Obstetrics and Gynecology. Edited by H-J. Prill and M. Stauber. 525 pp. New York, Springer-Verlag, 1982 $36.

Conquering Infertility. By Stephen L. Corson. 182 pp. illustrated. Norwalk, Conn., Appleton-Century-Crofts, 1982. $12.95.

Everywoman: A gynaecological guide for life. Third edition. By Derek Llewellyn-Jones. 411 pp. illustrated. Boston, Faber and Faber, 1982. $16.95 (cloth); $4.95 (paper). (Distributed by Harper and Row, New York.)

Gynecology. (Concise Textbook Series.) Edited by Ralph W. Hale and John A. Krieger. 419 pp. illustrated. New Hyde Park, N.Y., Medical Examination Publishing, 1982. $21.

Instrumental Insemination. (Clinics in Andrology. Vol. 8.) Edited by E. S. E. Hafez and K. Semm. 231 pp. illustrated. The Hague, Martinus Nijhoff, 1982. $79. (Distributed in the U.S. by Kluwer Boston, Hingham, Mass.)

Metabolic Toxemia of Late Pregnancy: A disease of malnutrition. By Thomas H. Brewer. 171 pp. New Canaan, Conn., Keats, 1982. $7.95.

SURGERY

Advances in Stroke Therapy. Edited by F. Clifford Rose. 330 pp., illustrated. New York, Raven Press, 1982 $58.

Cellular Communication during Ocular Development. (Cell and Developmental Biology of the Eye.) Edited by Joel B. Sheffield and S. Robert Hilfer. 196 pp. illustrated. New York, Springer-Verlag, 1982. $32.50.

Color Atlas of Cardiac Surgery: Acquired heart disease. By James L. Monro and Gerald Shore. 165 pp. illustrated. Norwalk, Conn., Appleton-Century-Crofts, 1982. $110.

A Colour Atlas of Foot and Ankle Anatomy. By R. M. H. McMinn, R. T. Hutchings, and B. M. Logan. 96 pp., illustrated. London, Wolfe, 1982. $35. (Distributed in the U.S. by Appleton-Century-Crofts, Norwalk, Conn.)

Complications in Anesthesiology. Edited by Fredrick K. Orkin and Lee H. Cooperman. 765 pp., illustrated. Philadelphia, J.B. Lippincott, 1982. $95. (Distributed in the U.S. by

Follow-up of the Cancer Patient. By Ben Eiseman, William A. Robinson, and Glenn Steele, Jr. 232 pp. New York, Thieme-Stratton, 1982. $38.

Patient management problems have been helpful in this regard because they attempt to simulate the unfolding, longitudinal nature of clinical problem solving and they attempt to assess selected decision-making skills at multiple points in the evolution of a case. However, because we have been bound to a paper-pencil technology, it has not been possible to create comprehensive clinical simulations that allow physicians the flexibility of investigating and managing problems as they would in an actual clinical setting. Because choices must be presented to examinees instead of requiring them to generate their own options, an element of cueing inevitably results that can shape and focus the performance of examinees in ways that do not accurately reflect their typical patterns of clinical decision making. Because the testing follows a paper format, the number of choices offered must be limited, to avoid developing a simulation that would be too cumbersome from a format point of view. It is also cumbersome to assess the sequence in which decisions are made, so that this important dimension of decision making can be judged in only a rather crude manner. The overall conclusion is that we *are* assessing skills in decision making today, although we are doing so incompletely and are relying on evaluation tools that provide rather gross measurements of some components of decision making and cannot provide assessments of other important components.

Several factor analytic studies have suggested that clinical problem solving can be divided into two phases: the diagnostic phase, in which problem-solving activities are directed toward the collection and evaluation of clinical data in order to reach one or more diagnostic conclusions; and the management/treatment phase, in which activities are directed toward the resolution of the patient's problems through the selection of and appropriate timing of therapeutic strategies, and the management of complications and secondary problems.[3-5]

For the past several years, the National Board has been designing and conducting preliminary field trials of a new evaluation format designed to assess the diagnostic phase of clinical problem solving. These simulations have been prepared for administration to senior medical students, although the development of more complex and subtle case material could make them appropriate for administration to experienced physicians.

Each simulation is designed to test four elements of diagnostic problem solving: the generation of an appropriate set of initial diagnostic hypotheses; the evaluation of specific findings from history, physical examination, laboratory tests, and investigative procedures in relation to these hypotheses; the reassessment of diagnostic hypotheses at multiple points in the simulation; and the formulation of a final assessment of the hypotheses and a diagnostic conclusion.

Two testing formats have been developed: a structured format in which examinees are presented with diagnostic hypotheses to choose from and predetermined lists of laboratory tests and investigative procedures from which to select; and a free response format in which examinees are required to generate their own initial list of diagnostic hypotheses, revise the set of hypotheses according to their evaluation of the data, and generate their own requests for laboratory tests and investigative procedures. In all other respects, the testing formats are identical and follow the same sequence of activities and presentation of data.

Each diagnostic simulation begins with an introductory description of the health care setting, the patient's presenting complaints, and in some instances a very small number of history and/or physical examination findings. With this set of cue presentations, examinees are asked to identify diagnostic hypotheses that might explain the patient's problems and to indicate on a four-point scale how likely they feel each hypothesis is. The four scale values are: highly probable; possible and likely; possible but unlikely; and highly improbable.

A summary of the positive findings and pertinent negative findings from the history are described. Each finding is then presented separately, followed by the list of diagnostic hypotheses, and examinees are asked to indicate whether the finding is evidence for, evidence against, or noncontributory to each of the diagnostic hypotheses. When the historical findings are evaluated, examinees are asked to reevaluate their list of diagnostic hypotheses and indicate the likelihood of each in light of additional available data. This same process of data presentation, data evaluation, and reassessment of diagnostic hypotheses is followed in relation to the findings from physical examination and from laboratory and investigative procedures. Once all of the clinical data have been presented, examinees are asked to make a final assessment of the diagnostic hypotheses and they are asked to select, from a rather long list, the management/treatment plan they would initiate. An examinee's answers are scored in relation to their distance from what has been judged by a group of experts to be the most appropriate responses. Hence, if a diagnostic hypothesis is judged by experts to be highly probable on the basis of the available clinical data, an examinee who indicates the hypothesis is highly improbable will receive a lower score than an examinee who rates the hypothesis as possible and likely. We believe that these diagnostic problem-solving tests provide reasonable simulations of the sequential and unfolding nature of problem solving and that they offer an opportunity of assessing the capabilities of medical students to think logically about clinical data.

Preliminary field trials of a limited number of these diagnostic simulations have shown very little correlation between performance on the structured response format and the free response format, and only slight correlations with performance on National Board examinations. The structured simulations do show modest correlations with tests of reasoning, whereas the free response simulations do not correlate with tests of reasoning. Estimates of internal consistency reliability on a limited number of structured format tests suggest that very acceptable reliabilities may be obtainable with a test of modest length. Studies of the consistency of performance across simulated cases have not yet been conducted, because of the limited number of problems that have been developed. Further field trials of the structured response simulations are being conducted and the results may lead to the introduction of these problem-solving tests into National Board examinations.

Although these diagnostic problem-solving simulations are designed to assess the accuracy with which medical students evaluate clinical data and consider diagnostic hypotheses, these simulations do not assess skills in the management and treatment of patients. The timing of key clinical decisions, the sequence in which tests, procedures, and therapies are ordered, the ability to respond quickly and effectively to unexpected complications or events in the patient's clinical course, are all fundamental aspects of effective problem solving. To assess these skills, evaluation methods must be developed to provide the degree of flexibility and fidelity needed to simulate clinical conditions and patient responses to the decisions physicians make.

For the past ten years, the National Board has been experimenting with the development of computer simulations to evaluate skills in decision making related to the management and treatment of clinical problems. We have been joined in this effort by the American Board of Internal Medicine, and the two Boards, along with funding from the Robert Wood Johnson Foundation and Charles E. Merrill Trust, have supported Dr. Richard Friedman at the University of Wisconsin in his efforts to develop complex computer based clinical simulations suitable for formal evaluations of clinical competence.

The first requirement for such computer simulations is that they be capable of providing credible clinical data to physicians and be capable of altering the simulated patient's course, consistent with the tests, procedures, and therapies ordered at whatever point in the interaction. The clinical material presented must not only be believable at the outset, but must continue to evolve in a believable manner. Once computer simulations of sufficient fidelity have been devised, scoring strategies must be developed to reflect accurately and reliably the qualitative differences in decision-making skills among physicians, and in particular to be effective in distinguishing those physicians who may have significant deficits in decision-making skills.

The result of these efforts has been the development of the Computer Based Examination known as CBX. The CBX model has been designed to simulate a health care episode in which physicians are presented with a clinical case and given the opportunity to investigate the case, order tests and procedures, and implement therapies in any manner they wish. Physicians may communicate their requests and orders via free language text entry or by consulting a reference volume that contains a comprehensive list of tests, procedures, and therapies. The patient's status is updated continuously as a function of whatever courses of action a physician has taken. A microfiche reader is used to display selected physical findings, roentgenograms, ECG tracings, and the results of invasive procedures. The patient's clinical course evolves in simulated time, and the physician controls the movement of time through various decisions. The patient is programmed to evolve in a predetermined way over a predetermined period of simulated time, and this clinical course can be altered only by the decisions the physician makes, and by the time frames in which those decisions are implemented.

The patient can be programmed to depict an uncomplicated case of a particular disease, or the patient can be programmed to develop certain complications and secondary problems to which the physician must also respond. Some complications and secondary problems arise regardless of the actions the physicians has thus far taken (assuming that those actions have not already resulted in the death of the patient). Other complications and problems arise directly out of the actions the physician has taken or has failed to take. The simulation model also depicts interactions between and among tests and drug therapies.

In some instances quick, definitive action is required; in others a wide spectrum work-up or a wait-and-see approach is appropriate. The simulated cases have been written to require the diversity of clinical decision making that is required in actual practice; every attempt has been made to avoid a stylized simulation that requires a stylized approach to decision making. The computer model documents which decisions are made by the physician, when, in simulated time, the decisions are made, and the sequence in which they are made.

One of the most complex challenges in developing CBX has been the creation of scoring strategies to evaluate the quality of decision making. At present, physician performance on the simulated cases is evaluated along the following dimensions:

- the patient outcome that has been achieved;
- the amount of unnecessary cost that has been generated during the simulation
- the degree of unnecessary risk the patient has been exposed to;
- the appropriateness of the decision logic that was followed at various nodal points in the evolution of the case;
- diagnostic and therapeutic omissions and the degree of harm incurred from those omissions; and
- diagnostic and therapeutic benefits and the degree of benefit accrued from the decisions made.

These computer simulations have been administered to practicing physicians in family practice and internal medicine, and moderately good correlations have been found between the decisions made on the computer and decisions made in actual practice, as assessed by a review of hospital records for patients with similar kinds of medical problems. The degree of overlap found between the computer simulations and medical records in four studies was 66%, 77%, 78%, and 81%. More challenging simulations have been administered to first- and third-year residents in internal medicine, and, with the exception of scores on diagnostic benefit, the third-year residents have demonstrated significantly better performance than the first-year residents. Third-year residents have achieved better patient outcomes, at less unnecessary cost and risk to the patient; they have made fewer diagnostic and therapeutic omissions, and they have demonstrated better decision logic. As would be expected, there is less variability in the performance of third-year residents than among first-year residents, although the distributions of scores indicates that a small number of third-year residents perform very differently from their peers. Of particular importance is the finding that expert clinicians reviewing printed records of a resident's performance on a case rate the performance in a manner that is similar to several of the numerical scores of performance derived from the scoring criteria specified by an expert committee. The strongest correlations have been found between scores and ratings of patient outcome, unnecessary costs, and unnecessary risk. The magnitude of these correlations has ranged from 0.65 to 0.73.

The results of the field studies conducted to date have provided very encouraging evidence for the validity and reliability of computer simulations. From a technical point of view, computer-based testing is feasible on a national scale. We have found it possible to train examinees in the use of the CBX model with a 20-minute audiovisual orientation package and a practice case. A great many improvements are needed in the man-machine interface, in the procedures for designing and debugging simulated cases, and in the procedures for scoring performance. It is certainly possible that these efforts will lead to the introduction of large-scale computer testing in national evaluation programs for licensure and certification, and that we will thereby enhance significantly our capabilities for evaluating skills in clinical decision making.

References

1. American Institutes for Research. The definition of clinical competence in medicine: Performance dimensions and rationales for clinical skill areas. Palo Alto, reissued, May 1976.
2. Hubbard JP. Measuring medical education: The tests and the experience of the National Board of Medical Examiners. 2nd ed. Philadelphia: Lea and Febiger, 1978.
3. Donnelly MB, Gallagher RE, Hess JW, Hogan MJ. The dimensionality of measures derived from complex clinical simulations. Proceedings, Conference on Research in Medical Education, Association of American Medical Colleges, 1974.
4. Juul DH, Noe MJ, Nerenberg RL. A factor analytic study of branching patient management problems. Paper presented at the annual meeting of the National Council on Measurement in Education, New York City, April 1977.
5. Skakun EN. The dimensionality of linear patient management problems. Proceedings, Conference on Research in Medical Education, Association of American Medical Colleges, 1978.

Section III. Clinical Decisions and the Clinical Laboratory

CHAPTER NINE

The Role of the Laboratory in Clinical Decision Making

D. S. Young, MB, PhD

INTRODUCTION

Except in unusual situations, physicians request clinical laboratory tests after they have taken the history of a patient's illness and completed a physical examination. The laboratory tests are ordered by physicians to assist them in decision making—usually to seek support for impressions gleaned from personal interaction with the patient. The data reported by most clinical laboratories are usually in numerical form. In few laboratories do the staff interpret the data and provide it in such a form that it would reduce the number of decisions that a clinician has to make. Although laboratory staff traditionally provide detailed interpretations of bone-marrow aspirates, they rarely provide a similar depth of interpretation for other tests; in some centers, though, the staff do interpret protein electrophoretic patterns or immunoelectrophoretic patterns.

However, some clinical decisions *are* made from data resulting from skilled laboratory decisions. Such decisions, which can be made by a technologist or physician or scientist, follow from the proper designation of a peak on a chromatographic strip-chart or spot on a plate, as with the identification of an unknown drug, or band on an electrophoretic tracing. Critical (but unrecognized) laboratory decisions are made many times a day in the matching of peaks on a strip-chart with the specimens analyzed in a batch and in the acceptance or rejection of batches of data depending on their acceptability by predetermined criteria for quality assurance.

Laboratory decisions may affect patient care in other ways. In many laboratories, "loops" have been developed so that follow-up of an abnormal result proceeds automatically. Such loops include the follow-up to an abnormal result obtained by a second-level, or screening type, instrument with the repeat of the test using a more sophisticated instrument. For example, a calcium result that is abnormal when obtained by a colorimetric method is often verified by a repeat analysis on an atomic absorption spectrometer. In many laboratories, a decision level has been established for several serum enzyme activities at which isoenzyme fractionation is automatically performed. In many of the screening programs for inborn errors of metabolism, a positive screening test is automatically followed by a test that may provide a definitive identification of the disease.

Important decisions also are made by laboratory staff when they use their knowledge of effects of drugs, or biological variability, on laboratory tests to provide information to a clinician that would allow him to interpret results properly. Yet the only times when a laboratory becomes directly involved in clinical decision making are when a laboratorian assumes responsibility for the care of a patient or when one actively consults with a clinician caring for a patient. These are roles which clinical pathologists have been urged often to accept, but which few do at present.

THE REASONS THAT TESTS ARE ORDERED

The reasons most tests are ordered are summarized in the accompanying tabulation. This summary is not organized either by importance of each application nor by number of tests used for each purpose. Although the table presents the applications as if they are discrete, there is, in actual practice, considerable overlap so that one test may be used to tell whether a disease exists and how bad it is. A test used to screen for disease is often at the same time able to exclude the presence of the disease.

Reasons for Ordering Laboratory Tests

    Diagnosis of disease
    Screening for disease
    Determination of severity of disease
    Determination of appropriate management of patient
    Monitoring progress of disease
    Monitoring therapy
    Monitoring drug toxicity
    Predicting response to treatment

A committee of the Intersociety Council of Laboratory Medicine of Canada[1] has identified areas in which clinical laboratories make important contributions to health care. These include the maintenance of a safe environment, and the screening of well people to detect potential or unrecognized disease. The committee also recognized the importance of the clinical laboratory in both diagnosis and the monitoring of treatment, and noted that teaching and research are important roles that affect laboratory usage. Finally, the committee concluded that the clinical laboratory can make an essential contribution to health care by providing quality control of the practice of medicine.

DIAGNOSIS OF DISEASE

In a study of 80 outpatients, Hampton et al.[2] found that the clinical history provided enough information to make an initial diagnosis in 82% of the patients. In only 9% was the physical examination useful in making the diagnosis although in another 31% it altered the confidence of the physician in the initial diagnosis he had developed from the history. In only 9% of the patients did laboratory tests alter the diagnosis initially derived from the history and physical examination. In a second study from the United Kingdom, Sandler[3] observed that 56% of diagnoses made on 630 medical outpatients were made from the history, while 17% were made from the physical examination. Laboratory investigations contributed to 23% of all diagnoses. However, the usefulness of the three procedures in the diagnosis of diseases of the different organ systems varied considerably. Thus 67% of all diagnoses of the cardiovascular system were made from the history, whereas the history enabled diagnoses in only 27% of the patients with disorders of the gastrointestinal system. In contrast, routine and special investigations contributed to only 9% of the diagnoses of the patients with cardiovascular diseases, but to 53% of the diagnoses of those with endocrine disorders. From a study by Franco[4] it is apparent that diagnostic procedures are of more importance in developing a diagnosis when a patient is evaluated at a periodic health examination when he does not present with an overt complaint than when he presents with a real complaint. Thus, the history contributed to only 34% of the diagnoses and the physical examination to 22%. The clinical laboratory tests contributed to about 14% of all diagnoses.

There is a general belief that American physicians are more dependent on laboratory data than their counterparts in Britain; it would be interesting to learn whether the clinical laboratory plays a greater role in the diagnostic process.

In a study of the practice of three German physicians, Gergely[5] noted that 6.1% of routine laboratory tests were important for the differential diagnosis, and 7.2% led to another diagnosis. Of tests that the physicians deemed to be necessary, 1.2% provided proof of the clinical diagnosis, 35.5% were of value in leading to the differential diagnosis and 8.9% pointed to another diagnosis. This study suggests an important role for the clinical laboratory, especially when physicians are selective in the tests ordered, in the diagnostic decision making. Yet, it should be noted that in the United States, at least, physician usage of the clinical laboratories is a function of background and training, as demonstrated by the study of Freeborn et al.[6]

In all the studies cited above, the role of the laboratory in diagnosis making is clearly less than that of the history and physical examination, but in certain situations the clinician becomes much more dependent on the clinical laboratory to establish a definite diagnosis. Examples of this dependency are the assessment of the acid-base status of a patient and the early determination of pregnancy. Other clinical diagnoses that can be made only from the results of laboratory tests are the detection of early renal disease, for which the examination of urine for protein, casts, and cells is essential. Detection of Hepatitis B_s antigen (Australia antigen) in serum is required to confirm that a liver disease is hepatitis, although liver disease might be readily apparent from the physical examination without any laboratory tests having been performed. Measurement of the various porphyrins (and relevant enzymes) in different tissues is necessary to establish the exact nature of a porphyria. To determine the causative agent of an allergy, the clinician must seek the measurement of the appropriate allergen specific IgE antibody in serum or undertake appropriate skin testing. The diagnosis of multiple myeloma and other gammopathies depends on appropriate laboratory tests having been performed.

SCREENING FOR DISEASE

Screening can be thought of as the search for disease in individuals in whom its presence has not been established previously. As the prevalence of different diseases varies in different age groups, the biochemical tests to be used to detect disease should be varied with the likelihood of a disease being detected. Screening is used to provide clues to the presence of a disease and need not be used to establish conclusively the nature or extent of a particular disease, which can be determined subsequently from definitive laboratory tests.

Henderson and Sherwin[7] have categorized screening for disease according to whether the approach is discrete, i.e., only a single test is used, or multiple, which involves several tests; whether the application is discriminate, i.e., limited to a previously selected population or more widely applied; and whether the tests are specific—targeted toward a single disease—or nonspecific—intended to detect disease in general that could be defined better subsequently by the history, physical examination, and specific laboratory tests. The measurement of phenylalanine in the serum of a newborn can be considered a specific discriminate test for phenylketonuria, whereas the hospital admission profile is a nonspecific indiscriminate multiple test for a variety of diseases.

Screening for disease is most often undertaken in early childhood, although the widespread hospital admission profile is used to exclude diseases that might be overlooked when an individual undergoes a periodic health examination, or is admitted to a hospital. Screening for disease in the child has now been broken down into prenatal screening and neonatal screening. Rarely is a physician more dependent on the laboratory than when attempting to detect a disease in the unborn child. Data from the National Registry Study of amniocenteses suggest that most amniocenteses are performed to detect Down's syndrome in the unborn child.[8] As most cases occur in the children of women aged 35 years or older where a child with Down's syndrome has been born in the same family, clear indications for amniocentesis are apparent. Other current applications include the detection of other cytogenetic disorders, x-linked disorders, and some metabolic diseases. It is probable that the number of amniocenteses will increase to detect neural tube defects and to examine the children of mothers who are carriers at risk of having an affected child.

Most screening for inherited metabolic disorders is done on children within a few days of birth. Many states have set up mandatory programs to screen for certain treatable diseases. The program in Minnesota is typical, with screening for phenylketonuria, galactosemia, and neonatal hypothyroidism. The incidence of neonatal hypothyroidism is about 1 in 8,000 births, and of phenylketonuria and galactosemia 1 in 10,000 and 1 in 33,000, respectively.[9] The diagnosis of any of these diseases is almost entirely dependent first on a laboratory screening test and then on a more definitive laboratory test. The initial blood spot test on filter paper for thyroxine is followed by a thyroid-stimulating hormone (thyrotropin) measurement before a diagnosis of hypothyroidism is made. Although cystic fibrosis has a prevalence of 1 case per 2,000 births, screening for the disease, while feasible (especially in older children), is not usually included as part of a screening program. Most of the diseases that are screened for are treatable, and their inclusion in screening programs has been justified because of the favorable benefit-to-cost ratio that results when the diseases are detected early and the patients are treated.

Even though it is not possible to screen for all metabolic errors, several objectives can be met through screening programs. These include the prevention or minimizing of irreversible damage, avoidance of expensive delay in diagnosis, reduction of exposure to harmful drugs or a harmful environment, and education of the parents of patients of the risks of recurrence.[10] For certain populations of older children, it is desirable to screen for lead poisoning. Once more, the diagnosis of lead poisoning is dependent on laboratory tests—a combination of the blood lead concentration and that of erythrocyte protoporphyrin.

Although laboratory tests are included as part of most periodic health evaluations or hospital admissions, few diagnoses are made from the group of tests that is usually administered, although the results may lead to further tests that are used to establish a diagnosis. Hayashi[11] in a study from Japan has discussed the usefulness of a urinalysis in leading to a diagnosis. The urinary glucose, done as part of the routine urinalysis, is probably the single test that leads to most diagnoses of diabetes mellitus. Of more than 6,000 successive urinalysis specimens examined in our laboratories about 1 in 30 demonstrated glycosuria but only 1 in 60 was from a diabetic patient. Ten new diabetics were diagnosed in this way, nine being maturity onset diabetics and one being a new patient with juvenile onset diabetes. The demonstration of glycosuria provides only a clue to the presence of diabetes but the final diagnosis also rests on laboratory tests. The National Diabetes Data Group[12] has now established criteria, mainly laboratory, that should be used for establishing the diagnosis of diabetes mellitus.

Heath et al.[13] have recently discussed the Mayo Clinic experience with the serum calcium measurement as a diagnostic aid for hyperparathyroidism. The apparent incidence of hyperparathyroidism increased sixfold when the serum calcium was first introduced as part of a battery of tests that were performed together, although it later fell to 3.5 times the prebattery incidence. At the same time the number of patients who presented first with urolithiasis decreased markedly. Although hypercalcemia is not caused by hyperparathyroidism only, the finding of a high serum concentration does enable a thorough work-up for a parathyroid tumor to be initiated early, so that the more severe consequences of hyperparathyroidism can be prevented.

The inclusion of uric acid, cholesterol, and urea nitrogen or creatinine as part of a group of tests used on a patient's admission to hospital or during a periodic health examination has also proved of value in screening for gout, cardiovascular disease, and some renal diseases respectively, although test results must be considered in conjunction with clinical findings before an unequivocal diagnosis can be made.

One application of laboratory tests that should be considered under the heading of screening tests is that of screening for risk factors. These, to date have been concerned primarily with identification of individuals at risk for cardiovascular disease and thus include lipid tests mainly. The lecithin/sphingomyelin ratio in amniotic fluid is performed as a test to determine fetal lung immaturity, to predict problems that may be encountered by the child shortly after birth. The serum alpha-antitrypsin concentration is used also to identify children who may develop respiratory problems.

Although most physicians use laboratory tests to screen for disease, the same tests can be used to rule out disease, and may be of great value in reassuring the worried well that they do not have a disease. Simple screening tests are usually adequate for this purpose as there is no need to follow up the normal screening test result with a more definitive test.

DETERMINATION OF SEVERITY OF DISEASE

In general the magnitude of the deviation of the serum concentration or activity of an analyte from normal is related to the severity of damage to an organ. As few of our current laboratory tests are tests of organ function, there need not necessarily be any correlation between the magnitude of the laboratory changes and the prognosis of the patient. Serial measurements of cardiac enzymes in serum have been used, in conjunction with knowledge of their half-lives, to estimate the size of a myocardial infarct. Many assumptions have to be made about the ability of enzyme released from cells to enter the circulation. These do not consider the release of enzyme that is known to occur with simple ischemia of tissues without actual irreversible damage having taken place.

Again for liver disease, there is a rough relationship between serum enzyme activity and extent of damage, although the nature of the liver disease must be known before valid conclusions can be drawn.

That there can be a poor correlation between laboratory tests and severity of disease can be seen in that even with the sensitive radioimmunoassay for prostatic acid phosphatase, certain patients will have normal enzyme activity, although they may have widely disseminated metastases at the same time. Small differences in serum concentration or activity of analytes occur as a manifestation of normal biological variability,[14] but it has not been established for most analytes whether this change is due to differences in organ function or size, or related only to genetic factors. Accordingly, it is difficult to correlate small changes in test values observed in different individuals with the extent of change in organ function. It should also be remembered that for many organs, no changes in laboratory test values need be observed until severe damage has occurred.

Nevertheless, it is still appropriate to consider that a large deviation of test values from normal probably reflects more severe organ damage than does a small change.

DETERMINATION OF APPROPRIATE MANAGEMENT

Measurement of risk factors could appropriately be considered under this heading, although it is difficult in many instances to convince a patient to modify his life style when such factors are identified and the patient is young and apparently healthy.

The most successful use of laboratory tests in determining appropriate management is in the measurement of estrogen and progesterone receptors in malignant breast tissue. The results of these assays are used to determine whether chemotherapy or hormone ablative therapy is more appropriate. The serum bilirubin concentration is used in newborn infants to determine whether an exchange transfusion is required; the test has been further refined by measurement of the bilirubin binding capacity. Measurement of the serum urea-nitrogen or creatinine concentration is used to determine the time at which dialysis should be undertaken for individuals with acute or chronic renal failure, and an increase of 0.3 mg/dL in the serum creatinine concentration has been used in patients who have had renal transplants, as an indication that rejection is taking place and as a signal to institute aggressive immunosuppressive therapy.

MONITORING PROGRESS OF DISEASE

In a recent study of the use of the laboratory in a large teaching hospital, Wertman et al.[15] observed that almost as many tests were requested by physicians for monitoring the progress of a patient's illness (33%) as for diagnosis (37%) or screening (32%). These reasons were much more common than the next most frequent, a previously abnormal result (12%).

Once a diagnosis has been established and treatment instituted, laboratory tests provide one of the most effective means for following the patient's response. Laboratory tests provide a quantitative indication of change that is often more reliable than the subjective impression provided by the patient. Yet, Sandler[3] has demonstrated that the history is still more important in managing a patient than laboratory tests or physical examinations. However, a patient may often feel well before laboratory tests have reverted to normal, and, conversely, laboratory tests may be normal although a patient may still feel unwell.

Nevertheless, the normal practice in hospital is for physicians to use one or more tests that have been used to demonstrate organ malfunction or damage, as measures to follow the progress of a disease in response to treatment. A single test to monitor the disease usually suffices. This can be a general test like total serum creatine kinase activity rather than its MB isoenzyme once the diagnosis of myocardial infarction has been established.

The major role for the measurement of tumor antigens may be in following surgery or other forms of treatment designed to remove or destroy the tumor. Following a successful outcome, the concentration of carcinoembryonic antigen in serum, which has been used to follow the treatment of many tumors of the gastrointestinal tract, usually decreases to a low value although this is often not observed immediately.

Elion-Gerritzen[16] has noted that many physicians interpret small changes in laboratory data that fall within normal analytical variability as being of clinical significance. It is important that physicians do not attach too much importance to small changes in laboratory data, as these can often be caused by either analytical or biological variability. The frequency of ordering tests to monitor a specific function should also be linked to the rate at which the data could be expected to change in a healthy individual. It is also important for physicians to be aware of the large influence that therapeutic drugs may have on the concentration of many constituents of body fluids.[17] For these reasons, physicians should be judicious in using laboratory data as their prime yardstick for monitoring the progress of a disease.

MONITORING THERAPY

Many of the drugs administered to patients are potentially toxic, yet also are ineffective at a low plasma concentration. For such drugs, it is important that their concentrations in plasma be measured at frequent intervals to ensure that a therapeutic concentration is maintained. Werner et al.[18] have developed a series of weightings based on both clinical and laboratory factors to determine which drugs should be monitored. Most of the drugs routinely measured in clinical chemistry laboratories have high weightings by these criteria. Pippenger[19] has pinpointed the usefulness of therapeutic drug monitoring in the clinical management of a patient. Noncompliance or individual variations in drug-disposition patterns can be identified. Altered drug utilization as a consequence of disease can also be determined. Therapeutic drug monitoring also allows altered physiological states to be compensated for, and modifications in dosage to be made, so that an efficacious serum concentration is achieved. Situations in which therapeutic drug monitoring is particularly desirable include drug administration to patients with renal disease when the drugs are eliminated through the kidney. Drug concentrations should be monitored when a patient demonstrates signs of toxicity that are drug related, or when a patient known to be receiving the drug fails to respond. Patients with diseases that may reduce the half-life of a drug, or patients who have an altered physiological state such as occurs with old age, pregnancy, the newborn state, fever, obesity, or an expanded or reduced plasma volume, should be subjected to therapeutic drug monitoring, even when this might not be considered for other patients.

Therapeutic drug monitoring has undoubtedly had a positive effect on patient care. Kutt and Penry[20] believe that therapeutic drug monitoring has been responsible for a reduction by as much as 50% in the number of epileptic patients with poor control of seizures. Duhme et al.[21] have confirmed that use of radioimmunoassay for digoxin improved the control of cardiac arrhythmias and reduces the number of adverse reactions to the drug. Nevertheless, Booker[22] cautions against the overdependence on reported serum concentrations of drugs, noting that the values tend with time to regress to published therapeutic concentrations. As a result, individuals with low serum concentrations may have their dose increased and individuals with high concentrations have the dose decreased, even though their clinical response has been satisfactory.

MONITORING DRUG TOXICITY

The use of highly potent drugs that are metabolized to some extent, at least, in the liver necessitates monitoring the function of the liver. Guidelines for detection of hepatotoxicity due to drugs have been established by an International Committee of experts in liver diseases.[23] Although these guidelines are oriented to new drugs, they are appropriate for monitoring drugs that are in routine use. The experts recommended that any aspartate aminotransferase activity value that was above the upper limit of normal, established with the same method, was cause for suspicion of liver disease, and any value more than twice this value should be considered to indicate hepatic injury unless this has been excluded by other studies.

Similarly, drugs that may produce renal damage should be monitored by periodic checks of renal function to ensure that treatment is stopped if damage occurs. It should also be recalled that the influence of disease may affect the amount of free drug. The amount of free drug, which is probably responsible for much of the toxic potential of the drug, as it is for its therapeutic action, should be monitored (although this is largely impractical). The free-drug concentration should be considered to be possibly increased even though the amount of total drug need not be increased in situations such as uremia that affect the protein-binding of drugs. Thus, drug toxicity can occur at very different concentrations of total drug in the serum of different individuals.

PREDICTING RESPONSE TO TREATMENT

Prediction of response of patients to a variety of treatments is obviously a desirable goal for any physician. If a model could be developed for each patient and the various candidate treatments evaluated, it would be of real benefit to patients in selecting early the appropriate treatment. This state has not yet been achieved, although the outcome of treatment of breast cancer is beginning to be affected by the determination of the estrogen and progesterone receptor activity of an excised tumor, and chemotherapy or hormone ablative therapy is then selected to follow the initial operation. It should be possible to simplify the procedure further by an initial tissue biopsy and in-vitro assessment of receptor activity on a small scale to determine the likelihood of response so that operative intervention could probably be avoided.

Sullivan et al.[24] have demonstrated that platelet monoamine oxidase activity may be used to predict the response of patients who have manic-depressive illness to treatment with lithium. The excretion of 3-methoxy-4-hydroxyphenyl-ethylene glycol appears also to be of value in predicting the response of depressed individuals to treatment with tricyclic antidepressants (A. H. Rosenbaum and T. P. Moyer, personal communication).

Although little research has been performed to date on establishing the predictable response of a patient's disease to treatment, and although we should recognize that this research is difficult to carry out, it is still likely to become a future area of considerable usefulness for the clinical laboratory.

OTHER PROBLEMS

The ready availability of laboratory tests to clinicians, while solving the need for some complicated clinical decision making, has created the need for this on other occasions. When physicians receive abnormal results from tests that they either did not order, or did not anticipate when they did order the test, they are faced with problems in deciding how to use the result. Sisson et al.[25] have discussed in some detail the hazards of using additional data, and most laboratory workers have experience with the problems posed for clinicians when they receive an abnormal test result and feel compelled to act on it.

The problem of the unanticipated abnormal result has become more acute since the introduction of multitest chemical analyzers with their capability of producing many results simultaneously from a single specimen when only a few tests were requested. Follow-up of such test results has shown that only a few of these test results lead to new diagnoses and most are not indicative of presymptomatic disease.[26] Indeed, a large number of these tests on reanalysis of the specimen become normal.

Nevertheless, the quantitative information that can be provided by a laboratory to clinicians is able to facilitate their decision making in many facets of patient-management, from the diagnosis to the treatment. The role of the laboratory in clinical decision making is likely to be augmented in the future. However, optimum use of the laboratory will occur only when clinical and laboratory decision makers work out together the appropriate strategies for use of the clinical laboratory.

References

1. Working group on laboratory services. Guidelines for the appropriate use of medical laboratory services in Canada. Report to the Intersociety council of laboratory medicine of Canada. Department of National Health and Welfare, Ottawa, Ontario, Canada, 1979.

2. Hampton JR, Harrison MJG, Mitchell JRA, Prichard JS, Seymour C. Relative contributions of history-taking, physical examination, and laboratory investigations to diagnosis and management of medical outpatients. Br Med J 1975;2:486-89.

3. Sandler G. Costs of unnecessary tests. Br Med J 1979;2:21-4.

4. Franco SC. The early detection of disease by periodic examination. Industr Med Surg 1956;25:251-7.

5. Gergely T, Kinhast H, Pointner H, Wegmann R, Gabl F, Deutsch E. Der Wert klinisch-chemischer Analysen. Dtsch Med Wochenschr 1980;105:406-9.

6. Freeborn DK, Baer D, Greenlick MR, Bailey JW. Determinants of medical care utilization: physicians' use of laboratory services. Am J Public Health 1972;62:846-53.

7. Henderson M, Sherwin R. Screening—a privilege, not a right. Prev Med 1974;3:160-4.

8. NICHD National Registry for Amniocentesis Study Group. Midtrimester amniocentesis for prenatal diagnosis: Safety and accuracy. JAMA 1976;236:1471-6.

9. Raine DN. Inborn errors of metabolism. In: Brown SS, Mitchell FL, Young DS, eds. Chemical Diagnosis of Disease. Elsevier: Amsterdam, 1979: 927-1008.

10. Holtzman NA. Newborn screening for inborn errors of metabolism. Pediatr Clin North Am 1978;25:411-21.

11. Hayashi Y. The value of qualitative tests of the urine. Asian Med J 1973;16:5-20.

12. National Diabetes Data Group. Classification and diagnosis of diabetes mellitus and other categories of glucose intolerance. Diabetes 1979;28:1039-57.

13. Heath H III, Hodgson SF, Kennedy MA. Primary hyperparathyroidism: incidence, morbidity, and potential economic impact in a community. N Engl J Med 1980;302:189-93.

14. Young DS. Biological variability. In: Brown SS, Mitchell FL, Young DS, eds. Chemical Diagnosis of Disease. Elsevier:Amsterdam, 1979:1-113.

15. Wertman BG, Sostrin SV, Pavlova Z, Lundberg G. Why do physicians order laboratory tests? A study of laboratory test request and use patterns. JAMA 1980;243:2080-2.

16. Elion-Gerritzen WE. Requirements for analytical performance in clinical chemistry. Ph.D. Thesis, Erasmus University, Rotterdam, 1978.

17. Young DS, Pestaner LC, Gibberman V. Effects of drugs on clinical laboratory tests. Clin Chem 1975;21:1D-432D.

18. Werner M, Sutherland EW III, Abramson FP. Concepts for the rational selection of assays to be used in monitoring therapeutic drugs. Clin Chem 1975;21:1368-71.

19. Pippenger CE. The rationale for therapeutic drug monitoring. American Association for Clinical Chemistry Therapeutic Drug Monitoring Program. July 1979.

20. Kutt H, Penry JK. Usefulness of blood levels of antiepileptic therapeutic drugs. Arch Neurol 1974;31:283-8.

21. Duhme DW, Greenblatt DJ, Koch-Weser J. Reduction of digoxin toxicity associated with measurement of serum levels. Ann Intern Med 1974;80:516-19.

22. Booker HE. Phenobarbital, mephobarbital, and metharbital: relation of plasma levels to clinical control. In: Woodbury DM, Penry JK, Schmidt RP, eds. Antiepileptic Drugs. Raven Press:New York, 1972:329-34.

23. Davidson CS, Leevy CM, Chamberlayne EC, eds. Guidelines for detection of hepatotoxicity due to drugs and chemicals. 1979. (DHEW. NIH publication no. 79-313).

24. Sullivan JL, Cavenar JO Jr, Maltbie A, Stanfield C. Platelet monoamine-oxidase activity predicts response to lithium in manic-depressive illness. Lancet 1977;2:1325-7.

25. Sisson JC, Schoomaker EB, Ross JC. Clinical decision analysis: the hazard of using additional data. JAMA 1976;236:1259-63.

26. Bradwell AR, Carmalt MHB, Whitehead TP. Explaining the unexpected abnormal results of biochemical profile investigations. Lancet 1974;2:1071-4.

CHAPTER TEN

Assessing the Effectiveness of Laboratory Test Selection and Use

William R. Fifer, MD

Presumably some laboratory tests are more useful than others. Given the immense number of tests available (all of which appear to have at least *some* value) and the increasing awareness of resource limitations, it becomes important to evaluate laboratory tests in terms of effectiveness, to guide their selection and use. This paper will present selected aspects of the problem of laboratory test evaluation.

"Assessment" is defined as "rating," "appraising," or "evaluating." Evaluation, which is the process of making a judgment about the worth of something, uses a referent or standard as the benchmark with which to compare the thing to be evaluated. Evaluation systems are often divided into those that are "norm-referenced" and those that are "criterion-referenced." The use of reference norms enables one to compare a given value with a statistical mean of like values. Criteria, by contrast, are expressions of optimal values often developed by experts.

Medical care evaluation models commonly use as referents criteria that Donabedian[1] categorizes into inputs, processes, and outcomes. Input criteria are sometimes called "structural" criteria, and specify desirable preconditions to performance that, when present, attest to the readiness or capability of a system to achieve a desired result. In medical care evaluation, process criteria specify the steps or processes that experts feel represent "best" performance; outcome criteria specify the optimal achievable results of the patient care process. Brook's classic paper[2] describes the great variation in evaluation results dependent on which parameter is used.

Another important consideration relative to the use of criteria for evaluation is *validity*. Although some criteria possess face validity (a clear picture speaks to the quality of a television receiver), others are often arrived at by expert consensus or, less commonly, are scientifically validated by well-designed studies that demonstrate high level correlation between the criterion and the desired result or value. The evolution of reliable systems of medical care evaluation has been frustrated by the general lack of scientifically valid criteria, usually attributed to the development of medical care practices through empirical means rather than through a series of randomized control trials. Consensus criteria are almost equally rare, owing to disagreement among experts, even about such an apparently doctrinaire practice as tonsillectomy.[3]

In assessing laboratory criteria for "effectiveness," the first task is to define "effectiveness," which Webster describes as "producing the intended result." What are the intended results of laboratory testing? At least some of the more important ones are

- screening to detect disease;
- aiding the processes of diagnosis and differential diagnosis in symptomatic individuals;
- prognostication, either of impending disease through identification of risk factors or of the course and/or outcome of known disease; and
- control or monitoring of physiologic parameters (such as blood glucose) or drug levels.

It becomes clear that laboratory tests have a number of intended results, and that evaluation of their effectiveness in "producing the intended result" will depend on a clear explication of what the intended result is to be.

Galen and Gambino, in their remarkably insightful analysis of laboratory test utility,[4] extended our understanding "Beyond Normality." They pointed out that a test possesses:

- *sensitivity* or "positivity in disease";
- *specificity* or "negativity in health";
- *predictive value*, which depends not only on a test's sensitivity and specificity, but also on the prevalence of the disease or condition identified by the test results; and
- *efficiency*, which they defined by this formula:

$$\frac{\text{true "positives"} + \text{true "negatives"}}{\text{grand total}} \times 100.$$

Further, they pointed out the enhancing effect of clinical judgment as exemplified by the increase in sensitivity of diagnostic tests for pheochromocytoma in patients with episodic hypertension, tachycardia, and flushing. They described the complexity of analyzing multiple tests or combination testing, as exemplified by the statistical treatment of weighted multiple risk factors in predicting coronary artery disease. Finally, they reminded test selectors that they might have to sacrifice one quality to get another, as few tests possess the happy combination of optimal sensitivity, specificity, predictive value, and efficiency.

How then are we to choose criteria to evaluate laboratory test effectiveness? First, we should have a clear idea of the intended result of the test to be evaluated. Next, evaluation criteria should be selected that "fit" the intended result. It is tempting to ask the experts what they do and evaluate performance in terms of compliance with their behavior. We find, however, that such process criteria become exhaustive ("cookbooks") if they try to anticipate the context of clinical decision, and that compliance with a cookbook is so context-related that widespread variation from the "best" model is demonstrated by competent clinicians. Greenfield[5] has adapted the algorithm approach to criteria specification, by constructing "criteria maps" consisting of a branching decision logic to display optimal behavior in sequencing clinical intervention, or decision nodes in the diagnostic process.

One could, for example, derive expert consensus as to the laboratory work-up and surveillance of the hypertensive patient on therapy. What is troubling about this approach to evaluation is the lack of correlation between "good" process and "good" outcome (the latter being control of blood pressure and prevention of morbidity in hypertensives) shown by the studies of Nobrega[6] and others. Does optimal use of the laboratory in treating the hypertensive patient constitute conformance with testing processes, or securing of good results for the patient? The lack of correlation between process-oriented and outcome-oriented evaluation is troublesome but at least partially explained by McAuliffe's analysis,[7] which concludes that faulty experimental design weakens the claim that process and outcome do not correlate as they should if the textbooks are correct.

The referent for laboratory test evaluation may be tissue, other laboratory evidence, opinions of experts, or an independent outcome. The validity of various serum enzyme abnormalities to accurately diagnose acute myocardial infarction may be determined, for example, by histologic proof at autopsy. Alternatively, such abnormalities may derive their diagnostic value by virtue of correlation with other laboratory tests (such as the erythrocyte sedimentation rate), electrocardiographic abnormalities, or conclusions by expert cardiologists based on a number of assessment parameters.

Finally, laboratory testing can and should be subjected to cost-benefit and cost-effectiveness analyses on the grounds that not every result is cost beneficial and that cheaper alternatives of equal effectiveness exist for many commonly used laboratory tests.

Let me close by providing some examples of laboratory test evaluation from the recent literature:

- Jacobson[8] reported on the efficacy of a large battery of laboratory tests commonly used in an attempt to identify the cause of chronic urticaria. He concluded that, with the exception of sinus x-rays, such tests were not helpful in uncovering an underlying cause for this distressing manifestation. Specifically, he concluded that examination of the stool for ova and parasites was a dreadful waste of time and money, inasmuch as none of the eighty such examinations yielded evidence of parasitism.
- Wheeler[9] compared the performance of test subjects with an algorithm developed by expert hematologists to evaluate the appropriateness of laboratory test selection in the evaluation of anemia. He found that lab-

oratory use was "inappropriate" 40 percent of the time in this situation, with 24 percent of the total representing underuse, 11 percent overuse, and 5 percent a mixture of overuse and underuse.

- George[10] illustrated the importance of the objective in evaluating the effectiveness of laboratory testing: After ten years of using radionuclide scans to diagnose brain tumors at Hopkins, he found that the interval between the onset of symptoms and operation fell from nearly four years to less than one year, making the test look very effective. However, the survival rate remained unchanged despite the decrease in surgical delay.
- Furth[11] used cost-benefit analysis to evaluate laboratory diagnoses of thyroid cancer, and concluded it cost $105,320 to identify each case. By contrast, the cost of detecting a single case of congenital hypothyroidism is $9, 300, which, added to treatment cost of $2,500, produces $105,000 worth of benefit for each $11,800 spent, a cost-benefit ratio of 1:8.9.
- Taylor[12] concluded that stool guaiac tests were "only valuable if six slides are prepared from three consecutive bowel movements while [a patient is] on a meat-free, high-residue diet."
- Galen and Gambino[4] cite many examples of worthwhile and worthless tests, such as alpha-fetoprotein (false positive rate of 30.2 percent), PKU screening (hobbled by low incidence of disease), metanephrines (high sensitivity, high specificity). They illustrate the relative value of the same test in different situations with the VMA test (highly sensitive and specific in pheochromocytoma, but crippled by low sensitivity and prevalence when used as a test strip for neuroblastoma).

In summary, there is great need for ongoing evaluation of the selection and use of laboratory tests, both because of their aggregate cost and because of the variability in their utility. Evaluation methods are varied in approach and effectiveness, and are capable of skewing the results of evaluation. Most clinicians who utilize the laboratory have only a rudimentary understanding of the sophisticated insights of Galen and Gambino, which probe the area "Beyond Normality." And, finally, evaluation efforts will continue to depend on a clear understanding of the objective or "intended result" of the test.

The arena of evaluation of laboratory test selection and use contains profound challenges and opportunities for continued development.

References

1. Donabedian A. Evaluating the quality of medical care. Milbank Memorial Fund Quarterly 1966;44:166-206
2. Brook RH, Appel F. Quality of care assessment: choosing a method for peer review. N Engl J Med 1973;288:1323-9.
3. Carden TS. Tonsillectomy—trials and tribulations: a report on the NIH consensus conference on indications for T. & A. JAMA 1978;240:1961-2.

4. Galen, RS, Gambino SR. Beyond normality—the predictive value and efficiency of medical diagnoses. New York: John Wiley & Sons, 1975.
5. Greenfield S, et al. The clinical investigation and management of chest pain in the emergency department: quality assessment by criteria mapping. Med Care 1977;15:898-905.
6. Nobrega FT, et al. Quality assessment in hypertension: analysis of process and outcome methods. N Engl J Med 1977;296:145-8.
7. McAuliffe WE. Studies of process-outcome correlations in medical care evaluation: a critique. Med Care 1978;16:907-30.
8. Jacobson KW, Branch LB, Nelson HS. Laboratory tests in chronic urticaria. JAMA 1980; 243:1644-6.
9. Wheeler LA, Brecher G, Sheiner LB. Clinical laboratory use in the evaluation of anemia. JAMA 1977; 238:2709-14.
10. George RO, Wagner HN Jr. Ten years of brain tumor scanning at Johns Hopkins: 1962-1972, non-invasive brain imaging: computed tomography and radionuclides. In: DeBlanc HJ Jr., Sorenson JA, eds. Soc Nuc Med New York 1975:3-16.
11. Furth ED. Quoted in: Kangilaski J. Medical progress—can we afford the cost? Forum on Medicine 1979 April:294.
12. Taylor R. Health care screening: not an end in itself. American Medical News 1980 March 28;4.

CHAPTER ELEVEN

Use or Misuse: Variations in Clinical Laboratory Testing

Werner A. Gliebe, MA

Increasing the effectiveness of laboratory test use is essential if we are to achieve maximal quality of medical care at the lowest possible cost. The significance of this component is readily apparent, since about $15 billion annually can be accounted for by clinical laboratory use. Focusing on increasing effectiveness does suggest, however, that substantial improvements could be made, an implication that may not be true ahistorically.

If the pressures to contain high health care costs were not so intense, it is quite conceivable that the clinical laboratory would be seen for its positive effects and its limitations given little emphasis. Indeed, the question becomes whether we should look at use or misuse, the glass as partially empty or full. Since we create our own history, but are also controlled by it, we will try to look at both sides of the argument.

Variations in laboratory testing are in and of themselves not characterized by misuse; rather the characterization is made in the context of external events. Since economic issues are currently paramount in the public consciousness, variations tend to be viewed as negative. However, misuse can only be confirmed if we document variations in laboratory testing occurring for other than clinically appropriate reasons.

But the clinical situation and the associated clinical reasoning are complex and difficult to evaluate. "This process of observation and reasoning used for these decisions is as diverse as the intricacies of human thought, and is performed differently by each clinician. Because so many different types of data are involved, because so many elements of the data are difficult to specify, and because clinicians and patients are so diverse, the process is usually regarded as an art-like, sometimes mystical, often intuitive procedure."[1]

The ideas presented in this paper were developed with and reflect the continued support of the National Fund for Medical Education, Hartford, CT.

MISUSE AND QUALITY ASSESSMENT

At the aggregate level of public policy, the term "misuse" in the context of medical care conjures up the notion of quality assessment and its measurement. For practical purposes, as most readers are aware, attempts to measure quality have concentrated on process and outcome indicators. These concepts have been applied to overall judgmental determinations about the entire medical care episode. Researchers have developed specific process criteria to assess care quality; others have elaborated outcome criteria to arrive at judgments. To address pragmatic policy issues (such as which kind of indicator to use in making assessments), others have attempted to correlate process and outcome measures to determine which indicators yielded the most correct picture of real clinical events. However some major relevant criticisms of these attempts at process-outcome comparisons have recently been made; "presently we know very little regarding the validity of methods being used to assess quality of care . . . . the ultimate success of quality regulation will hinge in part on the soundness of its assessment methods."[2]

Since the initial emphasis on quality, review of care has been assigned an additional goal, namely cost containment. The success or failure of PSROs will be determined by the money saved from such activities. But quality and cost are inextricably related. Misuse of services such as the clinical laboratory, which is also poor quality care, can be documented only if we understand what appropriate use is in a given clinical context. In view of the limitations of these overall judgmental techniques commonly used in process and outcome assessment, such techniques must also be seen as inadequate for validly defining misuse. In other words, general medical care evaluation techniques whose level of specificity ends with a diagnosis (perhaps of a given severity) must treat all patients identically. The patient management process for individual cases cannot be understood.

One promising attempt to understand the logical, stepwise process relevant to an individual case is criteria mapping. "This method shifts the focus of the evaluation from the disease to the individual patient, emphasizing the actions taken as patient-specific clinical information is elicited in the course of the workup."[3] The system is set up in such a way that "when criteria are individualized through branching logic, physicians are not penalized for appropriate omissions."[4] Criteria mapping is, however, designed for quality assessment; it identifies sets of treatment paths that, when taken, satisfy minimal process criteria. Their goal is to develop acceptable process measures that will more closely correlate with outcome. Although important, such a technique does not help to identify misuse. After auditing a case through criteria mapping, we can make the judgment whether an acceptable treatment path for this diagnosis has been followed; in the words of the authors, "physicians are not penalized for appropriate omissions."[4] But no information is gained about any "inappropriate commissions" that may have been rendered along the way. Documentation of misuse, therefore, remains elusive.

If we have not quite returned to the beginning, we at least feel like a turtle trying to run like a hare as we try to respond rapidly to public concern. We must return to the reality of variations, try to understand it, and use this understanding toward the goal at hand. The remainder of this paper will try to answer three questions in some detail in the hope that we can approach these ends.

1. Can variations be understood through a meaningful classification of real or imagined behavioral correlates?
2. Can a system to identify misuse be developed that has sufficient validity and resource economy for widespread application?
3. Can both issues be reconciled within a model of clinical behavior that can capture misuse and foster cost-effective, high quality clinical laboratory use?

VARIATIONS IN LABORATORY TESTING I

Toward a Meaningful Classification of Correlates

In returning to the concept of variation and whether it can be dealt with meaningfully, we begin by examining how variations have been classified and analyzed by other researchers. Traditionally, variations have been studied along the dichotomy of medical versus nonmedical factors or correlates. This still represents perhaps the most common way to classify much of the research to date. Some of the more comprehensive studies illustrate the correlates commonly used in studies of clinical laboratory use.

One research report found a slight relationship between physician age and clinical laboratory use, older physicians tending to be lower utilizers. Variation was related also to when and where physicians attended medical school. However, there was no relationship between patient load and laboratory use. The authors concluded that much more research needed to be done and recognized the need for "a conceptual framework to guide further analysis."[5] The finding that older physicians were lower utilizers had also been reported a decade earlier by researchers in Scotland; the explanation suggested was that younger physicians had been trained in a higher technology environment.[6] The findings on patient load contradicted the hypothesis that busy physicians might order laboratory tests to save time rather than use clinical skills.[7] The study by Freeborn also wondered "whether or not the rising cost associated with increased laboratory use has resulted in commensurate benefits to the patient."[5] This question was partially answered by one study that found "no positive association between a physician's frequency of laboratory use and either clinical productivity or outcomes of care."[8] Another widely quoted study reported "no predictive characteristics permitting identification of 'high cost' or 'low cost' physicians."[9] Another study examined physician specialty in some detail and reported internists used more services than family physicians.[10] A later study of specialty practice found that modal specialists provided the most cost-effective care for selected diagnoses.[11]

Sociologists have often studied patient-provider relationships in the hospital and reported differences in treatment patterns. Traditional teaching patients were often older, indigent, and, it was argued, subjected to more unnecessary laboratory testing. A recent study has provided some evidence that patients with certain characteristics, that is, nonwhite females under thirty-five and without their own physician at admission are used more often as educational subjects.[12] Other studies have elaborated the varied ways "good" patients versus "problem" patients are treated in the same hospital.[13]

All the studies have limitations; some did not try to assess the care provided at all. Some studies examined the clinical process of medical care in detail and then tried to explain variations using theoretically suggestive correlates. However, those that assessed care used process or outcome quality measures to then correlate other variables, but as we have seen, these quality measures may have little validity independently and no relationship to one another. Further, and not surprisingly, the correlates then tested to "account for" laboratory use variations explain small portions of total variance. None of these studies looked at the actual clinical situation as the unit of analysis. No dynamic model of identifying misuse, calculating costs, and monitoring clinical encounters is identified.

How could information about the clinical situation be derived? Can the individual case rather than the aggregate somehow be understood?

If we focus on the individual case, much of the previous research that dealt with aggregate cases and correlates becomes inadequate. Rather, we must examine those correlates that directly or consciously influence a physician's thought process when making a clinical decision. From this perspective, the number of relevant correlates are reduced; those indirect correlates such as age or specialty become tangential or irrelevant. The important set of correlates becomes those that can be collectively classified as related to the physician's "definition of the situation." These reflect the physician's intentions or reasons for ordering particular tests at a particular time. The key concept in determining misuse in the individual clinical case is intentionality. If intentionality can be communicated, determined, and assessed, a precise judgment as to the existence of misuse can be made. Given this concept, a more useful dichotomy to classify reasons for variations in clinical behavior would focus on unconscious versus conscious factors or correlates.

The conscious-unconscious dichotomy within the context of individual clinical situations has now become our framework for analyzing variations, identifying misuse, and calculating its costs. Synthesizing the literature from this perspective will provide us with the state of the art; we can then proceed to develop a dynamic evaluative system derived from this framework.

Unconscious vs. Conscious Correlates

Unconscious correlates as conceptualized here include many of those often thought of as nonmedical. However, some nonmedical correlates will shift under the new dichotomy since they can be relevant to the particular clinical situation. As such, they can be seen as conscious factors that may directly impinge on the thought process of the physician in the individual clinical situation. Unconscious correlates or factors include the following:[14]

1. Socioeconomic characteristics of patients
   a. social class
   b. income
   c. ethnic background
   d. sex
   e. age
2. Background of physician
   a. specialty
   b. age
   c. professional status
3. Physician relationships with other providers
   a. type of practice
   b. location of practice
   c. other spatial variables affecting access
4. Physician-patient encounter

Although such factors have been linked to variations in laboratory use, none of them have done so with substantial explanatory power. Such factors may correlate with or even influence laboratory use variations, but this association can be determined only after we identify misuse in the clinical situation. For this identification, we must first examine conscious factors that can directly affect how a physician behaves in a particular clinical context. Such factors are fewer in number and have been systematically studied less often although anecdotal observations often appear in the literature.[15]

Conscious factors directly affect a physician's thought process in ordering laboratory tests. Such factors can be medical or nonmedical and may or may not define an action as laboratory misuse. For example, a physician may order a brain scan when the patient complains of a headache, not because his clinical judgment deems it necessary, but to avoid possible malpractice claims. Defensive practices, while nonmedical, are nonetheless conscious factors in the clinical decision-making process. Tests ordered for educational purposes also constitute a conscious choice in clinical decision making.

The clinical situation is an appropriate focus since it constitutes the relevant purview of decision making from the physician's perspective. Any critique of a physician's patient management will have greatest legitimacy and credibility when focused on the clinical context of decision making. In other words, if we accept the profession's disease specific orientation toward medical problems, the so-called medical model of illness also known as scientific medicine, then to analyze, understand, and change clinical behavior demands focus on the clinical context. This constitutes, if not the path of least resistance, the path of most readily understandable and changeable behavioral focus. How is the biomedical thought process (or clinical decision-making process) affected by the medical event? How can that process be altered if necessary? Is alteration necessary, that is, is misuse so prevalent?

For analytical purposes, conscious factors operating in the clinical arena represent the most accessible foci to foster decision-making changes. Unconscious factors can later be examined to determine whether the misuse documented by the clinical situation varies in any systematic way with such factors. Unconscious factors may yield correlations but may provide few direct avenues or rationales for attacking behavioral change.

What are some of these conscious factors that enter into a single clinical decision? Several can be cited:[15,16]

Legitimate use

1. Diagnosis consistent with previous results
2. Monitoring consistent with previous results
3. Research if agreed to by concerned parties

Misuse (administrative remedy)

4. Malpractice fears—positive defensive medicine
5. Need to reorder—previous results not yet available

Misuse (personal remedy)

6. Educational purposes—tests assessed under particular conditions
7. Inexperience/learning—complete documentation syndrome
8. Diagnosis but misinformed strategy—lack of understanding of specificity and sensitivity
9. Personal habit—magic of the trinity (routine ordering by threes)
10. Time saver

Intentionality: Problems of Measurement

Having identified several conscious factors in the clinical decision-making process, the difficulty now becomes one of measurement. In any given clinical case, the distribution of conscious factors or correlates cannot be precisely established without asking the physician responsible. The issue has been stated more elaborately and clearly elsewhere and bears repetition.

The issue of measurement validity in research of this type warrants some comment. The method used here takes into account the circumstances that can affect a treatment choice at one point in time. There are as yet no expert-developed criteria by which an outsider can evaluate a patient's care and determine with certainty whether a test or procedure was done for diagnostic, educational, or defensive reasons. Information derived from the beliefs of other physicians as to what should have been done and a further assessment of why other things were done is twice removed from the actual treatment situation.

It would seem that the physician responsible for the patient is in a much better position to say why he has done something since he is familiar with the context of that treatment situation and aware of his own management logic. As such, he appears to be a more useful source of the type of data examined here. He can best tell us why he did what he did. Further, understanding an individual physician's patient management logic is essential if strategies for effecting individual behavioral changes are determined to be desirable.[17]

Such a suggestion is consistent with the more recent statement by Eisenberg that: "Further investigation is needed into how the clinician does behave. Various methods of sociologic research could be used to provide the data for these studies—participant observation, record review, questionnaires, interviews, case studies, or direct recording of the interaction."[14]

But such research methodologies are expensive to implement, difficult to coordinate, and, perhaps most important, may intrude on the very process that is being measured. Heisenberg referred to the limits of measurement in his principle of uncertainty at the level of atomic physics; the idea certainly is applicable many times over when we try to measure something like the clinical situation.

With these limitations in mind, we can refer to very few studies that have used this method for our purposes. Sociologists have used this method to look at characteristics of the physician-patient encounter, but have not dealt with the reasons or logic behind clinical decision making. In other words, they have not tried to measure intentionality. Other studies have used questionnaires or simulated/hypothetical conditions that try to measure intentionality, but do not use the true clinical situation. Few studies have tried to satisfy both criteria but two studies involving this author can be noted.

The first presented results on how frequently residents ordered clinical laboratory tests for defensive reasons.[17] The results demonstrated that 9% of all diagnostic tests (including x-rays) the residents ordered for their patients were acknowledged to have been done for defensive reasons. The evidence was accumulated by asking the residents to maintain diaries of their management decisions especially prepared by the investigators. One of the authors served as preceptor and could therefore monitor completion of the diaries. This attempt satisfied both our criteria: it tried to measure intentionality and focused on the clinical situation. A separate paper published from the same project[18] reported 11% of all tests ordered to be done for educational purposes, or what we have termed inexperience/learning in our listing of conscious factors. Such a study permitted some focus on identified, specific contexts that might demand some behavioral change. The study also permitted some assessment of the costs of educating physicians in teaching hospitals. The latter issue is often addressed by aggregated, indirect measures of cost comparisons.

However, such studies have the practical limitations mentioned above as well as measurement difficulties. Further, even if intentionality were completely measurable, we would then want to introduce other unconscious correlates to help us design the most effective possible change strategies. The other long-term difficulty would be gradual replication in enough locales to arrive at some estimate of the external validity of any relationships uncovered.

Since so few studies have successfully measured intentionality in the clinical situation, and few efforts can be anticipated in the near future, what if anything can be done to identify misuse on a less limited scale? Can misuse be documented through some other mechanism more suited to the demands of large scale evaluation necessary to contribute to public policy issues?

VARIATIONS IN LABORATORY TESTING II

A System to Efficiently Identify and Analyze Misuse

The system outlined below is being designed conceptually toward the goal of cost containment and to satisfy two objectives: (1) as a prospective feedback mechanism for attending physicians; and (2) as a retrospective feedback mechanism for attending physicians.

A. A Dynamic Evaluative System

We are coming full circle, returning to the problem of assessment and what is being measured. Previous studies have used process or outcome indicators, with either or both implicit and explicit criteria. But these have been shown to have difficulties. Criteria mapping shows promise as a dynamic system but focuses on quality assessment; it has not been designed to achieve cost containment.

Any system that is acceptable and useful must be (a) dynamic rather than static; must (b) focus on the clinical situation; and must (c) measure intentionality. To have all these characteristics, the system must be conceptualized not as process, not as outcome, but as a vital series of process-outcome, process-outcome decisions. The clinical situation is not static but changes with the condition of the patient and with the results of previous clinical decisions. As results of clinical laboratory tests arrive, these are seen as outcomes of an earlier process. The outcomes in turn create a new process that will create its own outcome. Fundamentally, it can be represented by the simplest communication model.

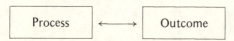

The incremental unit in the suggested model is one day. Clinical decisions made on day 1 (process) should then be evaluated in the context of results (outcome) available by day 2. At that point, day 2 begins with another series of clinical decisions (process) that will generate further results (outcome).

To consider large scale implementation of such a system, it must be computerized. The key hospital unit in such a system must be laboratory medicine and pathology, where personnel would feed the results into the system. When the system addresses the objective of a prospective feedback mechanism to the attending physician, for effective information flow, terminals and printers would be desirable on selected floors and/or patient units throughout the hospital. Computer printouts containing the process and outcome data will then be available to the physician at the start of each new day.

The essential elements for such a system include (1) the tests ordered and dates; (2) the test results, (3) the charges for each test, and (4) relevant clinical/diagnostic information.

Summary data for each time unit (day) would then include the above elements plus cumulative and day by day charge profiles, as well as an area for physician self-assessment as to the clinical necessity or importance of each day's decisions (intentionality). Tables 1 and 2 give a preliminary illustration of how this system might appear. Obviously, the reasons or intentions for ordering a test can be programmed in whatever varieties or combinations are desired.

When such a system is used only as a retrospective feedback mechanism, the capital resources needed by the hospital diminish but the logic and the model remain the same. Staff persons will need the same data elements but can obtain them through an itemized patient bill, and the test results from the patient chart. These can be programmed to yield the profile of the complete hospital stay as illustrated by Tables 1 and 2. Retrospective judgments can then be made as to specific instances or ongoing patterns of misuse by the attending physician. The costs of misuse will then be computed by the system on a case by case basis.

B. The Synthesized Model: Possibilities

Although it is only in the preliminary stages, such a dynamic system can focus on the clinical situation and enable judgments about intentionality. Such a system also compacts all these requirements into a format that is readily usable by physicians. The extent of misuse and its economic effect can then be documented.

Some may argue that such a system is too expensive, as is direct questioning of the physician about his decisions. However, this system, once in place, provides for minimal intrusion into the physician's practice pattern. As such it has the potential for long-term viability. Most important, it can be used as a device through which precise, focused strategies can be developed to monitor, control, and decrease by programmatic interventions, the extent of misuse in clinical laboratory testing.

Figure 1 represents in summary form the framework presented, its constituent elements, and their dynamic interrelationship. We have also presented one possible technical mechanism to implement this model. Other technical tools may be developed that can do the job better; we hope this will in fact happen. Critical to the issue at hand, however, is that intentionality within the clinical situation become the dynamic basis for documenting misuse.

References

1. Feinstein AR. Clinical judgment. Baltimore: Williams and Wilkins Co., 1967.
2. McAuliffe WE. Studies of process-outcome correlations in medical care evaluation: a critique. Med Care 1978; 16:907-30.
3. Greenfield S, Nadler MA, Morgan MT, Shine KI. The clinical investigation and management of chest pain in an emergency department: quality assessment by criteria mapping. Med Care 1977;15:989-905.

Table 1. Computer Printout of Laboratory Tests, Results, and Charges

TEST REPORT FOR: CASE B.G.

First Hospitalization – Feb. 20, 1973
Diagnostic Work-Up with Results from Feb 20 to March 2, 1973
DATE:

TEST DESCRIPTION	TOTAL CHG	2/20 DAY 1 RESULT	2/21 DAY 2 RESULT	2/22 DAY 3 RESULT	2/23 DAY 4 RESULT	2/24 DAY 5 RESULT	2/25 DAY 6 RESULT	2/28 DAY 7 RESULT	3/2 DAY 8 RESULT
LAB CBC	12.30								
LAB WHITE BLD CNT		9.4							
LAB RED BLD CNT		4.12							
LAB HGB HCT		11.2/34							
LAB DIFFERENTIAL C		70/28/1/0							
LAB PLATELET COUNT		ADEQUATE							
LAB SED RATE	6.20	43/40			/36	25/22	23		
LAB ASO TITER	14.20	125							
LAB CRP LATEX QUAL	6.20	1:5					POS. UNDILUTE		
LAB LE PREP	8.20						1:8		
LAB ANTINUCL ANTIBOD	20.40		NEGATIVE						
LAB VDRL	4.10		NEGATIVE						
NCL T 3 TEST	10.70		7.7					30.4%	
NCL T 4 TEST	15.00							6.5	
LAB ELECTROLYTES	24.80					136/4./97/25			136/4./96/22
LAB HAA	24.50		NEGATIVE						
LAB URINALYSIS	4.10								
LAB PH UR		6							
LAB-SPECIFIC GRAV		1.017							
LAB PROTEINS		TR							
LAB GLUCOSE UR		0							
LAB KETONES UR		0							
LAB OCCULT BL UR		0							
LAB UR MICROSCOPIC		RARE WBC							
LAB EMP FEC O/P/CULT	13.50	NEGATIVE			NEGATIVE				
LAB PIN WORM TAPE	4.10				NEGATIVE				
LAB EMP NO5TH CULT	14.20	B-ST,GP 14SH		POSITIVE NO B-STREP					
LAB BLOOD CULTURE	12.30	NEG AT 48HRS							
XR CHEST 1 VW	14.20	WNI							
NCL HEART SCAN	60.00						MIN CARD IMP		
ELECTROCARDIOGRAM	14.90				ELG-LT.R&LUT				

TOTAL NO. OF TESTS/DAY:		8	5	2	2	5	4	1	2
TOTAL CHARGE/DAY:		$ 88.00	$ 66.60	$ 18.30	$ 78.50	$ 65.90	$ 47.00	$ 10.70	$ 39.80
CUMULATIVE NO. TESTS/DAY:		8	13	15	17	22	26	27	29
CUMULATIVE CHARGE/DAY:		$ 89.00	$ 154.60	$ 172.90	$ 251.40	$ 317.30	$ 364.30	$ 375.00	$ 414.80

PAUSE

Table 2. Cost-Benefit Analysis of Laboratory Tests

First Hospitalization – Feb. 20, 1973

Cost-Benefit Analysis of Diagnostic Work-Up from Feb. 20 to March 2, 1973

TEST REPORT FOR: CASE B. G.

TEST DESCRIPTION	TOTAL CHG	2/20 DAY 1 RESULT	IMP	2/21 DAY 2 RESULT	IMP	2/22 DAY 3 RESULT	IMP	2/23 DAY 4 RESULT	IMP	2/24 DAY 5 RESULT	IMP	2/25 DAY 6 RESULT	IMP	2/28 DAY 7 RESULT	IMP	3/2 DAY 8 RESULT	IMP
LAB CBC	12.30		UN														
LAB SED RATE	6.20		UN										NUNN				
LAB ASO TITER	14.20		UN														
LAB CRP LATEX QUAL	6.20		UN		NUNN												
LAB LE PREP	8.20										NUNN						
LAB ANTINUCL ANTIBOD	20.40				NUNN												
LAB VDRL	4.10										UN						
NCL T 3 TEST	10.70												UN		NUNN		
NCL T 4 TEST	15.00												NUNN				NUNN
LAB ELECTROLYTES	24.80				NUNN												NUNN
LAB HUA	24.50				NUNN						NUNN						
LAB URINALYSIS	4.10		UN						UN								
LAB EMP FEC O/P CULT	18.50		UN				NUNN		UN		NUNN						
LAB PIN WORM TAPE	4.10						NUNN										
LAB EMP NO&TH CULT	14.20		UN								NUNN						
LAB BLOOD CULTURE	12.30		UN						NUNN				NUNN				
XR CHEST 1 UN	14.20																
NCL HEART SCAN	60.00								NUNN								
ELECTROCARDIOGRAM	14.80				NUNN												

	2/20	2/21	2/22	2/23	2/24	2/25	2/28	3/2
TOTAL NO. OF TESTS/DAY:	8	5	2	2	5	4	1	2
TOTAL CHARGE/DAY:	$88.00	$66.60	$18.30	$78.50	$65.90	$47.00	$10.70	$39.80
CUMULATIVE NO. TESTS/DAY:	8	13	15	17	22	26	27	29
CUMULATIVE CHARGE/DAY:	$88.00	$154.60	$172.90	$251.40	$317.30	$364.30	$375.00	$414.80

CUMULATIVE NO. OF TESTS/DAY:

	2/20	2/21	2/22	2/23	2/24	2/25	2/28	3/2
USEFUL & NECESSARY	8	8	8	9	10	11	11	11
USEFUL BUT NOT NECESSARY	0	0	0	0	0	0	0	0
NOT USEFUL & NOT NECESSARY	0	5	7	8	12	15	16	18

	TESTS	PERCENT		CHARGES	PERCENT
TOTAL	29	100.0		$414.80	100.0
I) USEFUL & NECESSARY	11	37.9		$118.90	28.7
II) USEFUL BUT NOT NECESSARY	0	0.0		$0.00	0.0
III) NOT USEFUL & NOT NECESSARY	18	62.1		$295.90	71.3

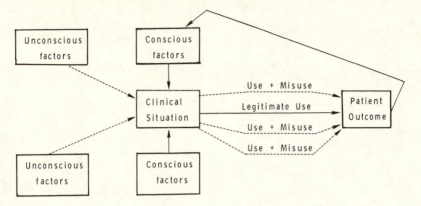

Figure 1. A model of cost effective clinical laboratory use or "The shortest distance between two points is . . . ."

4. Greenfield S, Lewis CE, Kaplan SH, Davidson MG. Peer review by criteria mapping: criteria for diabetes mellitus. Ann Intern Med 1975;83:761-70.
5. Freeborn DK, Baer D, Greenlick MR, Baily JW. Determinants of medical care use: physicians' use of laboratory services. Am J Public Health 1972;62:846-53.
6. Morrison SL, Riley MM. The use of hospital diagnostic facilities by general practitioners. Med Care 1963;1:137-42.
7. Gellman DD. The price of progress: technology and the cost of medical care. Can Med Assoc J 1971;104:401-6.
8. Daniels M, Schroeder SA. Variation among physicians in use of laboratory tests II: relation to clinical productivity and outcomes of care. Med Care 1977;15:482-7.
9. Schroeder SA, Kenders K, Cooper JK, Piemme TE. Use of laboratory tests and pharmaceuticals: variation among physicians and effect of cost audit on subsequent use. JAMA 1973;225:969-73.
10. Garg ML, Mulligan JL, McNamara MJ, Skipper JK, Parekh RR. Teaching students the relationship between quality and cost of medical care. J Med Educ 1975;50:1085-91.
11. Garg ML, Mulligan JL, Gliebe WA, Parekh RR. Physician specialty, quality and cost of inpatient care. Soc Sci Med 1979;13C:187-91.
12. Gliebe WA. Unnecessary educational experimentation: patients in a teaching hospital. Sociol Symposium 1978;23:1-16.
13. Lorber J. Good patients and problem patients: conformity and deviance in a general hospital. J Health Soc Behav 1975;16:213-25.
14. Eisenberg JM. Sociologic influences on decision-making by clinicians. Ann Intern Med 1979;90:957-64.
15. Krieg AF, Israel M. Why physicians order too many laboratory tests. Med Lab Observer 1977 Feb:46-51.
16. Benjamin DR. The role of the laboratory in clinical diagnosis. J Continuing Educ Pediatr 1979;21(3):13-26.
17. Garg ML, Gliebe WA, Elkhatib M. The extent of defensive medicine: some empirical evidence. Leg Aspects Med Pract 1978;6(2):25-29.
18. Garg ML, Gliebe WA, Elkhatib M. Diagnostic testing as a cost factor in teaching institutions. Hospitals 1978;52(14):97-100.

CHAPTER TWELVE

Factors Leading to Appropriate Clinical Laboratory Workload Growth

Donald P. Connelly, MD, PhD,
Philip N. St. Louis, BS, and Lynn Neitz, BS

INTRODUCTION

The rapid and continued expansion of health care costs has focused attention on the efficiency of use of our nation's medical resources. Ten percent of the nation's health care dollar is spent for clinical laboratory services, and by 1985, if present trends continue, the annual laboratory service cost will be nearly $50 billion.[1] It is becoming clear that "small ticket items," in the aggregate, account for much more of health care costs than do the high technology, "large ticket items" such as the CT scanner.[2] A commonly held view among physicians, health insurance payers, and policy makers is that much of the expansion in clinical laboratory workload has not contributed to improved health care for the patient,[3-4] but firm evidence to support or refute this view is difficult to acquire. The linkage between test and diagnosis is a tenuous one; the linkage between test and outcome is, for the most part, unmeasurable.

Policy makers are proposing two general approaches to limit the expenditure for laboratory services: (1) decreasing the per unit cost and, (2) decreasing the test volume.[5-8] The latter course requires special caution. The factors affecting laboratory workload growth are many and complex.[9] The current tendency is to identify those factors that might indicate ineffective utilization; however, a number of factors, in concert, might be expected to contribute to a significant but appropriate growth in laboratory testing. An increase in the number of patients presenting to a medical center, a shift in case mix toward patients requiring more intensive medical services, and additional testing allowing more rational clinical decisions all lead to additional but appropriate laboratory workload growth. Efforts to limit the volume of laboratory tests must be applied discriminately so that appropriate and necessary testing is not hampered. Thus, it is important to break down the laboratory workload carefully, defining those portions resulting from appropriate and inappropriate growth influences. We have assessed the effect of an increase in patient volume and changing case mix in clinical chemistry workload in one hospital setting.

METHODS AND PROCEDURES

For the years 1970 to 1978, annual summary data regarding case mix and clinical laboratory workload were collected at the University of Minnesota Hospitals, a 750-bed tertiary care facility. Total clinical chemistry workload for each year was partitioned into a count of those tests most often used for purposes of patient monitoring (serum electrolytes, creatinine, urea nitrogen, glucose, and blood gases) and all other chemistry tests. Annual test volume data for the coagulation laboratory were also obtained. On the basis of annual summary data obtained from the hospital's business office records, the portion of the clinical chemistry and coagulation laboratories' workload attributable to inpatient care was calculated. Annual mortality figures for the hospital were also collected.

Along with the number of annual inpatient admissions, the count of discharged patients with a primary diagnosis among the 50 most frequently encountered diagnoses for each year was tabulated. This group of diagnoses accounted for 36 to 43 percent of annual admissions. To develop a composite list of most frequent diagnoses for the nine years, some adjustments were required because of changes in diagnosis coding conventions over the period. In 1975, the coding system was changed from ICDA-8 to H-ICDA-2. Those few common diagnoses for which there was no exact one-to-one mapping were grouped with new very similar diagnostic codes. After adjustment for coding scheme change, the yearly lists of frequently encountered diagnoses were combined into a single composite list. Ninety-three diagnoses were represented in this list.

Next, the laboratory records of 2,262 patients consecutively discharged over a two-month period during the fall of 1978 were grouped by diagnosis. The mean number of chemistry tests per admission were calculated for each of the diagnoses represented on the composite list. To calculate the mean chemistry test volume for those diagnoses that occurred less than three times in this two-month sample, one or more additional cases (to make a total of at least three cases per diagnosis) were drawn from patients discharged during the first half of 1978. Seventy additional cases were examined for this purpose. Based on the mean chemistry test volume and the relative frequency of each of the 50 most frequent diagnoses in each year 1970 to 1978, we predicted the chemistry laboratory workload per inpatient admission accounted for by these diagnoses.

The frequent diagnoses were also grouped as requiring less than 20 (Group 1), 20 to 40 (Group 2), or more than 40 (Group 3) clinical chemistry tests per admission, figures based on the mean number of chemistry tests per admission calculated from the sampling period data. These three groups represented diagnoses expected to lead to a small, moderate, and large chemistry test volume. The test volume criteria were chosen so that, for 1978, the number of cases in each group would be approximately equal.

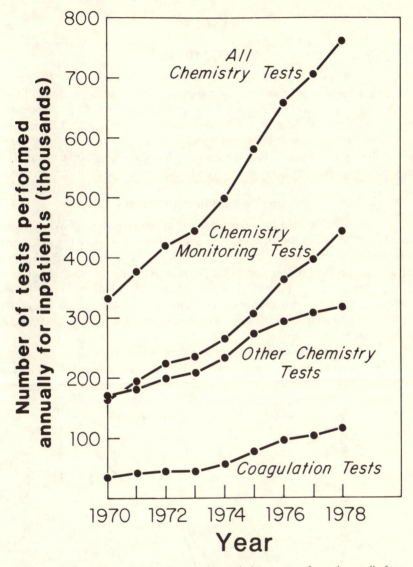

Figure 1. Number of clinical chemistry and coagulation tests performed annually for inpatients for the years 1970 to 1978. Clinical chemistry tests have been factored into a group of frequently used monitoring tests (serum electrolytes, creatinine, urea nitrogen, glucose, and blood gases) and all other clinical chemistry tests.

RESULTS

Workload Growth

Figure 1 shows the workload in clinical chemistry test volume. The yearly growth is large and the rate of growth appears to be steadily increasing. From 1970 to 1978 the overall clinical chemistry test volume increased by 128 percent. The number of tests commonly used for monitoring increased by 172 percent, while the number of other chemistry tests increased by 87 percent. In this same period the tests of the coagulation laboratory have grown by 309 percent. The bulk of the coagulation laboratory's workload is related to patient monitoring.

Changing Workload Influences

From 1970 to 1978 the annual number of inpatient admissions has grown from 17,163 to 22,229, for an overall increase of 30 percent. Since there has been a continuous shift in case mix, the predicted number of clinical chemistry tests for the average inpatient having one of the 50 most frequently encountered diagnoses has increased by 34 percent since 1970 (Figure 2). This change in service intensity related to case mix change does not appear to be slowing. The composite predicted change in test volume over the period due to changes in patient volume and case mix is 73 percent.

Table 1 lists diagnoses as related to a light, moderate, or heavy laboratory workload according to the average chemistry test volume observed among the

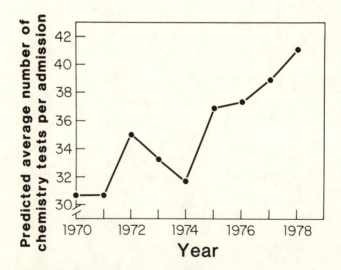

Figure 2. The predicted average number of chemistry tests per inpatient admission from 1970 to 1978 for patients with the 50 diagnoses most frequently encountered each year.

Table 1. Mean Chemistry Tests Performed per Admission
for 50 Most Common Primary Diagnoses

Diagnosis	No. of Cases	Mean	SEM
Group 1			
Single, term newborn—spontaneous delivery	54	3.7	.5
Detachment of retina	51	5.0	.04
Uncomplicated delivery	20	11.4	4.4
For radiation aftercare	20	16.4	2.5
Cataract—not otherwise specified	19	6.7	1.4
Lumbar disk displacement	18	13.0	1.7
Clinical research exam/normal	14	2.1	1.1
Medical exam	13	19.1	2.6
Chronic serous otitis media	13	17.2	13.3
Chemotherapy	11	11.3	1.2
Headache	11	16.2	5.0
Chronic otitis media—not otherwise specified	11	4.0	0.4
Spinal paraplegia	10	19.4	8.0
Mandible and maxilla size anomaly	10	4.9	1.0
Trigeminal neuralgia	10	13.0	1.4
Single, term newborn—Caesarian section	9	19.6	11.3
Osteoarthritis	9	16.4	4.7
Impairment of hearing, unspecified	9	5.6	1.2
Angina pectoris	9	20.0	4.2
Hematuria	8	14.4	1.5
Kidney donor	8	13.0	1.1
Symptoms referable to nose and sinus, other	8	7.0	2.6
Syncope and collapse	8	13.1	1.8
Urethral stricture due to unspecified causes	8	17.8	3.8
Behavior disorder of child, adolescent	8	11.0	4.3
Group 2			
Pain in back	25	21.1	6.6
Epilepsy—not otherwise specified	21	32.1	3.6
Abdominal pain	17	20.6	4.3
Bowel anastomosis status	15	21.1	1.8
Clinical research investigation	13	38.1	21.2
Malignant neoplasm corpus uteri	11	36.7	10.6
Follow-up, chemotherapy	10	27.7	16.9
Chest pain	9	33.1	11.1
Single, preterm newborn	8	36.5	18.3
Essential benign hypertension	8	22.9	3.0
Lung	8	30.3	5.1
Obesity not specified as endocrine	8	37.3	8.3
Group 3			
Chemotherapy aftercare	84	45.6	7.0
Chronic renal failure	31	157.7	22.9
Chronic ischemic heart disease	30	52.3	5.5
Complication of transplanted organ	19	182.9	42.8
Respiratory distress syndrome	16	142.8	27.1

Table 1—Continued

Diagnosis	No. of Cases	Mean	SEM
Group 3 (continued)			
Pneumonia—not otherwise specified	12	74.7	30.9
Fever of unknown origin	11	81.1	40.8
Congestive heart failure	10	103.5	34.0
Lymphosarcoma	9	64.0	33.4
Abdominal aortic aneurysm	9	68.7	10.9
Aplastic anemia	8	115.0	55.3
Acute lymphocytic leukemia	8	194.9	46.2
Peripheral vascular disease	8	42.8	8.4

Group 1 constitutes those diagnoses for which the mean number of chemistry tests per admission observed during a two-month sampling observed during a two-month sampling period in 1978 was less than 20. For Group 2 diagnoses, the mean number of chemistry tests per admission was from 20 to 40. Each Group 3 diagnosis had a mean of more than 40 chemistry tests per admission

cases sampled in 1978. Figure 3 shows the trends among the three groups of diagnoses leading to small, moderate, and large laboratory test volumes. Among inpatients with the 50 most frequently encountered diagnoses the proportion of patients with a Group 1 diagnosis (a diagnosis with a mean number of chemistry tests per admission of less than 20), except for 1974, shows a steadily falling trend from 52 percent of the cases with the 50 most frequently encountered diagnoses to 36 percent in 1978. The corresponding annual incidence of Group 2 diagnoses (mean number of chemistry tests per admission from 20 to 40) steadily rose until 1976 and then began to fall. The annual incidence of Group 3 diagnoses (mean number of chemistry tests per admission greater than 40) has risen rapidly since 1974. In the sample period, patients in the three groups underwent an average of 10.1, 29.7, and 84.0 chemistry tests per hospitalization. Thus, an increase in the number of Group 3 cases affects the overall workload eight times more than a similar change in Group 1 cases. The proportion of annual inpatient admissions represented by patients with a diagnosis among the fifty most frequently occurring diagnoses ranged from 36 to 43 percent during the eight-year period.

Patient mortality as a percent of annual admissions is plotted in Figure 4. The mortality rate shows a nearly steady fall from 3.8 percent in 1970 to 2.3 percent in 1978. This improvement is in the face of a shift in case mix toward a group receiving more intensive laboratory services.

DISCUSSION

A commonly offered explanation for the increase in laboratory volume over the last decade has been the advent of highly automated multichannel instrumenta-

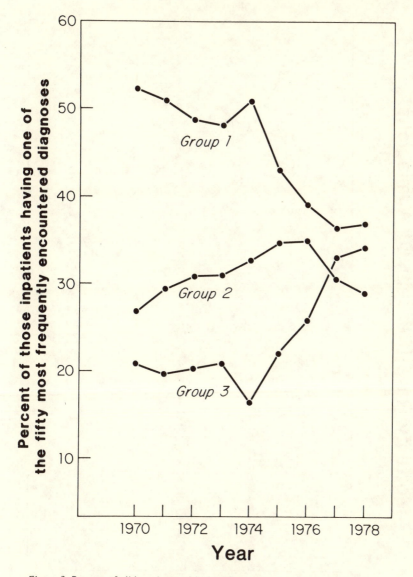

Figure 3. Percent of all inpatients with the 50 most frequently encountered diagnoses for diagnostic groups leading to light (Group 1), moderate (Group 2), and heavy (Group 3) chemistry test volume for the years 1970 to 1978.

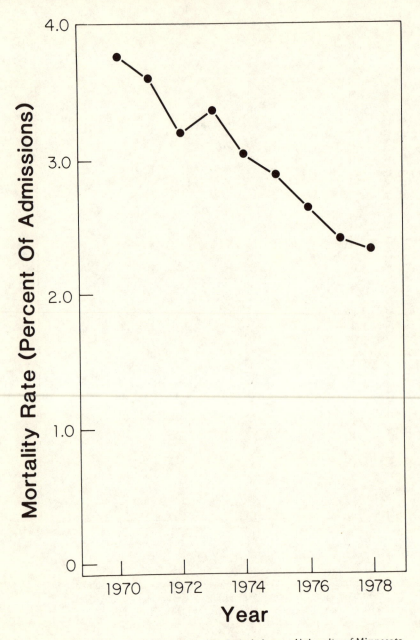

Figure 4. Annual death rate as percent of admissions at University of Minnesota Hospitals.

tion in the laboratory.[10,11] Our study shows that although the more highly automated chemistry procedures grew at a more rapid rate than less automated or "single-channel" chemistry procedures, the rate of growth was far below the coagulation laboratory test volume, where procedures have been manual throughout the study period. Similarly, Finkelstein, studying the change in laboratory test volume from 1969 to 1977 in 204 hospitals, demonstrated that a nonautomated laboratory area (bacteriology) underwent a large test volume growth comparable to that of more highly automated areas (chemistry and hematology).[12] The growth in the volume of manually performed coagulation laboratory tests and automated chemistry tests may reflect, at least in part, a change in case mix toward a patient population requiring more intensive laboratory service for purposes of monitoring patient progress.

That is not to say that automation is a negligible influence in increasing laboratory volume in general. In the hospital setting studied, very large multichannel chemistry analyzers have been avoided, and such questionable practices as multicomponent admission profiling based on multichannel analyzers have not been encouraged. In a setting where highly automated chemistry analyzers are introduced and used in a less restrained manner, the impact of automation on laboratory volume could be considerable.

The effect of changing case mix on laboratory workload is difficult to assess. Many approaches to correlating the patient mix to hospital resource use have been proposed,[13-15] but laboratory test volume is not often included in these studies. For that reason, we devised our own measure of anticipated test volume, based on a direct analysis of a sample of cases. The variation of test volume among patients with a common primary diagnosis was often quite large. Given a much larger data base with which to work, some of the variation could perhaps be minimized by grouping patients by additional factors such as secondary diagnoses, major procedures, and age.[16]

We are drawing inferences regarding the entire patient population in a particular hospital from a subset of patients, those having a primary diagnosis among the 50 most frequently encountered diagnoses. This subset of patients accounts for approximately 40 percent of the hospital's annual admissions. From this subset of patients, a sample of patients discharged over a two-month period was studied to arrive at an estimate of laboratory use. The frequency of particular diagnoses occurring in the sample period even for the diagnoses among the 50 most frequently encountered for each of the nine years studied was often quite low. In a number of instances, cases found in the sampling period were augmented by additional samples to bring the minimum number of cases inspected for any diagnosis to three. Again, given a much larger data base, additional diagnostic groups could be included in the analysis.

An influence we cannot readily measure directly is the effect of increased rational care decisions made possible by more frequent and more specific laboratory tests. In the face of case mix changes that suggest increasingly complex cases are being encountered, patient outcome appears to be improving, as indicated by the decreasing in-hospital mortality rate. This improvement in outcome is due to a multitude of changes in the health care system, including those of the clinical laboratory. Another influence that this approach does not measure is a change in test ordering patterns for a particular diagnosis over the years. Scitovsky has shown that this shift can be considerable.[17] Such a shift may represent changes in physician patterns of laboratory use.[12] It might also reflect a change in case severity over the period for a particular diagnosis. For instance, in the hospital studied, an increasing number of renal transplants were performed on diabetic patients whose postoperative course is generally more complex, requiring more extensive use of monitoring tests.

In the hospital setting studied, the composite effect of an increase in both the number of patients and the intensity of service required for the average patient leads to a predicted appropriate volume increase of 73 percent over a nine-year period. An amount of growth appropriate because it reflects more rational care decisions probably does exist but its volume is unknown. Put in this perspective, much of the observed 87 percent change in diagnostic chemistry test volume as represented by the nonmonitoring tests may be medically appropriate. Case mix changes might not have equal effect on monitoring and diagnostic test volume. For instance, an increasing number of cases of renal transplantation would be expected to affect the volume of monitoring tests far more than the number of diagnostic tests. Still, allowing for the possibility that the number of diagnostic tests might increase at a somewhat lower rate than the change in laboratory workload related to case mix, a substantial portion of the increase in diagnostic chemistry testing appears to result from appropriate growth influences.

Chemistry monitoring test volume has grown far faster than the 73 percent change predicted. Again, an unknown portion of the unexplained growth would be expected to be appropriate because it leads to more rational care and perhaps contributes to better outcomes. However, the large discrepancy between actual and predicted volume changes suggests that if inappropriate growth factors exist, the use of monitoring tests is the more likely area to investigate for their effect. This approach concurs with the findings of a number of investigators studying laboratory utilization.[4,18,19]

We have shown that a large portion of the increase in laboratory workload growth over a nine-year period in one hospital setting was due to appropriate growth influences. The greatest discrepancy between observed and predicted growth was in the use of monitoring tests. These observations should be useful to those planning actions designed to influence the clinical laboratory workload volume.

References

1. Clinical Chemistry News 1980;6(2):22.
2. Moloney TW, Rogers DE. Medical technology—a different view of the contentious debate over costs. N Engl J Med 1979;301:1413-19.

3. Relman AS. The allocation of medical resources by physicians. J Med Educ 1980;55: 99-104.

4. .Griner PF, Liptzin B. Use of the laboratory in a teaching hospital: implications for patient care, education and hospital costs. Ann Intern Med 1971;75:157-63.

5. Schwartz WB, Joskow PL. Medical efficiency versus economic efficiency: A conflict in values. N Engl J Med 1978;299:1462-4.

6. Fineberg HV. Clinical chemistries: The high cost of low-cost diagnostic tests. In: Altman SH, Blendon R, eds. Medical Technology: The Culprit Behind Health Care Costs? Washington: US Department of Health, Education, and Welfare (DHEW publication no. (PHS) 79-3216).

7. Kassirer JP, Pauker SG. Should diagnostic testing be regulated? N Engl J Med 1978; 299: 947-9.

8. Sheinbach J. The clinical laboratories: Problems of cost containment as a challenge. In: Benson ES, Rubin M, eds. Logic and Economics of Clinical Laboratory Use. New York: Elsevier, 1978.

9. Connelly DP, Steele B. Laboratory utilization: Problems and solutions. Arch Pathol Lab Med 1980;104:59-62.

10. Lester E. The machines are taking over. Lancet 1979;2:949-50.

11. National summary. Lab Management 1979;17:34-5.

12. Finkelstein SN. Technological change and laboratory test volume. In: Benson ES, Rubin M, eds. Logic and Economics of Clinical Laboratory Use. New York: Elsevier, 1978.

13. Luke RD. Dimensions in hospital case mix measurement. Inquiry 1979;16:38-49.

14. Horn, SD, Schumacher DN. An analysis of case mix complexity using information theory and diagnostic related grouping. Med Care 1979;17:382-9.

15. Thompson JD, Fetter RB, Mross CD. Case mix and resource use. Inquiry 1974;12: 300-12.

16. Mills R, Fetter RB, Riedel DC, Averill R. AUTOGRP: An interactive computer system for the analysis of health care data. Med Care 1976;14:603-15.

17. Scitovsky AA. Changes in the use of ancillary services for "common" illness. In: Altman SH, Blendon R, eds. Medical Technology: The Culprit Behind Health Care Costs? Washington: US Department of Health, Education and Welfare (DHEW publication no. (PHS) 79-3216).

18. Liptzin BA, Williams JS. Laboratory utilization on a university surgical service. Surgery 1972;71:247-53.

19. Dixon RH, Laszlo J. Utilization of clinical chemistry services by medical housestaff: An analysis. Arch Intern Med 1974;134:1064-7.

CHAPTER THIRTEEN

Reducing the Use of the Clinical Laboratory: How Much Can Be Saved?

Stan N. Finkelstein, MD

I. INTRODUCTION

The recent increases in health care costs have led many to offer possible strategies for moderating the rate of growth. Ancillary services have been seen as a potential target for cost containment because some observers believe that a substantial portion of their utilization is unnecessary. Efforts directed toward achieving a more discerning use of ancillary services would also be consistent with an objective with which many clinicians would sympathize, a more reasoned practice of medicine.

The clinical laboratory is one aspect of ancillary services in which some cost containment strategies are being proposed and tested. In general, two different kinds of interventions have been discussed. The first set of strategies are regulatory in nature, and certificate of need control represents an example.[1] In the clinical laboratory, these interventions would potentially limit the technological capacity to perform tests. Those who espouse this kind of intervention believe that in limiting capacity, clinical judgment will need to be exercised to establish priorities for access to technologies. The hopeful result would be a decline in the volume of tests ordered.

An alternative set of strategies that have been or are being investigated in some clinical laboratories addressed directly the behavior of practitioners who order tests.[2-5] A considerable number of reports in the journal literature have suggested that a primary reduction in laboratory test volume has been or could be effected by means of educating practitioners in appropriate test ordering behavior, revising the reimbursement structure to reflect the need to carefully consider the number and types of tests ordered, or creating other incentives designed to reduce test volume.[6]

Proponents of the regulatory and behavioral approaches to contain costs make the plausible assumption that, if volume of tests ordered can be decreased, costs will decline. It is of interest to be able to predict, however, the extent of the cost response to changes in test volume.

In this paper, we describe an approach to estimating the magnitude of cost-reduction or "cost-behavior" that might be observed in response to hypothetical changes in the use of a clinical laboratory. We approached the problem by first deriving the operating costs for a hypothetical laboratory and its functional sub-divisions. The cost savings to be realized, assuming a hypothetical reduction in the number of tests ordered, was estimated and found to be less than expected. A sensitivity analysis is reported to consider the variability in cost savings as a function of the assumptions made.

II. METHODS

A. Development of the Approach

To develop our approach we gained access to laboratory cost and test volume data from a large major metropolitan teaching institution. In 1977, the year for which the most complete data were available for this analysis, this hospital with more than 500 beds served more than 20,000 inpatient admissions and well in excess of 300,000 outpatient visits. The clinical laboratory is one of the larger hospital laboratories in the country. In the sensitivity analysis to be described later, it will be necessary to consider applicability to smaller facilities.

The chemistry laboratory we initially studied is organized into 10 rooms, each with a specialized function. Table 1 provides an overview of this functional specialization and describes, for each named room, the kinds of tests performed and the principal analytical instruments used. As seen in the table, the level of technology in use by the laboratory in 1977 to perform chemistry tests was typified by the dual channel continuous flow automated analyzer. The laboratory did own a four-channel continuous flow instrument that it did use to perform electrolytes; however, extensive use was not made of the multichannel continuous flow analyzers or of the large-batch analyzers during the period of our study. The laboratory also had a computer system in place that was used regularly for the storing and reporting of test results as well as for other administrative functions. Chemistry laboratory tests volumes from 1977 were taken from financial records of the hospital and verified using information from the laboratory instrument records. Test volume figures used in our analysis were not subjected to any of the weighting schemes sometimes used. In the rare instances in which a test included duplicate or replicate determinations, the tests were broken down to the smallest available units and counted in that manner for consistency. Counts for a single run on the four-channel continuous flow analyzer were coded to reflect the actual number of tests ordered. The growth in volume of tests performed in the laboratory from 1976 to 1977 was 2%.

For our planned cost analysis, we needed to arrive at the "production

Table 1. Organization of the Chemistry Laboratory According to "Rooms"
Performing Specialized Function*

Specialized Laboratory "Room"	Examples of Major Tests Performed	Representative Analytical Instrument
1. Autonalyzer	BUN, glucose creatinine, calcium	Dual-Channel Continuous Flow Analyzer
2. Electrolyte	Sodium, potassium, chloride	Four-Channel Continuous Flow Analyzer
3. Liver Function	Bilirubin, albumin, amylase	Spectrophotometer
4. LKB	LDH, SGOT	Enzyme Analyzer
5. Iron	Iron, TIBC, CPK, thyroxine	Continuous Flow Analyzer
6. "Odd Job"	Ammonia, fibrinogen, barbiturates, isoenzymes	pH-meter, spectrometer, fluorometer
7. Cholesterol	Cholesterol, triglycerides	Dual-Channel Continuous Flow Analyzer
8. Steroid	17-OH-steroids, VMA, magnesium	Spectrophotometer
9. Electrophoresis	Protein electrophoresis, 5'-nucleotidase	Electrophoresis unit
10. GLC	Diphenylhydantoin	Gas-liquid chromatograph

*Table appears in *Human Pathology Symposium*, September, 1980, and is reproduced here with permission of the editor.

function" for the chemistry laboratory as a whole and for the functionally specialized testing rooms. It would not have been valid to use laboratory test charges for the rates at which patients were billed for the tests performed. For this hospital and most others, the billing rate for laboratory tests, the so-called "charge," is paid only by patients without health insurance and by the commercial insurance carriers. State and federal hospital reimbursement programs and the Blue Cross agencies reimburse the hospitals in some proportion to actual costs that, in most instances, would be expected to be considerably lower than the billing rates.

Our approach for determining the production function for the overall laboratory depended on the categorization of all expenses incurred by the laboratory as either supplies, general overhead, salaries, equipment, and services. Examples of the kinds of line-items provided under each expense category are as follows. Supplies include supplies for tests (93% of all supplies), personnel support supplies (6%), and office supplies (1%). Within general overhead, the building space allocation accounted for 32% of the overhead costs whereas the overhead in the laboratory amounted to 68%. Salaries were those of technical (58%), administrative staff (28%), and support personnel (14%). Equipment included instrumentation used to perform laboratory tests (84%), and general equipment used to support the laboratory such as refrigerators (16%). Finally, services included maintenance costs of equipment (11%), personnel support services (89%) such as glass washing, and contracting expenses for the performance by outside laboratories of certain tests not usually done in the laboratory.

To determine the cost response to declining laboratory utilization, it is necessary to determine which categories described above are fixed and independent of volume and which others vary in relation to volume. To make this tentative determination, we reviewed laboratory cost records for the years 1964-1976 in addition to the detailed analysis using 1977 data. During the entire year for which detailed data were collected and analyzed, the equipment/manpower configuration of the laboratory did not significantly change.

For purposes of this preliminary analysis, the dependence of the specified categories of laboratory costs on test volume will be treated as follows. Supplies for tests are variable with respect to volume and support supplies are indirectly variable. Support supplies are variable with respect to personnel, which in turn is variable with respect to volume. For our analysis, the entire category of supplies will be treated as variable. Overhead expenses are considered fixed and will be treated as such in our analysis. They are assigned to the laboratory by the central hospital accounting office on the basis of floor space utilized and other considerations only peripherally related to test volume. The space requirements did not change during 1977.

Salary costs are sometimes referred to as being semivariable with respect to volume. Voluntary hospitals are generally not known for massive layoffs of their staff and the most common means of achieving a desired reduction of level of staffing is by transfer or attrition. Salaries can realistically be considered variable in the long run. Even though a year might,or might not be quite enough time to achieve a staff reduction in this manner, salaries will be treated as variable in this analysis.

Because we assumed that the equipment configuration of the laboratory did not change during the year studied, equipment costs will be treated as fixed, at the replacement value of the instruments in use. Service costs may in some instances be indirectly dependent on laboratory test volume. Under other circumstances it might have been a difficult decision as to whether to treat service costs as fixed or variable. In this instance because they will be seen to represent a rather small percentage of total laboratory costs, we make the arbitrary decision to treat service costs as fixed. Table 2 summarizes the magnitudes of the fixed and variable costs of performing tests in the Chemistry Laboratory in 1977.

We were cognizant of the possibility that those tests contributing to the largest costs in the laboratory were not necessarily those being performed at the highest volume. To allow for the capability, in our analysis, of accounting for differences in rates of decline among individual tests to yield an overall twenty percent decline in laboratory test volume, it was necessary to consider the costs associated with performance of different categories of tests. The categories of tests represented by the ten specialized laboratory workrooms represented a natural framework in which to consider costs at levels of aggregation beneath the whole laboratory. We determined the fixed and variable costs of performing tests in each of the functionally specialized laboratory work rooms as well as in the laboratory as a whole. Personnel requirements used to calculate costs of operating the various work rooms were based on actual time studies conducted in the

Table 2. Fixed and Variable Costs of Performing Tests
in the Chemistry Laboratory in 1977*

Costs	Percentage of Total Laboratory Costs
Fixed costs	
Equipment	4.1%
Overhead	16.0
Services	2.5
Total fixed costs	22.6%
Variable costs	
Supply costs	15.0%
Salaries	62.4
Total variable	77.4%

*Table appears in *Human Pathology Symposium*,
September, 1980, and is reproduced here with
permission of the editor.

laboratory. These were compared with and found to be generally consistent with the standard work load reporting scheme used by the College of American Pathologists.[7] The dollar value used for an average full-time equivalent member of the technical staff was estimated to be $10,500 in 1977.

B. Sensitivity Analysis

Having developed our approach with data obtained from an actual laboratory, the next task was to ascertain how our results would change as a function of the assumptions we made. The hospital laboratory we chose to study was probably atypical in a number of respects. First, it was probably among the highest 5% of all hospital laboratories in terms of annual volume of tests. Probably more important for our analysis is the observation that the laboratory made relatively little use of the current generation of automated laboratory analyzer equipment that is available.

We developed a straightforward simulation model to consider how the resulting expected cost savings for a laboratory would vary according to our assumptions. We continue our assumption of the organization of the laboratory into functional work rooms, as this assumption seemed transferable to laboratories with a wide range of characteristics. Our model is linear, so that a 10% reduction in laboratory test volume would be expected to give half the cost savings as a 20% reduction, all else remaining the same. The model is driven by the change, from one case to the next, in the percentage of all laboratory costs that are variable. This is reflected in the ratio of labor to capital, or personnel costs to equipment costs, a parameter whose variation from one laboratory to another is of interest. The model was implemented on an IBM 370 computer using the APL language.

III. DISCUSSION OF THE LABORATORY WE STUDIED

Table 3 reports, for each functionally specialized room, the percentage of the chemistry laboratory's total volume and cost accounted for in 1977. Note that the Autoanalyzer "room" and the Electrolyte "room" are the highest ranking in both their shares of laboratory test volumes and costs. But, other test groupings contributing significantly to test volume make relatively less of a contribution to the total costs and vice versa. For example, tests conducted in the "Odd Job room" account for nearly 12% of total laboratory costs and just over 2% of the total volume. Note also that over 90% of the laboratory test volume is accounted for by the tests conducted in the five rooms performing the highest volume.

Next, we attempt to illustrate our approach by examining the cost behavior of declining utilization of the chemistry laboratory. A hypothetical 20% decline in utilization was assumed. This assumption would not be inconsistent with the magnitude of use decline, reported in the published literature, that resulted from educational and administrative interventions.

By way of illustration, cost savings in response to decline in test volume utilization are estimated according to three scenarios, with each succeeding scenario representing a refinement over the previous case. The first scenario is our reference case, in which we assume that all costs are variable with test volume in an elastic fashion. A 20% drop in utilization across the board will, therefore, result in a 20% decline in laboratory costs. Our assumption a priori is that this scenario is not realistic; however, it is included to serve as a reference against which the later scenarios can be compared. Using these assumptions and the costs of performing tests in the laboratory, a cost reduction of slightly more than $298,000 dollars would have been effected. This can also be expressed as an average saving

Table 3. Percentage of Total Laboratory Volumes
and Cost Accounted for by Each Functional Work Room*

Functional Work "Room"	% Total Volume	%Total Costs
Autoanalyzer	37.5%	29.6%
Electrolyte	32.3	22.4
Liver Function	12.0	11.0
LKB	7.8	5.0
Iron	3.5	5.9
"Odd Job"	2.3	11.9
Cholesterol	2.1	3.2
Steroid	1.5	5.6
Electrophoresis	0.6	2.7
GLC	0.4	2.7
Total chemistry laboratory	100%	100%

*Table appears in *Human Pathology Symposium*, September, 1980, and is reporduced here with permission of the editor.

of almost 28 full-time equivalent technical personnel. (For illustration, dollar savings are expressed as average FTE personnel. We do not mean to suggest that the laboratory could actually reduce its staffing level by 28 persons, even if this scenario were to hold true.)

The second scenario represents a refinement in the cost allocation methods, in which fixed costs are tentatively differentiated from variable costs in the laboratory. Variable costs are assumed to vary linearly with test volume and the assumptions of a 20% across the board decline in test volume is used in this case as well. The assumption of linearity in the variable costs are certainly an improvement over the reference case. In this scenario, the cost-savings of 20% of the 77.4% of total laboratory costs that are variable. Using these assumptions and the actual costs of performing tests in the chemistry laboratory, the annual savings would be only about $227,000 dollars or fewer than 22 full-time equivalent members of the technical staff. When variable costs are differentiated from fixed costs, the annual cost savings associated with a decline in utilization is less than observed in the reference case.

In the third and final scenario, we continue to assume that the average decline in the volume of laboratory tests performed is, as in the other cases, 20%. However, we assume differential rates of decline among the range of tests offered to give this average value. We treat the tests performed in the five highest volume laboratory work "rooms" as high volume tests and assume that their rate of decline is 21.5%, whereas low volume tests are assumed to show no decline at all. The average volume decrease for the entire chemistry laboratory will still be approximately 20% These high volume tests account for over 90% of the total laboratory's volume, but a lesser percent of total costs. In this scenario, the cost savings resulting from changing utilization would derive from the variable cost avoidance of the 21.5% decline in high volume tests ordered. Using these assumptions and the costs of performing tests in the chemistry laboratory, the cost savings is even less than that observed in the earlier cases and amounts to only $178,000 dollars or about 17 full-time equivalent technical staff members.

The results of this scenario analysis are summarized in Table 4. We have moved from the straightforward but highly unrealistic scenario of overall elastic cost decline in response to volume decrease, to scenarios that represent some degree of refinement as to the treatment of fixed and variable costs and those which differentiate tests performed in high and low volume. In the setting we chose to study, the magnitude of the dollar savings in response to test volume decline becomes progressively smaller as these factors are accounted for. From the illustrative numbers presented above, it appears that the dollar savings associated with a hypothesized 20% decline in chemistry laboratory utilization would be at most about 12% of dollar cost or about 60% of the "expected cost savings," were it not important to consider the effect of fixed costs and variable decline in volumes. Administrative staff of the hospital and laboratory in question have expressed their belief that any savings would, in fact, be considerably less than that.

Table 4. Cost-Behavior of Declining Laboratory Use in Three Alternative Cases

Case	Assumed Decline in Test Volume			Fixed and Variable Costs Differentiated	Resulting Cost-Savings		
	Overall	High Volume Tests	Low Volume Tests		Dollars	FTE Technical Staff	% Expected Savings
I	20%	20%	20%	No	$290,000	28	100%
II	20	20	20	Yes	$227,000	22	78
III	20	21.5	0	Yes	$178,000	17	61

IV. GENERALIZABILITY TO OTHER LABORATORIES

To explore the generalizability of the magnitude of the cost-savings one observed, we undertook the sensitivity analysis described earlier. Of particular interest was to examine the effect of relaxation of two assumptions that were made for our "base case" laboratory. First, the ratio of labor to capital or personnel to equipment in our "base case" laboratory was about 15:1. We were interested in how the expected cost savings would change under labor/capital ratios that more closely approximated the actual situation in hospital laboratories that made greater use of available automated equipment. The other assumption we wished to explore was the one that 10% of the tests performed by the laboratory were done in sufficiently low volume that their volumes and hence the associated costs would change little even if strategies to reduce the use of the laboratory as a whole were successful.

Table 5 reports the "expected cost savings" as a function of the simulated change in labor/capital ratio from our "base case" assumptions. As the labor/capital ratio changes greatly from 15/1 to nearly 1/1, the observed change in "expected cost savings" is from slightly more than 60% to about 40%. From Table 6, one observes that little difference is made when the fraction of tests

Table 5. Percentage of Expected Cost Savings as a Function of Labor/Capital
Ratio in Which 90% of Tests Are "High-Volume" (Simulation)

Labor/Capital Ratio (approx.)	All Variable Costs (approx.)	% Expected Cost Savings	Comments
15/1	75%	61%	Base case
3/1	67	51	
2/1	60	47	"Most likely" case
1/1	50	40	

Table 6. Cost-Savings as a Function of
Percentage of Hypothetical Laboratory Tests
Considered "High Volume" (Simulation)

Labor/Capital Ratio (approx.)	% Expected Cost Savings if 90% "High Volume"	% Expected Cost Savings if 80% "High Volume"
15/1	61%	60%
3/1	51	59
2/1	47	45

considered "low volume" and not subject to volume, or cost reduction is increased from 10% to 20%.

V. SUMMARY

In this analysis, we have examined the extent of cost-response to changes in test volume that might be observed in response to one of a number of measures designed to reduce the use of the clinical laboratory. A first inclination would have been to determine if one would be justified in assuming the variation is "elastic." Were that to be the case, a hypothetical 10% reduction in the number of laboratory tests ordered would lead to a similar 10% decline in costs incurred. The analysis was refined to account for effects of the fixed component of laboratory costs and the observation that some tests, performed in high volumes, would likely be more responsive to a reduction. The expected cost savings were seen to be less than might have been otherwise predicted. A sensitivity analysis was performed to consider the variability of findings as a function of the different mix of personnel and equipment in the use in different laboratories to perform the tests. Over a broad range of assumptions, 40-60% of "expected cost savings" were recovered in response to hypothetical declines in laboratory utilization.

References

1. National Health Planning and Resource Development Act. Public Law 93-641. January, 1975.
2. Dixon RH, Laszlo J. Utilization of clinical chemistry services by medical house staff. Arch Intern Med 1974;134:1064-7.
3. Eisenberg JM. An educational program to modify laboratory use by house staff. J Med Educ, 1977;52:578-81.
4. Griner PF. Use of laboratory tests in a teaching hospital: Long-term trends. Ann Intern Med 1979;90:243-8.
5. Schroeder SA, Kenders K, Cooper JK, Piemme TE. Use of laboratory tests and pharmaceuticals, variation among physicians and effect of cost audit on subsequent use. JAMA 1973;225:969-72.
6. Moloney TW, Rogers DE. Medical technology—A different view of the contentious debate over costs. N Engl J Med 1974;301:1413-19.
7. College of American Pathologists. Laboratory workload recording method. 1978 edition.

Section IV. Medical Education and Effective Laboratory Use

CHAPTER FOURTEEN

Teaching Effective Use of the Laboratory to Medical Students

M. Desmond Burke, MD,
and Donald P. Connelly, MD, PhD

INTRODUCTION

Physicians are said to order laboratory tests for the following reasons: to detect disease, to confirm or exclude diagnostic hypotheses, to estimate prognosis, and to monitor therapy.[1] The process is a simple one: Laboratories issue request forms complete with names of tests and designed to facilitate easy ordering. All the physician need do is make the appropriate check mark(s) — or have an intermediary do so — and in due time test results appear in a format designed for easy readability. Laboratories neither demand nor expect a statement of the clinical problem. By the same token, physicians neither expect nor seek interpretative comments. This arrangement carries the implicit assumption that medical graduates are skilled in test strategies and interpretation of results. The assumption is reasonable, particularly in the light of modern medicine's increasing reliance on technology — a phenomenon borne out by the annual increases in laboratory tests ordered and duly performed.[2]

It should come as a surprise, therefore, to learn that formal courses of instruction in effective use of laboratory services are the exception rather than the rule in United States medical schools. The surprise should be greater when one considers that medical technology in general and laboratory testing in particular are regarded as major contributors to the ever-increasing costs of medical care.[3]

In 1968, a course of systematic instruction in the interpretative aspects of laboratory medicine was offered as an elective course to senior medical students at the University of Minnesota. In 1968, one student enrolled. By 1974, the number had increased to 150. At that time, it became necessary (mainly for logistical reasons) to limit further enrollment. This course is now offered to 50 senior medical students three times during the academic year. This report describes instructional goals, course content, teaching methods, and the results of several approaches to course evaluation, with particular attention to recently developed patient management problems (PMPs) specially adapted to test strategy and interpretation of results.

COURSE DESCRIPTION

A description and evaluation of the first five years of the laboratory medicine course were reported in 1976.[4] Five hours of formal instruction and case discussion are scheduled daily for six weeks. Since 1976, more time has been devoted to case discussion, with greater emphasis on critical appraisal of the daignostic value of test innovations—particularly in the area of chemical pathology. This has been made possible by the development of more comprehensive course materials designed to provide background information. Since April, 1978, a description of course content has appeared in a series of monthly articles published in *Postgraduate Medicine* and coordinated by one of the authors of this report (MDB). The series was scheduled to be completed by July, 1981.

Instructional Goals

The general goals of the course are that students should develop a logical approach to ordering and interpreting laboratory tests for the diagnosis and management of the more common clinical problems. Process objectives may be articulated in more formal terms as follows: (1) in given clinical situations the students should be able to (a) identify the laboratory tests that will potentially yield the most useful diagnostic information, and (b) identify the appropriate sequence in which tests should be ordered; (2) for specified laboratory tests, the students should be able to interpret the results.[4]

Course Content

A broad outline of course content is given in Table 1. At the beginning of each course, students are made aware of the hypothetico-deductive process.[5] Distinctions are made between screening, case-finding, and diagnosis.[6] It is empha-

Table 1. Course Content

Instructor A	Instructor B	Instructor C
Immunologic Principles	Clinical Problem Solving	Anemia
Immunologic Diagnosis	Clinical Enzymology	Leukocyte Disorders
Serologic Diagnosis	Clinical Endocrinology	Renal Function
Coagulopathies	Risk Factor Assessment	Synovial Fluid
Blood Banking	Electrolytes and Blood Gases	Cerebrospinal Fluid

sized that the worth of a test (or test strategy) depends ultimately on clinical usefulness— usefulness in the sense that the patient benefits—and that, although vital prerequisites to clinical usefulness, neither technical validity nor diagnostic value are useful in themselves.[7] The predictive value concept, as enunciated by Galen and Gambino[8] and an informal version of the threshold probability concept of Pauker and Kassirer[9] are combined to provide a conceptual framework for test strategy that is used throughout the course.[10,11]

As a rule, the remaining topics listed in Table 1 are introduced by formal lectures and/or course materials dealing with underlying pathophysiology, with emphasis on pathogenetic reasoning. This is followed by the reverse process, presentation of relevant clinical problems appropriate to each topic with emphasis on diagnostic reasoning.[12,13] A critical appraisal of the technical validity, diagnostic value, and clinical usefulness follows. Ultimately, test strategies and interpretation of results are discussed and a case discussion reinforces the learning.

Instructional Approaches

Each instructor has his own inimitable style. All three use the Socratic method to generate dialog. Liberal use is made of mini-histories. In accordance with the hypothetico-deductive method, students are asked to generate hypotheses from the clinical story, to modify those hypotheses after hearing profile results, and to formulate further test strategies if necessary. The approach is based on the authors' concept of the role of laboratory testing in clinical problem-solving and is shown diagrammatically in Figure 1. In recent years, algorithms in flow-chart form have been used to illustrate test strategies.[14-17] Figure 2 shows one example.

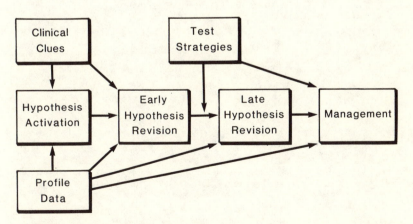

Figure 1. Diagrammatic representation of the role of the clinical laboratory in diagnosis and management.

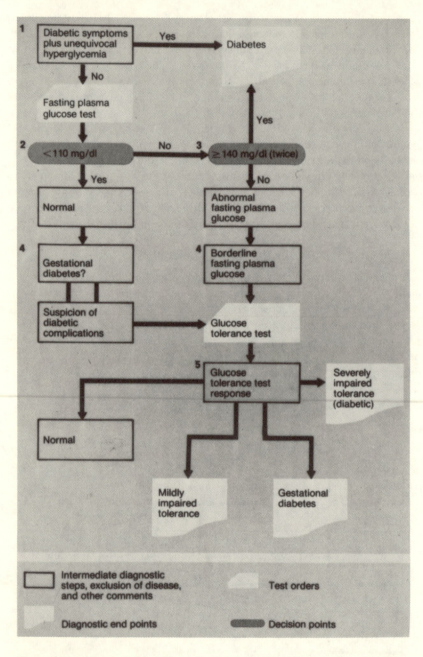

Figure 2. Algorithm depicting a diagnostic strategy for the evaluation of suspected diabetes mellitus. The steps in the decision-making process are numbered sequentially. From Burke.[16]

COURSE EVALUATION

Since the early seventies, a detailed evaluation form has been used to elicit student reaction to the specific aspects of the course. Students use a five-point scale to rate their overall educational experience as well as specific aspects of the elective. The course continues to be rated among the more popular in the medical school—to such an extent that the team of instructors has received Distinguished Teaching Awards for the years 1978 and 1979.

Multiple-choice examinations designed to measure student achievement with respect to course objectives are administered at the end of each elective period. Pretest and posttest multiple choice examinations were given during the spring of 1975 in the content areas of endocrinology, clinical enzymology, and fluid and electrolytes. Each test consisted of 30 questions matched for difficulty level. The pretest mean was 15, and the posttest mean was 24.5 ($N = 50$). This difference is significant at the .001 level as measured by a matched pairs t test.[18]

Patient Management Problems (PMPs)

In 1978, the authors designed a series of simulated laboratory diagnostic problems patterned after the PMP format introduced originally by Rimoldi[19] and further developed by McGuire and her associates.[20] Since 1979, several PMPs have been administered as precourse and postcourse examinations to several medical student groups. The purpose was threefold: (1) to provide some insight into the students' clinical decision-making processes; (2) to evaluate the effects of systematic instruction in laboratory medicine on student problem-solving performance; and (3) to test the hypothesis that prior clinical experience is an important requirement for the successful teaching of laboratory utilization. In 1977, Ward et al. expressed the view that clinical experience on the part of the students was one of the more important prerequisites to the successful teaching of the interpretative aspects of laboratory medicine.[18]

The PMP format consists of a six-page booklet that begins with instructions to study a clinical vignette that includes history, physical examination, and the results of a few routine laboratory tests (see Figure 3). The students are then directed to list their clinical hypotheses (ranked in order of likelihood) and to link those impressions to clinical clues detected in the case presentation. Next, they select laboratory tests from a specially prepared laboratory test selection and report form that accompanies the test booklet. Before obtaining test results, they are directed to link the tests selected to the hypotheses already held. Once this procedure is completed, the results are "reported" by using a latent image marker applied to the result field of the specially prepared laboratory test-selection report form. They are asked to rank a revised list of hypotheses and to link the "reported" results explicitly to those revised hypotheses. They are then given the opportunity to order a second set of laboratory tests. Finally, students

---

PROBLEM 1

You are an intern on general medicine in a local veterans hospital. A 50-year-old white male is admitted. He complains of ill-defined upper abdominal pain of about six days' duration. The pain is mild to moderate in degree. He has had similar pains for shorter periods of time in the past. He also complains of increasing tiredness over the previous two weeks.

There is no significant history other than the foregoing. Specifically, no history of alcoholism or previous jaundice is elicited. Neither does the patient admit to recent or previous anorexia, diarrhea, bloody stools, or weight loss.

Physical examination is negative except for the presence of mid-upper abdominal tenderness without rebound and a questionably palpable liver.

Oral temperature—99°F; pulse—80/minute; blood pressure—130/80.

Urinalysis: Normal except for a slight amount of bilirubin and increased urobilinogen.

CBC: Hemoglobin 13.5 g/dl; WBC—6000/mm³; differential WBC—normal; MCV—83μ^3; MCH and MCHC—normal.

Figure 3. Text of Problem 1.

are asked to list their final hypotheses linked to the second set of laboratory test results.

Thus, following presentation of the clinical problem, three cycles of hypothesis generation, data interpretation, hypothesis evaluation, and data acquisition take place—patterned after the hypothetico-deductive model.[5] The first cycle (Stage 1) is represented by the logging of clinical impressions linked to specific clinical clues and followed by the first laboratory test selection. The second cycle (Stage 2) is represented by the logging of revised impressions (hypotheses) linked to the first set of laboratory tests selected, followed by selection of the second set of laboratory tests. The third cycle (Stage 3) is represented by the final hypothesis (or, ranked list of hypotheses) linked to the second set of laboratory test results contributing to final hypothesis revision.

Hypotheses were scored on three scales: *specificity, appropriateness,* and *diagnostic goal.* The hypothesis specificity index refers to the hierarchical level of disease classification represented by any particular hypothesis. The diagnostic goal index is a measure of the proximity of a particular hypothesis to the correct diagnosis. The appropriateness index is a measure of how well suited any particular hypothesis is to the clinical vignette. A data-hypothesis matrix was constructed that specified the appropriateness of each clinical clue for each hypothesis. For each laboratory test and hypothesis, the matrix specified both the appropriateness of selecting the test for that hypothesis and the interpretation appropriateness of the test result. The scoring criteria and encoded examination data for each student were used as input to a FORTRAN program that computed derived measures of decision performance for each stage of the process (Table 2).

Students were classed as experienced if they had elected at least two clinical rotations in either internal medicine or pediatrics or both before electing the course; otherwise, they were classed as inexperienced. With the use of various linear combinations of the group means of changes in precourse-to-postcourse examination performance for each derived measure, effects of the course, examination differences, and clinical experience were evaluated.[21]

So far, PMPs have been constructed in the areas of clinical gastroenterology and endocrinology and administered in precourse and postcourse format to several student groups. Preliminary results for Problems 1 and 2 (clinical gastroenterology) indicate significant precourse-postcourse improvement ($p < 0.001$) on several derived performance measures. Results thus far support the hypothesis that prior clinical experience is a prerequisite to learning the interpretative aspects of laboratory medicine; experienced students improved significantly on 12 of the 18 derived performance measures, whereas the inexperienced group exhibited improvements of similar significance ($p < 0.001$) on only 3 of the 18 measures.[22]

Of particular interest is the finding that interproblem differences account for some of the precourse-postcourse changes. Pretest hypothesis specificity and

Table 2. Derived Performance Measures (Group Means)

Stage 1

Number of hypotheses
Hypothesis appropriateness
Hypothesis specificity
Hypothesis goal state
Hypothesis—clinical clue interpretation appropriateness
Number of tests selected
Appropriateness of tests selected
Percentage of tests selected that are appropriate

Stage 2

Number of hypotheses
Hypothesis specificity
Hypothesis goal state
Number of tests selected
Appropriateness of tests selected
Percentage of tests selected that are appropriate

Stage 3

Number of hypotheses
Hypothesis specificity
Hypothesis goal state
Test interpretation appropriateness

diagnostic accuracy (goal state) scores were higher for Problem 1—a case of hepatitis B surface antigen (Hb_sAG) positive chronic active hepatitis—than for Problem 2—a case of acute alcoholic hepatitis. This phenomenon is illustrated in Figure 4 in which the increasing goal state exhibited by Cohort 1 when presented with Problem 1 (chronic active hepatitis) in precourse format, may be due to the pathognomonic nature of a positive Hb_sAG test result. The failure of Cohort 2 to alter the diagnostic goal index of their hypotheses, when confronted with the problem of acute alcoholic hepatitis in pretest format, may reflect the fact that the laboratory clues—a pattern of several enzyme elevations of varying magnitudes combined with markedly elevated prothrombin time—although indicative of acute alcoholic hepatic disease, are not as well known as Hb_sAG and lack the latter's inherent diagnostic accuracy.[22] This finding has important implications for the teaching of laboratory medicine, specifically that we should strive to develop multivariate test indexes that have the same high impact value as that of the Hb_sAG.

Outcome Measures

Foregoing precourse-postcourse differences may be interpreted as a meaningful gain in cognitive knowledge. Nonetheless, the question still remains as to whether students who have taken the laboratory medicine elective can be distinguished from those who have not, in terms of their ability to function effectively in clinical situations. To answer this question, a study was designed by Ward et

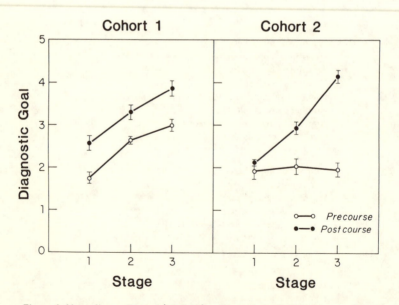

Figure 4. Mean diagnostic goal (±S.E.M.) at Stages 1, 2, and 3 for precourse and postcourse examinations in Cohort 1 and Cohort 2.

al.[4] to compare the clinical performance of students who had taken the elective with those who had not in each of two subsequent clinical electives, pediatrics and internal medicine. Students were ranked by clinical faculty on each of six dimensions of clinical performance: synthesis of information, appropriateness of therapy or treatment program, use of library and literature in study of patient problems, medical knowledge, and overall clinical potential (ability, judgment, attitude). Ratings were based on observations of student performance over the six-week period of the clinical electives. Within the pediatrics elective, the experimental group had significantly higher mean ratings on both "appropriateness of laboratory tests" and "overall clinical potential" when compared with two control groups—one of which had taken an alternative, less structured laboratory medicine elective and another exposed to no such elective ($p < 0.05$).[4] Within the internal medicine elective, however, no significant differences were found among the three groups on any of the six dimensions of clinical performance studied. To explain the foregoing findings, the authors hypothesized that skill in ordering and interpreting laboratory tests is given greater priority in pediatric than in internal medicine electives. Consequently, differences among students in laboratory utilization are more likely to be observed and reflected in pediatric ratings.[4]

CONCLUSIONS

It is ironic that despite the evidence of increasing reliance on medical technology as an adjunct to clinical problem solving, neither clinical decision making nor the role of laboratory tests in that process are taught in systematic fashion in most medical schools. Our evaluation of such a course of instruction at the University of Minnesota over the past several years using a variety of techniques—most recently, the PMP approach in precourse and postcourse format—suggests to us that those students with a minimum of three months' prior clinical exposure show significant improvement on several derived performance measures relating to appropriate use of laboratory tests. Although some evidence shows that postcourse improvement extends beyond the confines of the course itself (in the form of improved performance on subsequent pediatric electives), the evidence is meager; more extensive evaluation of behavior patterns in residency programs and clinical practice is required.

References

1. Young DS. Why there is a laboratory. In: Young DS, Hicks J, Nipper H, Uddin D, eds. Clinician and chemist: the relationship of the laboratory to the physician. Washington, DC: American Association for Clinical Chemistry, 1979.
2. Bailey RM Clinical laboratories and the practice of medicine—and Economic Perspective. Berkeley: McCutcheon, 1979.
3. Moloney TW, Rogers DE. Medical technology—a different view of the contentious debate over costs. N Engl J Med 1979;301:1413-19.
4. Ward PCJ, Harris IB, Burke MD, Horwitz CA. Instruction in interpretative aspects of laboratory medicine. J Med Educ 1976;51:648-56.

5. Elstein AS, Shulman LS, Sprafka SA. Medical problem solving: an analysis of clinical reasoning. Cambridge: Harvard University Press, 1978.
6. Sackett D, Holland WW. Controversy in the detection of disease. Lancet 1975;2:357-9.
7. Burke MD. Laboratory tests: basic concepts and realistic expectations. Postgrad Med 1978;63:53-60.
8. Galen RS, Gambino SR: Beyond normality: The predictive value and efficiency of medical diagnosis. New York:Wiley, 1975.
9. Pauker SG, Kassirer JP. Therapeutic decision-making: a cost benefit analysis. N Engl J Med 1975;293:229-34.
10. Burke MD. Focusing on utilization of laboratory data in teaching clinical pathology. Pathologist 1978;32:624-7.
11. Burke MD. Clinical decision-making: the role of the laboratory. In: Benson ES, Rubin M, eds. Logic and economics of clinical laboratory use. New York: Elsevier, 1978.
12. Feinstein AR. An analysis of diagnostic reasoning. I. The domains and disorders of clinical macrobiology. Yale J Biol Med 1973;46:212-32.
13. Feinstein AR. An analysis of diagnostic reasoning. II. The strategy of intermediate decisions. Yale J Biol Med 1973;46:264-83.
14. Burke MD. Clinical enzymology. II. Test strategies and interpretation of results. Postgrad Med 1978;64:149-56.
15. Burke MD. Hypertension: test strategies for diagnosis and management. Diagnostic Medicine 1979;2:72-84.
16. Burke MD. Diabetes mellitus: test strategies for diagnosis and management. Postgrad Med 1979;66:213-18.
17. Burke MD. Hypoglycemia: strategies for laboratory investigation. Postgrad Med 1979;66:131-8.
18. Ward PCJ, Horwitz CA, Burke MD. Teaching proper laboratory use to medical students and physicians. In: Clinician and chemist: The relationship of the laboratory to the physician. Young DS, Uddin D, Nipper H, Hicks J, eds. American Association for Clinical Chemistry, Washington DC, 1979.
19. Rimoldi HJA. The test of diagnostic skills. J Med Educ 1961;36:73-9.
20. McGuire CH, Solomon L. Clinical Simulations. New York: Appleton-Century-Crofts, 1971.
21. Nie NH, Hull CH, Jenkins JG, et al. Statistical Package for the Social Sciences. 2nd ed. New York: McGraw-Hill, 1975:422-6.
22. Burke MD, Connelly DP. Systematic instruction in laboratory medicine: effects on the clinical problem solving performance of medical students. Hum Pathol 1981;12:134-44.

CHAPTER FIFTEEN

Training House Staff in Effective Laboratory Use

Paul F. Griner, MD

Educational strategies designed to meet the needs of residents concerning laboratory test use must recognize the different purposes for these tests and other diagnostic procedures. Strategies to influence physicians' use of tests to monitor patients after diagnosis (i.e., the use of tests in patient management) may be quite different from those to influence use of tests in arriving at diagnoses. Both issues are equally important but the payoffs may be different. Strategies designed to reduce superfluous testing, which relates largely to test use in patient management, if successful, should result in some degree of cost savings. On the other hand, successful strategies designed to promote quantitative clinical reasoning may not reduce costs, but certainly should lead to improved quality of care. Both are desirable objectives; but in the teaching of house officers, if these objectives are not cleanly separated and identified as such, it is possible that the educational strategies will not be properly received. So, for the purpose of this symposium, I would like to orient my remarks according to these separate objectives, make some comments about existing strategies, and then suggest some additional approaches.

I. TEST USE IN PATIENT MANAGEMENT

Let us initially examine the issue of test use in patient management, with particular attention to the hospital setting. What is the nature of the problem and its determinants; what are some of the strategies that have been designed to address it, and how successful have they been; and what might be considered as additional rational strategies?

A. The Problem of Excessive Use

Finkelstein has shown that about three-fourths of all chemistry and hematology tests performed by hospital laboratories in this country are accounted for by automated multichannel test packages[1] and Benson has demonstrated that of these, between 75 and 80 percent are follow-up tests used for patient monitoring.[2] Most physicians are probably not aware that the liberal use of commonly available tests and procedures contributes more to the annual growth in medical expenditures than do high-cost technologies.[3] Moloney and Rogers have recently discussed this issue.[4] Studies of patterns of laboratory utilization at the University of Rochester Medical Center in the early 1970s have reinforced their conclusions.[5,6] Of even greater importance is the suggestion from these and other studies such as those conducted by Schroeder[7] and Eisenberg[8] that the increasing use of such commonly available tests has not been accompanied by any measurable improvement in outcomes of care. If one were to plot a relationship between the number of laboratory tests and patient benefit, current practices suggest that many physicians' patterns of laboratory test use are at the flat part of the curve where costs of diagnostic studies increase out of proportion to benefits. In addition to costs, one should not lose sight of the implications of excessive repetitive testing for laboratory efficiency. Since many such follow-up tests are ordered on an urgent basis, the deployment of phlebotomists and laboratory personnel necessary to handle large urgent loads may result in delayed turn-around times for those tests ordered as routines. The net effect is the tendency to order more routine tests on an urgent basis so that the results will be available before the house officer leaves for the day; this procedure compounds the problem.

B. Determinants of Excessive Test Frequency

The increasingly repetitive use of common tests and procedures in patient management is probably due to phenomena that are almost ubiquitous in clinical medicine. Some of these phenomena are given in the tabulation below. The identification of these factors and the clinical examples that reflect them are important in developing the necessary remedial strategies. This list is by no means complete. First is the insecurity of the young physician. One must recognize and expect that a certain amount of excess testing will inevitably occur when the most junior members of the patient care team are delegated the responsibility for test ordering. Some of the patterns of follow-up tests occasioned by insecurity, however, discount important knowledge gained in physiology. The ordering of daily electrolytes in patients receiving parenteral fluids whose electrolytes were initially normal and whose clinical problems do not place them at risk for subsequent abnormalities is a case in point.

- Insecurity of the young physician (Example: Daily serum electrolytes)
- Test routines (Examples: Daily chest x-ray on RCU patients; PT/PTT in preoperative evaluation; Serial hematocrits after liver biopsy)
- Penchant for overdocumentation (Example: Serum osmolality)
- Lack of knowledge of the expected rate of measurable change in the disease process after successful treatment (Example: Serial chest x-rays in the patient with pneumonia)
- Low priority assigned to bedside observations.

A second phenomenon is that of test routines. One does not have to observe a house officer in a busy teaching hospital for very long to understand why so many routines are developed. They help to simplify life in a complex and demanding environment, but they do so at the expense of individualized thinking. Some of the examples listed under this heading are common among teaching hospitals and cannot be shown to be very logical.

Third, the natural penchant of physicians, schooled in the physical and biological sciences, is to document and to quantitate even when it is unnecessary. The common practice of measuring the serum osmolality when it can be rapidly calculated within 5 percent of its true value from the results of an SMA-6 is a good example of a superfluous practice.

Fourth is the implication of the lack of knowledge of the expected rate of measurable change in a disease process after successful treatment. This results, for example, in the routine practice by some physicians of ordering an unnecessary chest x-ray every 2 or 3 days for a satisfactorily convalescing hospitalized patient with uncomplicated pneumococcal pneumonia.

Finally, the assignment of a low priority to daily follow-up information obtained at the bedside of the hospitalized patient may be the greatest determinant of excessive follow-up testing.

C. Strategies to Reduce Excessive Test Use in Patient Management

These determinants of excessive test use in patient management have brought about some strategies designed to alleviate the problem. Let us look at some of these strategies and how they have fared. Table 1 lists those gleaned from the literature and from personal communication.

Policy changes have ranged from the elimination of standing orders for daily tests and procedures to restrictions on the numbers of weekly laboratory tests permitted by each house officer.[6,9,10] Although the latter is successful as determined by short-term studies, such a policy does not, in my opinion, begin to address the educational needs.

A variety of cost awareness strategies have been used at both the medical

Table 1. Strategies Designed to Reduce Repetitive Test Use in Patient Management

Strategy	Result	Source (Ref. #)
A. Policy changes	Successful	6,9,10
B. Cost awareness	Probably successful	6,11
C. Fiscal incentives	Unsuccessful	12
D. Guidelines	Successful; require reinforcement	6,13,14
E. Departmental leadership involvement	Probably successful	6, 12
F. Audit followed by education	Successful	15,12

student and house staff level.[6,11] These have included providing manuals of charges for procedures and tests, education of house officers concerning the mechanisms of hospital reimbursement, and the distribution of individual, itemized patient bills to house officers. I did this for a number of years at Strong Memorial hospital and the medical house staff indicated that it was an effective method of pointing out the cumulative effect of repetitively ordered tests.

Fiscal incentives, such as providing money for house staff funds if tests are reduced by a fixed percentage, have not been shown to be effective means of lowering the number of repeat tests ordered.[12] Orientation of new interns concerning the proper use of the laboratory, the dissemination of information pertaining to specific tests (i.e., laboratory newsletters), and the distribution of broad guidelines concerning healthy test practices are strategies that have proved successful, at least in the short term.[6,13,14] Such approaches, however, require reinforcement on a regular basis if the effect is to be sustained.

It is likely that when the leadership of a clinical department is committed to the task of reducing unnecessary laboratory test use, regardless of the strategy, the effort will be successful.[6,12] This incentive has not been studied in any systematic way, however, to my knowledge.

A formal audit system, where specific examples or patterns of inappropriate test use are identified and then reviewed with the house officer in an educational setting is in my opinion likely to be the most effective long-term strategy. Such a system should not only accomplish a reduction in the numbers of repeat tests but should improve the use of tests and procedures in the diagnostic process as well. Schroeder, while at George Washington University, showed this strategy to be effective[15] and is mounting such a program in his new location at the University of California at San Francisco. Martin has just published the results of a similar study at the Peter Bent Brigham Hospital showing that an audit process proved successful there as well. The formal audit approach has the advantage of pinpointing specific educational needs of individual house officers and addressing them in an informal, nonpunitive fashion.

D. Factors Not Yet Addressed

Although I have no supporting data, it is my opinion that other determinants of excessively frequent follow-up testing include: lack of knowledge by house officers of the limits of reproducibility of tests or the likelihood that a given test result is significantly different from the last; factors other than disease that may influence the results of sequential tests; and less than optimum methods of displaying sequential data. On this latter point, Donald Connelly has suggested that the expression of sequential data in graphic rather than tabular fashion may help to reduce unnecessarily frequent repeat testing. Collaborative efforts between faculty in clinical disciplines and in laboratory medicine should be encouraged to study these questions. Are they significant or not? If so, what needs to be done to remedy the problem? Currently, Dr. Dean Arvan, Director of

Clinical Laboratories at Strong Memorial Hospital in Rochester, New York, and I are studying the clinical significance of differences in nondiffusible blood analytes induced by changes in the position of the patient to determine whether these *statistically* significant differences are recognized *clinically*, or are misconstrued and result in inappropriate follow-up testing.

These, then, are some observations concerning the problem of excessive test use in patient management and the resultant educational challenges. Let me turn now to the subject of the education of house staff about test use and interpretation in clinical problem solving as opposed to patient monitoring.

III. TEST USE IN CLINICAL DIAGNOSIS

Much has been written on the subject of medical problem solving, including the application of quantitative methods such as Bayesian and regression models. Many of the leaders in this field have spoken at this symposium. As a clinician/teacher with an interest in promoting the rational use and interpretation of diagnostic tests and procedures in the clinical setting, I have found that it is a difficult task indeed for house officers to move beyond an understanding of the principles of quantitative clinical reasoning to the application of these principles in their day-to-day evaluation of patients. Perhaps one way to address this problem, at least for the purposes of this symposium, is to examine the support systems that are necessary to promote this objective. Insofar as test interpretation is concerned, if we break down the Bayesian model, we can perhaps examine the component strategies and information necessary for the practical application of the model. Since you are all familiar with Bayes' theorem, its components will be shown in narrative rather than mathematical form. They are, simply: (1) an estimate of the probability of disease that is based on the information available prior to obtaining the test; (2) knowledge of the tests available for the disease in question and the operating characteristics of those tests; and (3), the necessary linkage of the test result with the prior probability to arrive at a revised estimate of the likelihood of the disease.

A. Estimate of Prior Probability of Disease

The accompanying tabulation outlines the requirements for a reasonably accurate estimate of the pretest likelihood of disease, the constraints to such accuracy at the house officer level, and some suggested short- and long-term strategies to remedy the problem.

1. Requirements
   a. Knowledge of disease
   b. Experience
2. Constraints
   a. Disease information base is deficient
   b. Lack of experience

3. Strategies
   a. Better information concerning the sensitivity and specificity of symptoms and signs of disease
   b. Organization of such data to accurately assess prior probability
   c. More intimate exposure to substitutes for explicit data (clinical expert)
   d. Broader mix of patients seen during training and the settings in which they are seen

During training, most house officers become fairly well informed about the characteristics of the diseases they will be dealing with in their specialties. Early in training, however, they suffer from the lack of information in textbooks and the published literature concerning the sensitivity and specificity of symptoms and signs. This is particularly the case in ambulatory medicine, where relatively little work has been done to clarify the operating characteristics of the symptoms of common medical illnesses. Much of ambulatory care deals with excluding rather than confirming specific diseases. Thus, the kinds of studies that Dr. Komaroff is conducting (see Chapter 24) should facilitate medical problem solving from the standpoint of both improved predictions of the presence or absence of disease before tests are applied and more appropriate test selection and interpretation.

Lack of experience is obviously the other major determinant of inaccurate assignment of prior probabilities. The work of Elstein, Sox (see Chapter 23), and others in applying such tools as linear regression to substitute for the predictions of the expert and putting them into programs of the kind described by Myers (see Chapter 26) should eventually assist in this component of problem solving. In the meantime, however, it will be necessary to apply more simple strategies to help house staff minimize the frequency of both over- and under-prediction. These strategies should include more intimate dialog between experienced attending physicians and junior house staff during the initial evaluation of hospitalized and ambulatory patients than exists in many teaching hospitals today. In addition, exposure to a broader distribution of patients and the settings in which they are seen should help to improve the perspective of the house officer when evaluating the significance of specific symptoms and signs in a given patient. Such perspective can probably substitute, in part, for experience in arriving at reasonable estimates of disease likelihood before tests are selected and their results interpreted.

B. Operating Characteristics of Tests and Procedures

The second component of the Bayesian approach concerns the operating characteristics of tests and procedures. Here is where I think a great deal of work needs to be done before the principles of quantitative clinical reasoning can be expected to be applied in a meaningful way by house officers. Some of the problem areas that must be addressed are:

- Lack of understanding of operating characteristics by those developing new tests and procedures;

- Problems of spectrum and bias in the determination of test characteristics;
- Lack of assurance that published test characteristics are operative in the laboratory that the physician uses.

First, there is an embarrassing lack of understanding of terminology among some who are developing or applying new tests and procedures. This is particularly true in the procedurally oriented fields such as radiology, despite the work of Lusted and McNeil. Little attention is paid to specificity and false-positive rates are often calculated incorrectly. The result is misleading information for the clinician.

Second, as Ransohoff and Feinstein have pointed out,[16] unless patients with and without the disease in question are properly selected and followed and an appropriate standard applied against which the new test or procedure can be compared, the published characteristics will be misleading—usually in the direction of a falsely high predictive value. One of the most consistent errors is the comparison of a test's value in discriminating between patients with the disease in question and those known to be normal. Such a comparison is satisfactory if the test is to be used for screening, but not when it is applied to a symptomatic patient. In the latter case, similarly symptomatic patients who do not have the disease must be included if an accurate assessment of specificity is to be made. These problem areas reinforce the need for insistence on proper methodology in determining the operating characteristics of new tests before publication and widespread application. Obviously, editorial boards and reviewers of major clinical journals must play a leadership role here.

A third problem is that published test characteristics may not be operative in the laboratory that the physician uses, particularly for special tests and procedures, where the methods used and skills of those performing and interpreting the procedure may vary widely from one hospital to another. I see no solution to this problem, short of having each hospital develop the systems necessary to determine the sensitivity and specificity of those tests and procedures that cannot be assumed to be uniform between hospitals.

Finally, house officers and practicing physicians will need to have readily available information about the characteristics of each test and procedure in relation to the specific diseases for which they are applied. This is no small task, and I am not aware of any teaching hospitals that have attempted to bring together this information from what is available in the literature, incomplete as it may be. In any case, until such information is provided to house officers in a practical way, it is difficult to see how they can apply the principles of quantitative clinical reasoning on a day-to-day basis even if they are well schooled in the principles.

C. Interpretation of Test Results

Strategies to improve the ability of residents to interpret test results, through the proper integration of prior probabilities with knowledge of test characteristics, is the last component for discussion. First, the educational process must begin before the residency years. Second, the editors of textbooks of medicine must encourage their contributing authors to begin weaving the principles of test interpretation into the content of their chapters. It is encouraging to see the application of these principles, increasingly, in articles in major clinical journals, particularly in the cardiology literature. Finally, the teachers of students and house staff must become more familiar with these principles and incorporate them into their teaching rounds and informal dialog with residents.

When all these components are in place and the principles regularly applied by residents, the ultimate question should be addressed. Does it make any difference in patient care outcomes or resource use? Intuitively, differences should indeed exist. To what extent they can be accurately measured is another question.

References

1. Finkelstein SN. Technological change and laboratory test volume. In: Benson ES, Rubin M, eds. Logic and Economics of Clinical Laboratory Use. New York: Elsevier North-Holland, 1978:225-34.
2. Benson ES. Strategies for improved use of the clinical chemistry laboratory in patient care. Ibid, 245-58.
3. Scitovsky AA, McCall N. Changes in the costs of treatment of selected illnesses, 1951-1964-1971. Washington, DC, Government Printing Office, 1976. (DHEW Publication No. (HRS) 77-3161).
4. Moloney TW, Rogers DE. Medical technology — A different view of the contentious debate over costs. N Engl J Med 1979;301:1413-19.
5. Griner PF, Liptzin B. Use of the laboratory in a teaching hospital: Implications for patient care, education, and hospital costs. Ann Intern Med 1971;75:157-63.
6. Griner PF. Treatment of acute pulmonary edema: Conventional or intensive care? Ann Intern Med 1972;77:501-6.
7. Schroeder SA, Schliftman A, Piemme TE. Variation among physicians in use of laboratory tests: Relation to quality of care. Med Care 1974;12:709-13.
8. Eisenberg JM, Williams SV, Garner L, et al. Computer-based audit to detect and correct overutilization of laboratory tests. Med Care 1977;15:915-21.
9. Dixon RH, Laszlo J. Utilization of clinical chemistry services by medical house staff. Arch Intern Med 1974;134:1064-7.
10. Gray G, Marion R. Utilization of a hematology laboratory in a teaching hospital. Am J Clin Pathol 1973;59:877-82.
11. Freeman RA. Letter: Cost Containment. J Med Educ 1976;51:157-8.
12. Martin AR, Wolf MA, Thibodeau LA, Dzau V, Braunwald E. A trial of two strategies to modify the test ordering behavior of medical residents. N Engl J Med 1980;303:1330-6.
13. Goldberg GA, Abbott Ja. Explicit criteria for use of laboratory tests. Ann Intern Med 1974;81:857-8.
14. McCoy KL. The providence Hospital Blood Conservation Program. Transfusion 1962;2:3.
15. Schroeder SA, Kenders K, Cooper JK, et al. Use of laboratory tests and pharmaceuticals: Variations among physicians and effect of cost audit on subsequent use. JAMA 1973; 225:169-73.
16. Ransohoff DF, Feinstein AR. Problems of spectrum and bias in evaluating the efficacy of diagnostic tests. N Engl J Med 1978;199:926-30.

CHAPTER SIXTEEN

Continuing Medical Education and Effective Laboratory Use

Stephen E. Goldfinger, MD

It is quite possible that the cause of effective laboratory use could be best served by abolishing all continuing medical education offerings for the next five years. Then, oblivious to what new round of costly and possibly dangerous technology was needed to remain up-to-date, physicians might start looking more sharply at their current testing practices to find out which ones really made a difference. A facetious suggestion, perhaps, but one that arises from deep concern that traditional programs of "show-and-tell" continuing medical education may give rise to the uncritical proliferation of newer techniques rather than to their rational use.

CONTINUING MEDICAL EDUCATION: AN OVERVIEW

Dissatisfaction with the present continuing medical education scene has been widely expressed;[1-3] the basic indictment is that current techniques are ineffective in producing the kind of learning that will be rapidly translated into improved patient care. Mandatory continuing medical education requirements have served only to cluster physicians into larger, more heterogeneous groups at courses such as those sponsored by medical schools and specialty societies. The inevitable dominance of the lecture format of teaching stifles the spirit of inquiry and initiative that learners should have; instead, they become passive receptacles for heaps of highly technical, plentiful information. Strategies for when and how *relevant* information should be sought are rarely thrashed out between the physicians and the faculty. A systematic assessment of real learning needs, based on a review of practice patterns, is not possible for these large programs. Evaluation of success is often expressed in terms of an attendance figure, occasionally as a measure of cognitive gain based on pretest and posttest scores, and virtually never as documentation of improved practice proficiency. Given this state of

139

affairs, it would be folly to suggest that traditional continuing medical education programs can, *in vacuo*, have a major effect on patterns of laboratory use. At best, they might serve as reinforcement, by echoing strongly worded explicit guidelines developed by expert panels organized at a national level, that might apply to such practices as mammography, preadmission screening tests, thallium scans, and so on.

There is a larger dimension to continuing medical education, though, that is rooted in adult learning theory and that embraces the totality of learning experiences occurring within the daily life of a physician, including reading, recommendations of consultants, participation in hospital rounds, clinical conferences and audits, exposure to mass media reports both directly and via patients' inquiries, and most important, the signals that emerge from each clinical encounter.[4] The challenge is to integrate these experiences into a coherent program of self-education. As George Miller proposed more than a decade ago, "it would seem that the time has come to try a different educational model—one built upon solid evidence about the way adults learn rather than upon the long-honored methods of teaching them. There is ample evidence to support the view that adult learning is not most efficiently achieved through systematic subject instruction; it is accomplished by involving learners in identifying problems and seeking ways to solve them. It does not come in categorical bundles but in a growing need to know. It may initially seem wanting in content that pleases experts, but it ultimately incorporates knowledge in a context that has meaning."[1] Knowles describes effective adult learning (which he terms "andragogy" in contrast to "pedagogy") as follows: it is instigated by self-diagnosis and aimed at solving fairly immediate problems rather than amassing a "reserve" information store for a lifetime; it is achieved in a spirit of equality, mutual respect, and joint inquiry between student and teacher; it is interactive, involving the learner as a seeker among a variety of educational resources; ultimately, evaluation occurs as the learner endeavors to validate improvement in his (her) competency.[5] Whether such a model can be easily and gainfully formalized within institutional continuing education programs remains to be proved. However, if physicians were queried individually, most would describe frequent, self-directed learning experiences, ones generated by clinical problems that were solved by practical help from respected colleagues and/or applied literature searches.

LABORATORY TESTS: AN OPPORTUNITY FOR NEW PROGRAMS

If we acknowledge the need to modify our understanding and approach to continuing medical education in the future, there are compelling reasons to place laboratory testing at center stage among programmatic themes for the 1980s. Concern for the cost and danger of testing has never been higher, for doctors are increasingly aware of their singular role in initiating these diagnostic studies. Many will admit uncertainty in the face of the complexity of choices now available. There are early signs that they will respond to educational efforts designed to sharpen their skills. Nearly 100 doctors enrolled in a three-day course in Decision Analysis in Clinical Medicine offered by Harvard Medical School and the Harvard School of Public Health last year, and its second session was over-subscribed. Alumni of the Strong Memorial Hospital medical residency program, when asked by questionnaire to choose topics most needed to supplement their traditional training (as they remembered it), rated issues of laboratory testing— sensitivity, specificity, predictive accuracy, etc.—as their top priority.[6] Thus, there is reason for guarded optimism that the first step in the process of effective learning—self-diagnosis of an area of deficiency—has occurred for many physicians. And it is encouraging that their perceived need to know more about laboratory testing relates to concrete, practical problems encountered on a daily basis, rather than to more abstruse fare such as immunological mechanisms or tumor biology. The opportunity to make decision analysis understandable to physicians by making it relevant to their practice, and to challenge those set behavioral patterns that become justified under the rubric of "clinical judgment," has an appeal that extends well beyond the narrower goal of improving laboratory use. A final, overriding reason for proposing that laboratory testing is uniquely desirable for future continuing medical education undertakings is that their impact could be measured fairly simply, by finding out whether laboratory use changes. Evaluation—often so elusive as to be forgotten in continuing medical education planning—would be feasible at relatively low cost, thus permitting ongoing assessment of which educational tactics really make a difference in upgrading physician performance. We might be surprised to learn, as Williamson did, that an improved response to abnormal screening tests (urinalysis, fasting blood glucose, and hemoglobin) was not achieved following a specially designed workshop, periodic newsletter reminders, and the introduction of an intern group to a hospital staff. Only after abnormal laboratory data were obscured by removable, fluorescent tapes did physician response to them change.[7] A sad lesson, perhaps, for those who would believe that rational persuasion in itself will bring about change, but an important one for those who wish to measure continuing medical education in terms of improved patient care.

GUIDELINES FOR THE FUTURE

Given the past inadequacies of continuing medical education, it would be presumptuous to set forth a detailed methodology for future programs directed to improving laboratory use. Yet, previous failures should be instructive enough to guide the broad planning strokes for such efforts. The following recommendations are expressed with full awareness that some fall well outside of traditional approaches to physician education, but there are no apologies for introducing more coercive techniques for behavioral modification when behavioral change is the desired goal.

1. *Programs should be locally designed and conducted.* Basing them within

specific institutions and organizations (e.g., hospitals, HMOs, group practices) would:

a. focus upon a defined cohort of physicians;
b. permit their involvement in identifying learning needs;
c. ensure relevance of educational messages to their practices; and
d. permit exploration of various modes of formal and informal communication within the group.

2. *Specific components of each program should begin and end by assessing patterns of laboratory use.* There is no adequate substitute for focusing on learning needs and corresponding achievement than by measuring such performance. It would be best to avoid controversy and "overkill" the product of too many previous audits—by restricting attention initially to the few most glaring examples of laboratory misuse, audits that are compulsively diffuse tend to displace emphasis from key areas of deficiency. As Ginzberg has stated, "It would better to obtain professional agreement about a few major types of bad medical practice and to take remedial action against them than to attempt to establish broad standards of quality."[8]

3. *Diagnosis should precede educational therapy.* The four generic reasons why a physician may deviate from desired testing practices are:

a. *Cognitive* —"I wasn't aware that prothrombin time was a poor way to determine heparin dosage."
b. *Attitudinal* —"I know that an ECG isn't needed on every visit, but my patients expect it and they pay for it."
c. *Psychomotor skill* —"Even though she has high fever and a stiff neck, I haven't done a lumbar puncture in so long that it just wouldn't go right."
d. *External constraints* —"Sure it's not needed here, but the hospital insists that skull films be taken on anyone coming to the emergency room with a head injury."

From these examples, it is obvious that appropriate therapy requires a correct diagnosis. Serving up straight information, per se, will probably have no effect on the last three cases.

4. *Leadership by clinical pathologists will play an invaluable role in identifying and achieving desired goals.* The effectiveness of focusing education on "educationally influential physicians" in communities was recently reported by Stross and Bole,[9] they found a significant improvement in the management of rheumatoid arthritis by *colleagues* after the influential physicians received special training based on group deficiencies revealed by record audits. There is no question that an enlightened, forceful, and communicative pathologist knows what is going on around him and is in a key position to do something about it. Some of the most successful educational programs in community hospitals have been generated by information on testing patterns emerging from the laboratory.

5. *Techniques other than "educational enlightenment" will most likely be*

necessary to modify practice patterns when doctors profit from excessive labora-tory use. Schroeder estimates that of eight variables (improved quality, patient demand, malpractice fears, fiscal incentives, practice variables, educational back-ground, knowledge of costs, medical teaching) fiscal incentive is the most impor-tant factor in influencing physician behavior in the use of clinical resources.[10] The most often-cited justification for what appear to be too many tests is the need to reassure patients. Given this argument, it would seem important to redirect our educational efforts to the lay public by launching a major campaign to inform people of the price they pay for such reassurance (including the worry generated by false positive results). Flagrant examples of laboratory overuse, as might oc-cur during routine check-ups, should be cited in detail. The July 1980 issue of *The Harvard Medical School Health Letter,* which has a subscribership of 300,000 lay persons, is devoted largely to this theme. More media attention to the prob-lem might have a greater influence on physicians than any number of journal articles or continuing medical education lectures. Another tactic would be the deployment of trustees, third party payers, and other members of the commun-ity in the planning and education of programs directed to improving laboratory use. More coercive strategies to change what doctors do fall even further outside the scope of what we generally regard to be continuing education. To the extent that physicians will consent to an environment in which positive reinforcements for proper actions and punishments for improper ones occur, we enter the do-main of behavior modification therapy. When consent is *extraneous* to the work-ings of such a system, we are dealing squarely with enforced regulation—the anathema to physicians that is the panacea for health planners. Its appeal is un-derstandable to those involved in continuing medical education, who are being held increasingly accountable to show that their efforts actually improve med-ical practice. When pitted against the fiscal incentive, though, even the most in-novative educational approaches will be apt to come out second best. Little has transpired since the Age of Athens to suggest that Plato was right in equating knowledge with virtue.

References

1. Miller GE. Continuing education for what? J Med Educ 1967;42:320-26.
2. Brown CR Jr, Uhl HSM. Mandatory continuing education—sense or nonsense? JAMA 1970;213:2660-8.
3. Lewis CE, Hassanein RS. Continuing medical education—an epidemiological evaluation. N Engl J Med 1970;282:254-9.
4. Goldfinger, SE. Continuing medical education and the primary physician. In: Noble J, ed. Primary Care and the practice of medicine. Boston: Little, Brown and Co., 1976: 247-59.
5. Knowles MS. The modern practice of adult education. New York: Association Press, 1970.
6. Griner P. Personal communication.
7. Williamson JW, Alexander M, Miller GE. Continuing education and patient care research. JAMA 1967;201:938-42.
8. Ginzberg E. Notes on evaluating the quality of medical care. N Engl J Med 1975;292: 366-8.

9. Stross JK, Bole GG. Continuing education for primary care physicians. Clin Res 1980; 28:300A.
10.Schroeder SA. Variations in physician practice patterns: a review of medical cost implications. In: Carels EJ, Neuhauser D, Stason WB, eds. The physician and cost control. Cambridge: Oelgeschlager, Gunn and Hain, 1980:23-50.

CHAPTER SEVENTEEN

Modifying Physician Patterns of Laboratory Use

John M. Eisenberg, MD, MBA

Efforts to contain medical care costs often emphasize the role of the physician in generating the demand for medical services. It follows that cost containment programs include attempts to decrease physicians' prescription of hospitalization, drugs, x-ray examinations, and laboratory tests. Therefore, implicit in those programs designed to change physicians' use of laboratory tests is the assumption that physicians currently use the laboratory inappropriately. Before reviewing methods of changing physician behavior, we need to ask the prerequisite question: "Are physicians misbehaving?" Before turning the hospital into a huge Skinner box to change physician behavior, we must ask "Do we have a behavior problem?"

The question of whether physicians' use of laboratory tests should be altered has three components: (1) What is the cost of laboratory tests in this country? (2) Will a reduction in the number of tests performed really reduce the cost of performing these tests? (3) What is the evidence for overuse of laboratory tests?

First, the cost of laboratory tests in the United States is considerable. During 1975 approximately $12 billion was spent for clinical laboratory services, approximately 10 percent of all expenditures on medical care.[1] During that year, it was estimated that 4.5 billion tests were performed; three years later, in 1978, approximately 5.7 billion laboratory tests were performed, an increase of 26.8 percent.[2] Clinical chemistries comprise 25 to 35 percent of all these laboratory tests.[3] Fineberg has pointed out that, although laboratory tests are generally not expensive diagnostic studies, they account for a large expenditure because of

Supported in part by the National Fund for Medical Education, the Prudential Foundation, Blue Cross of Greater Philadelphia, and the National Health Care Management Center (National Center for Health Services Research grant HS02557).

the frequency of their use, what Fineberg described as "the high cost of low-cost diagnostic tests."[3]

Second, laboratory tests *are* expensive to perform. All too often, we envision the cost of a diagnostic study as miniscule. The reasoning goes, "Why, all they have to do is stick the serum in the auto-analyzer. The only cost is the machine and they've already paid for that. One more test won't cost anything." In fact, the cost of such capital equipment as an auto-analyzer is a relatively small part of a laboratory's budget. A study performed at the George Washington University Hospital laboratory showed that nonprofessional salaries accounted for 39 percent of the clinical laboratory's operating expenses; professional salaries, 12 percent; consumable supplies, 26 percent; overhead, 19 percent; and, surprisingly, capital equipment expenditures, only 4 percent of the clinical laboratory's expenditures.[4] Therefore, personnel and supply costs constitute the bulk of the cost of running a laboratory. Despite the advances of mechanization, the laboratory remains work-intensive.

These personnel and supply costs are directly related to the number of tests performed. They are what the economists describe as variable costs, since these costs vary directly with the volume of activity. Indeed, when most costs are fixed and not variable, an additional unit is not costly to produce, but when most costs are variable, as they are with laboratory tests, the additional unit does impose significant costs. For example, the costs of reagents is closely related to the number of tests performed. Furthermore, although new staff will not be hired because of a few additional tests, if each physician were to order one or two more tests daily, the need for personnel would increase. Conversely, a reduction in the number of tests performed has the potential to decrease the cost of supplies and personnel and, therefore, save money.

Of course, the charge for a given test is not always the same as the cost of performing it. Generally, routine electrolyte profiles cost little to perform because they require little personnel time, and the actual cost will be less than the charge. However, unusual or emergency tests may be very expensive to perform and may cost more than the charge. Thus, one type of test may subsidize another. In addition, hospital laboratories often help to support other divisions of the hospital that do not generate revenue, such as nursing, or the laundry. On average, hospital administrators often describe their sense that laboratory charges are only about 25 percent greater than costs. However, cost accounting methods to determine the true cost of performing a laboratory test for a hospitalized patient have not been widely adopted, since hospital reimbursement is usually on a per diem basis.

Third, does overutilization occur? Little empirical data is available, but several studies indicate that physicians do use laboratory tests inappropriately. At the Hospital of the University of Pennsylvania, we have studied the use of multiple determinations of a test, using explicit criteria developed by an expert panel to guide chart audit in judging whether these tests were appropriate. In our study, about 50 percent of patients who underwent multiple testing had unnecessary tests performed.[5,6] Furthermore, certain tests are used frequently, despite data that indicate that they are useless. For example, we showed that approximately 30 percent of prothrombin time determinations obtained on admission to a Veterans Administration hospital were not necessary.[7] Finally, the wide variation in laboratory use among physicians[8,9] suggests that some physicians may be performing unnecessary tests, whereas others may be omitting necessary studies.

In summary, laboratory tests represent a large proportion of medical care expenses; therefore, a reduction in their numbers would save money; and overutilization does occur. We need to consider ways in which we might modify physician use of laboratory tests to make their use more appropriate.

CHANGING PHYSICIAN BEHAVIOR—STATE OF THE ART

Six principal methods have been used to alter physicians' use of diagnostic studies: (1) education, (2) feedback, (3) administrative changes, (4) participation, (5) rewards, and (6) penalties.

Education

Those who have proposed educational strategies to change laboratory use have concentrated on providing physicians with information about the tests. This strategy assumes that the acquisition of cognitive knowledge will make the physician a wiser, and therefore more parsimonious, consumer of diagnostic technology.

Is it true that physicians need this knowledge to use tests more wisely? Most investigators who have studied physicians' knowledge regarding the cost of laboratory tests have found it to be deficient. House staff at the Medical College of Ohio in Toledo knew the approximate price of only 30 percent of services such as laboratory tests and x-rays. Faculty knew the approximate charge for 45 percent of medical services.[10] Only two percent of house staff at Miami's Jackson Memorial Hospital knew more than 50 percent of the correct charges for tests, and most tended to underestimate charges.[11] At New York Hospital, both attending physicians and house staff generally knew the approximate charge for a semiprivate room, but less than half the attending physicians and about a quarter of the house staff knew the price of an electrolyte profile.[12] Community physicians do not fare better; Roth found that when 40 doctors in community hospitals were questioned, only 14 percent of medical care costs were estimated correctly.[13]

Efforts to remedy these deficiencies and improve physicians' knowledge have had two foci: knowledge of the charge for tests; and knowledge of the usefulness of the test and its indications. According to the Association of American Medical Colleges, in 1977, 34 percent of American medical schools had cost containment education programs for medical students, residents, or both.[14] Griner and Liptzin published the results of one of the first of these educational programs and reported that they were able to reduce the rate of increase in the use of laboratory tests for several months.[15]

We conducted a study at the Philadelphia Veterans' Administration Hospital[16] to reduce overuse of the determination of the prothrombin time. Separate medical services were working in the hospital, from each of two local medical schools, and both had the same high use of the prothrombin time—85 to 90 percent of all admissions had prothrombin determinations obtained. An intensive educational program on the appropriate use of prothrombin time, using posters, conferences, and mailings to the residents on one service, was associated with a significant decrease in test use, a decrease that did not occur on the other service. When the program was withdrawn, test use returned to its baseline level in the intervention group within six months. Similarly, Rhyne and Gelbach found that changes in physicians' ordering of thyroid profiles were temporary.[17] The major lesson to be learned from these studies is that an educational program may have temporary effects, but without a continued program, physicians will lapse into their old habits. These results are in keeping with the principle of behavior modification that states that newly learned behavior generally requires reinforcement to become installed as a regular part of behavior.

A second study by Griner has shown that long-term changes can occur. However, in this study, these changes were principally seen in the use of two tests often used inappropriately—the icterus index and the prothrombin time.[18] Furthermore, Griner used several strategies of intervention in conjunction with education, such as administrative changes. Therefore, it is difficult to know how much of the reduction in laboratory testing was due to new knowledge.

The assumption of these studies has been that improved knowledge leads to improved test use, but few data support this assumption. The American Board of Internal Medicine has shown that candidates who score well on multiple choice questions request fewer inappropriate diagnostic tests in the patient management problems than their less knowledgeable counterparts.[19] Although Greenland and associates were able to show that the use of diagnostic tests decreased as residents progressed through the three years of graduate medical education, no clear correlation was seen between test use and knowledge when measured by a questionnaire.[20] Similarly, we have shown that interns and residents perform fewer inappropriate tests as the year progresses. However, we were unable to show that a specific didactic educational program influenced this maturation.[5]

Therefore, residents may show a natural maturation toward more appropriate and parsimonious use of laboratory tests, but there is doubt about the long-term efficacy of didactic educational programs focused on the cost or utility of diagnostic tests.

Several recent educational programs have reported success, however. Martin and his colleagues at the Brigham and Women's Hospital have described success in reducing the use of laboratory tests,[21] as have Klein et al. in the use of antibiotics[22] and Lyle et al. in several aspects of patient care.[23] Each of these studies shares a common educational strategy—the preceptorial. In each program a respected physician, senior to the house staff, has conducted individual conferences with the residents. The greater success of these individualized programs contrasts with the modest success or lack of success of the more traditional didactic programs aimed at the use of a number of diagnostic services. The question must be asked then — are these individualized programs more successful at imparting knowledge, or is their success due to the charisma of the teacher, who becomes the change agent, who alters the attitudes and perhaps the knowledge of the physicians?

The striking decrease that we and the Rochester group have found coincident with the progression of the house officer through the course of his training, but not necessarily related to didactic education, raises the question of whether it is really the acquisition of information that induces the improvement. Perhaps it is the maturation of the resident, which transforms information to knowledge and then to wisdom. The problem we face may have been best stated by T. S. Eliot in his poem, "The Rock" when he wrote, "Where is the knowledge we have lost in information? Where is the wisdom we have lost in knowledge?"[24]

If we are willing to accept the conclusions of some investigators that education may induce behavior change among physicians, then we must identify the appropriate timing for introducing that education. If habits are formed in medical school and residency training (if Wordsworth was correct that "the child is father to the man"[25]), then we need to initiate these programs as early as possible. But teaching medical students without developing educational programs for residents and continuing education for practicing physicians may be futile if the experiences of residency and practice overwhelm habits developed in medical school.

Feedback

The second major strategy for changing physicians' use of laboratory tests is feedback. A number of programs have been established to provide physicians with information regarding their use of medical services, including laboratory tests. Indeed, feedback is a method used by Professional Standards Review Organizations (PSROs) for utilization review.

Several experimental programs have included chart audit to determine whether physicians' laboratory use has been appropriate,[5,6] but the methods for determining which tests are unnecessary are not well developed. Other feedback programs have compiled profiles of physicians' laboratory use and have shown each physician how he or she compares with peers.[8,26,27] Some of these programs have claimed success in reducing utilization.[26,27] Still others have given physicians copies of their patients' bills, in hopes that they would become more aware of the charges for services and the volume of services used.

Administrative Changes

Both the educational and the feedback strategies depend on physicians' making voluntary changes in their behavior. An alternative strategy to changing physician behavior is to institute administrative rules that mandate change. At Strong Memorial Hospital, several administrative changes, as reported by Griner,[18] may have contributed to the decreased use of tests. In that program, the hospital eliminated routine admission chest x-rays and required that residents write out all of the laboratory requests. At Stanford University, medical residents also were required to fill out their own requests.[28] In another experimental program, residents at the Durham, North Carolina, Veterans Administration Hospital were limited to eight tests per day.[29] Each of these experimental programs has been reported to induce decreases in laboratory use. Similarly, in many hospitals, certain diagnostic tests such as computed tomography scans cannot be obtained without the approval of a consultant. Blue Cross has requested that its local plans refuse to pay for admission screening tests unless they are specifically requested by the physician.

Participation

Another method of reducing laboratory use among physicians is to involve them in the cost containment program itself. A number of PSROs anecdotally report that the physicians who seem to respond the most dramatically to utilization review programs are those who are involved in the program. Similarly, dramatic decreases in the use of laboratory tests have been described (but not published) at Jackson Memorial Hospital, where residents developed their own program. At the Hospital of the University of Pennsylvania, we have found residents to accept a utilization review program more willingly when they are involved in its planning.

Financial Rewards

Several attempts have been made to change physician behavior by offering financial rewards. The Health Insurance Plan of New York showed that financial rewards induced physicians to reduce the use of the hospital,[30] as did Pennsylvania Blue Shield in a recent small experimental program.[31] Although residents in the Jackson Memorial Hospital cost containment program were probably influenced by educational and participation strategies, it is important to note that many residents understood that reductions in laboratory use would be followed by increases in house staff salaries. This same principle of financial rewards is used by prepaid medical care programs, such as health maintenance organizations, in which physicians may receive bonus payments if the organization is able to save money by limited utilization.[32]

In contrast to these reports of success, residents at the Brigham and Women's Hospital did not reduce laboratory use in response to financial incentives.[21] Residents at the Hospital of the University of Pennsylvania rejected the idea of rewards as an option in their program.[5]

Financial Penalties

The converse of rewards is penalties, and this strategy has also been used to modify physician behavior. The New Mexico Experimental Medical Care Review Organization showed a decrease in office injections when penalties were imposed for overuse, although this method was combined with an educational program.[33] Similar findings were reported by the San Joaquin Foundation for Medical Care when billing claims were adjusted by peer review for overutilization.[34] Blue Shield has recently instituted its Medical Necessity Project, in which payment is denied for outdated diagnostic tests. The effectiveness of the Medical Necessity Project is not yet apparent.

THEORETICAL CONSIDERATIONS

These six methods of altering physician use of laboratory tests presume that physicians are using the tests inappropriately and that their behavior should be modified to improve the quality of care and contain costs. In attempting to change physicians' use of laboratory tests, the fields of behavior modification and management theory offer principles that are relevant.

Behavior Modification

A preliminary step in many behavior modification programs is to search for clues to help identify factors responsible for maintaining the behavior, whatever the behavior may be.[35] Sherman describes this search as a "functional analysis" and points out that a behavior modification program should be aimed at addressing these "maladaptive behaviors." In keeping with this principle, in order to determine the reasons for overuse of laboratory tests, we have conducted a survey of resident and faculty physicians at the Hospital of the University of Pennsylvania and internists in the Philadelphia area.[36] We found that faculty and residents agreed that the principal reasons for overuse at their teaching hospital were inexperience, habitual ordering of groups of tests, and pressure from other physicians. In contrast, community physicians identified the principal reasons as routine screening for disease, habitual ordering of groups of tests, and concern about medical malpractice. Faculty and residents had listed concern about medical malpractice as the least important reason for potential overutilization of laboratory tests. Therefore, it becomes apparent that programs to modify the use of laboratory tests need to address different issues for academic and community physicians. A standardized approach to physician change may be appropriate in certain settings and inappropriate in others.

A second important principle of behavior modification is the use of feedback.[35] In general, in encouraging a new behavior, these reinforcements should be rewards. Penalties may be able to extinguish undesired behavior. When feasible, reinforcements should immediately follow the performance of the desired behavior. At first, each instance of the desired behavior should be reinforced. Eventually, as the desired behavior increases in frequency, it may be rewarded less frequently but often enough to reinforce it. Such an intermittent schedule for reinforcement will increase the strength of the response and make it more resistant to extinction. These principles of operant conditioning imply that reinforcement should continue for a long time, in contrast to the frequent one-shot interventions described in the literature regarding physician behavior.

It is also important that the reinforcement being used be meaningful to the recipient[35] perhaps even one that the recipient has chosen. These rewards and penalties need not be tangible. Indeed, medical audit may provide both direct feedback, which captures the physician's desire to perform well, and profiles, which compare the physician with peers. This feedback capitalizes on doctors' concern about their performance compared with that of their peers. These intrinsic rewards may be more important than extrinsic or tangible rewards and may explain the lack of response to financial rewards by residents in the Brigham and Women's study and the reluctance of residents to accept rewards in the University of Pennsylvania study.

A final point of importance with regard to behavior modification is the role of individualized instruction. In the Stanford Three-Community Study to reduce the risk of cardiovascular disease, Farquhar has reported that in a study of three towns in California, those individuals who were exposed to personalized instruction were able to improve their health habits more than those exposed to a mass media program.[37] These results imply that individualized instruction may be more potent in changing behavior and may help to explain the greater success of physician change programs that have used individual preceptorials with residents compared with those that have used more formal didactic educational strategies.

Management Theory

In addition to adapting the principles of behavior modification, programs that attempt to change physicians' use of laboratory tests might consider the experience of other organizations in influencing the way in which members of the organization operate. The field of management theory, and in particular organizational psychology, offers data from research studies that may be useful in modifying physician behavior. A major area of study in management theory is that of organizational change; a number of its principles are relevant to attempts to change the utilization of laboratory tests.

First, Lewin has described a successful strategy for change as having three components: unfreezing, changing, and refreezing.[38] In the unfreezing stage, old patterns of behavior are reevaluated and a sense of dissatisfaction with these patterns is generated. In addition, the system that previously supported the undesired behavior is dismantled. Next, a respected individual introduces a new pattern of behavior and the desire for this new behavior is internalized throughout the organization. Last, the new behavior is reinforced.

Second, the marketing literature emphasizes the role of leadership is disseminating a new pattern of behavior. In a classic study, Coleman, Katz, and Menzel showed that the use of a new antibiotic among physicians in a community was largely dependent on the acceptance of the new drug by professional leaders.[39] Stross and Bole have reported a successful program that induced physicians to change their patterns of caring for patients with rheumatoid arthritis by educating physicians who were leaders in the medical community and encouraging these physicians to convince other physicians to change their behavior.[40]

Third, the principle of contingency theory suggests that the appropriate way to initiate change in an organization is contingent on the work and the people involved. Lawrence and Lorsch have shown that decision making by researchers is best decentralized, that is, left up to the individual, because of the uncertain nature of the task and the professional nature of the people involved. In contrast, routine tasks such as those of an assembly line are best centralized.[41] Similarly, others have found that a hierarchical organization is best suited for repetitive simple tasks, whereas for complex tasks, an organization that enables participation in planning and operation by the workers is preferable.[42,43] It is not surprising, then, that Neuhauser has found that in a group of Chicago hospitals, physicians were most satisfied in an organization that used participatory strategies of management, whereas departments such as laboratory and dietary were best organized in a hierarchical fashion.[43]

These three principles of management theory imply that a successful program of changing physicians' use of laboratory tests will involve physicians in the planning of the program, identify certain physicians as pace-setters, convince physicians that their current behavior is not optimal, remove the old support system, and reinforce the new and desired behavior.

METHODOLOGIC ISSUES

As new programs incorporating these principles of behavior modification and organizational psychology in changing physicians' use of laboratory tests are initiated, investigators should consider a number of methodologic issues that remain unresolved and that should be addressed by subsequent experimental programs.

One difficult methodologic issue has been the development of satisfactory measures of laboratory use that can be used as indicators of the success of the intervention. Although the goal of these programs generally has been the reduction of unnecessary testing, the total use of diagnostic tests is the outcome often measured. However, it has not been demonstrated that only *over*use of the laboratory decreases as total use decreases. Since it is difficult to judge which tests are unnecessary, programs that attempt to detect inappropriate use will require the development of explicit criteria for appropriate use and will necessitate costly review of medical records.[44]

Another difficulty in determining measures of appropriate laboratory use is that many of the programs are oriented toward students, who rarely order diagnostic studies independently and, therefore, whose actual use patterns cannot be measured. Less satisfactory alternatives have been tried, such as patient management problems, simulated cases and written tests, but it is unclear whether these outcome measures really reflect changes in the way the student would use the laboratory.[14]

Another methodologic issue in the development of outcome measures is whether there are surrogates for overutilization. Is there some other measure of laboratory use that will indicate overutilization without requiring chart review? Experimental PSRO ancillary services review programs have used profile analysis and concentrated their review on physicians whose use of certain services was unusual when compared with that of their peers. Other review programs, such as that of Pennsylvania Blue Shield, have used the method of paired analysis, in which the use of two services for the same patient is reviewed to detect overutilization. For example chest roentgenograms for patients who have undergone normal deliveries might be investigated. Another possible surrogate for overutilization is the ratio of abnormal to normal test results. Although a physician whose testing generates few abnormal test results may be overusing the laboratory, this outcome is largely dependent on his or her patient mix and the reasons for using the test. Therefore, the ratio of abnormal to normal tests has not yet been evaluated as an appropriate surrogate for measuring actual overutilization.

In addition to the methodologic difficulty in determining when overuse occurs, there is the risk that the programs to change physician behavior will induce underuse of laboratory tests as well as reduce overuse. Since most experimental programs have only reported overall reductions in laboratory use, it is impossible to know whether these programs have reduced overutilization. Obviously, a program that reports decreases in overall use of the laboratory may have indiscriminantly reduced both appropriate and inappropriate tests, and a program that reports decreases in overutilization may have also caused decreases in necessary or appropriate testing. Again, explicit criteria need to be developed to distinguish appropriate from inappropriate testing.

Another methodologic issue is the definition of the "unit of measure." Since the physician is the subject of these programs, it is the use of laboratory tests by the individual physician that should be evaluated. When total laboratory use for an entire medical service or hospital is reported, individual differences among physicians are obscured. It may be, for example, that a few physicians respond to the program and that their reductions in laboratory use are so profound that overall use by the hospital is reduced significantly. An appropriate statistical analysis will use the individual physician as the unit of analysis to determine whether the program's impact was significant. Studying the physicians individually has the additional potential advantage of determining which kinds of physicians respond to the program.

On the other hand, studying physicians as individual units of analysis ignores the interaction that occurs among physicians in determining plans for diagnosis and management, particularly in a teaching hospital where these issues are often discussed by the intern who orders the test with his resident, attending physician, and consultants. Coser[45] has shown that medical services in teaching hospitals use this participative style of decision making more than surgical services, in which decisions are often made by a senior physician and merely implemented by the resident. If teams of physicians can be identified and are stable for a reasonable period of time, it may be that the team is the appropriate unit of analysis rather than the individual, the entire service, or the hospital.

Another methodologic issue in assessing the effectiveness of these physician change programs is that of determining which intervention was successful — education, feedback, administrative changes, participation, rewards, or penalties. There is reasonable evidence, which has been reviewed in this chapter, that physician behavior can be altered. However, the fundamental question is which, if any, of these strategies is effective. The next research question is the definition of the cost-effectiveness of the various approaches. Unless the strategies are clearly defined in experimental programs, it is difficult for others to use the methods of these trials to develop their own effective and efficient programs to reduce inappropriate laboratory use. Randomized controlled or quasi-experimental trials will help to distinguish the effective and noneffective strategies.

The pertinent methodologic issues in the development of educational strategies have been reviewed, but it is important to emphasize them. Should these educational programs address medical students, house officers, attending physicians, practicing physicians, or all of them? Will individualized instruction prove to be more effective than formal, didactic education? If so, is it cost-effective? Is it really education in the sense of information transfer, or does physician change depend on the charismatic ability of the teacher to alter attitudes? Will education about several tests or about laboratory use in general be as effective as education that focuses on one test, such as prothrombin time determinations or thyroid profiles?

The role of the reimbursement system raises other unresolved problems. Can any strategy to reduce physicians' laboratory use be effective in the context of a reimbursement system that rewards the use of medical technology? In the language of behavior modification, will students and house officers extinguish their newly learned behavior of cost-effective laboratory use when, as practicing physicians, they are exposed to the positive reinforcement of being paid to perform diagnostic studies? Can we study the impact of reimbursement systems on physician behavior or even alter the systems to reward appropriate use of the laboratory?

In establishing feedback programs, what will be the appropriate type of feedback? Should it be positive, pointing out what the physician has done correctly, or should it be negative? How soon after physicians order a test should they receive feedback? The principles of behavior modification indicate that feedback should occur as soon as possible.[35] Should the feedback review the physicians' use in reference to peers or should it independently describe their own performance?

Another methodologic issue in the development of physician change programs is the problem of long-term follow-up. Few programs have studied the effect of their attempts to reduce laboratory use beyond a few months, and the amount of continued education or feedback needed to maintain the new behavior has not been defined.

In addition, control groups of physicians are necessary to insure that the manifest change in behavior was actually due to the intervention. Controls within the hospital risk being contaminated by communication among the experimental and control physicians. Using physicians as their own controls, by studying laboratory use before and after an intervention, neglects the natural evolution of physicians' development and the effect of concurrent influences on them. Even studying a separate group of physicians as a control group may not be satisfactory if the control group knows that its performance is being reviewed (the Hawthorne effect).

Finally, in developing these experimental programs to change physician behavior, we seldom ask whether we need to obtain the permission of our subjects. Although investigators are required to obtain the informed consent of other subjects whom they may study, physicians generally are not given any choice about participating in programs designed to change the way they practice medicine.

For almost a decade now, we have experimented with changing the use of laboratory tests by physicians. We have made some progress, but many questions remain unanswered. As utilization review programs such as the PSROs begin to institute ancillary services review, methods that have been developed in the sheltered environment of the teaching hospital are being transcribed to broader use. Whether the state of the art is sophisticated enough for broad scale programs to be started may be irrelevant; the need to reduce the overuse of diagnostic tests is too pressing. Our hope is that the evaluation of these large programs, as well as the continued development of truly experimental programs, will be designed carefully enough that we can answer some of our questions about how to change the way that physicians decide to use diagnostic technology.

References

1. Conn RB. Clinical laboratories. Profit center, production industry, or patient-care resource. N Engl J Med 1978;298:422-7.
2. National survey of hospital and non-hospital clinical laboratories. Laboratory Management 1979 (March);17:33-48.
3. Fineberg HV. Clinical chemistries: the high cost of low-cost diagnostic tests. In: Altman S, Blendon R, eds., Medical Technology: The Culprit Behind Health Care Costs? Proceedings of the 1977 Sun Valley Forum on National Health. (DHEW Publication No. (PHS) 79-3216, pp. 144-65.)
4. Werner M. Economics of microassays in the clinical laboratory. In: Werner M, ed., Microtechniques for the Clinical Laboratory. New York: John Wiley and Sons, Inc., 1976: pp. 405-16.

5. Eisenberg JM, Williams SV, Poyss LF, Pascale LA. Changing diagnostic test overutilization. Clin Res 1980;28(2):294A.
6. Eisenberg JM, Williams SV, Garner L, Viale R, Smits H. Computer-based audit to detect and correct overutilization of laboratory tests. Med Care 1977;15:915-21.
7. Eisenberg JM, Goldfarb S. Clinical usefulness of measuring prothrombin time as a routine admission test. Clin Chem 1976;22:1044-7.
8. Schroeder SA, Kenders K, Cooper JK, et al. Use of laboratory tests and pharmaceuticals: Variation among physicians and effect of cost audit on subsequent use. JAMA, 1973; 225:969-73.
9. Rose H, Abel-Smith B. Doctors, patients and pathology. Occasional papers on social administration. London: G. Bell and Sons, 1972:1-79.
10. Skipper JK, Smith G, Mulligan JL, et al. Physicians' knowledge of costs: the case of diagnostic tests. Inquiry 1976;13:194-8.
11. Dresnick SJ, Roth WI, Linn BS, Pratt TC, Blum A: The physician's role in the cost containment problem JAMA 1979;241:1606-9.
12. Nagurney JT, Braham RL, Reader GG. Physician awareness of economic factors in clinical decision-making. Med Care 1979;17:727-36.
13. Roth RB. How well do you spend your patients' dollars? Prism, September, 1973.
14. Hudson JI, Braslow JD: Cost containment education efforts in the United States medical schools. J Med Educ 1979;54:835-40.
15. Griner PF, Liptzin B. Use of the laboratory in a teaching hospital. Ann Intern Med 1971; 75:157-63.
16. Eisenberg JM. Educational program to modify laboratory use by housestaff. J Med Educ 1977;52:578-81.
17. Rhyne RL, Gelbach SH. Effects of an educational feedback strategy on physician utilization of thyroid function panels. J Fam Pract 1979;8:1003-7.
18. Griner PF and the Medical House staff, Strong Memorial Hospital. Use of laboratory tests in a teaching hospital: long term trends. Ann Intern Med 1979;90:243-8.
19. Webster G. Presentation at Association of Program Directors in Internal Medicine Meeting, Kansas City, MO, April 5, 1981.
20. Greenland P, Mushlin AI, Griner PF. Discrepancies between knowledge and use of diagnostic studies in asymptomatic patients. J Med Educ 1979;54:863-9.
21. Martin AR, Wolf MA, Thibodeau LA, Dzau V, Braunwald E. A trial of two strategies to modify the test ordering behavior of medical residents. N Engl J Med 1980; 303:1220-6.
22. Klein L, Charache P, Johannes R, Lewis C. Effect of physician tutorials on prescribing patterns and drug cost in ambulatory patients. Clin Res 1980;28(2):296A.
23. Lyle CB, Biarchi RF, Harris JH, Wood ZL. Teaching cost containment to house-officers at Charlotte Memorial Hospital. J Med Educ 1979;54:856-62.
24. Eliot TS. "The Rock."
25. Wordsworth W. "My Heart Leaps Up When I Behold."
26. Wennberg JE, Blowers L, Parker R, et al. Changes in tonsillectomy rates associated with feedback and review. Pediatrics 1977;59:821-6.
27. Dyck FJ, Murphy FA, Murphy JK, et al. Effect of surveillance on the number of hysterectomies in the province of Saskatchewan. N Engl J Med 1977;296:1326-8.
28. Dohring E, Marton K, Sox HC. Spontaneous and induced changes in laboratory test ordering in a general medical clinic. Clin Res 1980;28(2):293A.
29. Dixon RH, Laszlo J. Utilization of clinical chemistry services by medical housestaff. Arch Intern Med 1974;134:1064-7.
30. Jones E, Densen PM, Altman I, Shapiro S, West H. HIP incentive reimbursement experiment: Utilization and costs of medical care, 1969 and 1970. Soc Secur Bull 1974;37: 3-21.
31. Markel GA. Per case reimbursement for Medicaid services. National Center for Health

Services Research Summary Series. (NCHSR-DHEW publication no. PHS 79-3230, October 1978, 31 pp.).

32. Luft HS. How do health-maintenance organizations achieve their "savings"? N Engl J Med 1978;298:1336-43.

33. Brook RH, Williams KN. Effect of medical care review on the use of injections: A study of the New Mexico Experimental Medical Care Review Organization. Ann Intern Med 1976;85:509-15.

34. Buck CR Jr., White KL. Peer review: Impact of a system based on billing claims. N Engl J Med 1974;291:877-83.

35. Sherman AR. Behavior Modification: Theory and Practice. Monterey, CA: Brooks/Cole Publishing Company, 1973.

36. Williams SV, Eisenberg JM, Pascale LA, Kitz DS. The reasons for unnecessary diagnostic testing. National Health Care Management Center Discussion Paper No. 19, Leonard Davis Institute of Health Economics, University of Pennsylvania.

37. Farquhar JW, Wood PD, Breitrose H, et al. Community education for cardiovascular health. Lancet 1977;1:1192-5

38. Lewin K. Group decision and social change. In: Newcomb TM, Hartley EL, eds. Readings in Social Psychology. New York: Holt, Rinehart and Winston, Inc., 1958.

39. Coleman JC, Katz E, Menzel H. Medical Innovation: A Diffusion Study. Indianapolis: Bobbs-Merrill Co., 1966.

40. Stross JK, Bole GG. Continuing education in rheumatoid arthritis for the primary care physician. Arthritis and Rheumatism 1979;22:787-91.

41. Lawrence PR, Lorsch JW. Organization and Environment. Cambridge, MA: Division of Research; Graduate School of Business Administration, Harvard University, 1967.

42. Lowin A. Participative decision making: A model, literature critique, and prescriptions for research. Organizational Behavior and Human Performance 1968;3:68-106.

43. Neuhauser D. The hospital as a matrix organization. Hosp Adm 1972;17:8-25.

44. Faulkner PL, Nevick R, Williams SV, et al. Concurrent utilization review of diagnostic testing: a medical audit program. Hospitals 1981;55:57-59.

45. Coser RL. Authority and decision making in a hospital: a comparative analysis. Am Sociol Rev 1958;23:56-64.

CHAPTER EIGHTEEN

Problem Solving in Medicine: Can We Teach It?

Lawrence L. Weed, MD

In the last analysis, we teach by example. People will do what is done in the real world of everyday practice—regardless of what they were "taught" in an "educational situation." High quality, efficient problem solving for most of the patients most of the time is not occurring. This is because in all types of medical settings, physicians and other medical personnel hear new data, recall memorized knowledge, formulate problems, generate plans, and record all the data in rapid sequence, without systematic use of appropriate aids to their senses and their intellectual capacities. So to varying degrees they may falter at every step. In today's standard literature in psychology, the limitations of the unaided human mind for solving complex problems have been repeatedly demonstrated and much in the medical literature of an empirical sort confirms it. The article from Duke on antibiotic usage,[1] the analysis from Harvard on the use of data in arriving at diagnostic conclusions,[2] and Elstein's book on problem solving in medicine[3] are just a few of the many studies that should long ago have destroyed our illusions.

A single human mind cannot grapple successfully with all the complexities involved in defining and solving medical problems in the total context of an individual patient's life any more than single-celled organisms can do what a sophisticated multicellular organism can do. The emphasis must shift from teaching single individuals all of problem stating and problem solving, to the development of the best combination of philosophy, systems, machines, and people with a variety of skills to bring the best of medical science to most of the people most of the time.

I am indebted to the staff of the PROMIS Laboratory without whom development and implementation of the ideas presented here would have been impossible.

This work has been funded primarily by the National Center for Health Services Research, Department of Health, Education and Welfare, under contract nos. 230-76-0099 and 233-78-301.

Furthermore, the emphasis must be on the precision of the connections among individuals, as opposed to the talents or contribution of any single individual. In a well-functioning multicellular organism, each cell type lacks the autonomy it may once have enjoyed before it joined other cells to achieve a larger goal.

PROMIS is a system of philosophy, machines, and people designed to overcome the coordination, logic, memory, and feedback problems that now plague the practice of medicine. Even the first approximation of a "nervous system" to connect human nervous systems in precise and reproducible ways can become complex very rapidly, even though its everyday use can be deceptively simple and straightforward—as the simple movement of an arm does not even vaguely reveal, nor should it reveal, the literally thousands of impulses and parts that make it possible. In this sense PROMIS already represents thousands of lines of code, thousands of computer displays, and an almost infinite number of pathways among precisely defined options. Before describing some of the present attributes of PROMIS, I shall review some of the philosophical notions that, in addition to the problem-oriented philosophy, underlie PROMIS' present form and future goals.

STRUCTURES AND PROCESSES IN THE HUMAN BODY

The structures and processes of the human body are the very substance of medical science and medical practice. If every structure and process in the human body were known and could be continuously monitored one could see precisely each primary derangement and keep track of the rapidly cascading consequences. In such a situation, problems and procedures to detect and correct problems could all be defined in terms of those well-defined structures and processes.

Even with a relatively small number of structures and interacting processes in a known system, the possible secondary effects of a single derangement can be very great and varied when the processes are always active and subject to environmental influences. In the human body, detailed understanding of the implications of any single derangement are particularly difficult because the number of structures and processes is very large, genetic variations in them are significant, and environmental influences on them extraordinarily varied. And in addition to the number of structures and processes being overwhelmingly large, they are not all yet known and we have very far to go in making them known. It would be extremely unlikely for two individuals to have identical derangements and consequences: each individual is unique and one's problems are unique combinations of specific scientifically identifiable derangements and other unknown factors. The more details one has on an individual, the more this uniqueness reveals itself.

It is important for all those functioning within the medical sciences—from the patient to the specialist—to have a picture of how medical science has developed and medical roles are developing in the face of these difficulties.

Since dysfunction was seen and written about in medicine long before the rudiments of anatomy, physiology, and biochemistry (the structures and processes) were understood, the human body and mind and spirit were treated as a "black box" exhibiting all sorts of difficulties on the surface (symptoms and signs) for which all sorts of remedies were devised with varying amounts of logic and understanding. Names were placed on various collections of signs and symptoms that recurred, and names were placed on various treatments for these collections.

A few people in each culture made it their business to study and manage the outer evidences of dysfunction and naturally developed and transmitted all sorts of notions as to what the dysfunctions are due to and how they should be managed. Some of these notions have turned out to be remarkably correct in the light of present understanding; others have proved wrong. We might laugh at a person from Mars who put nickels in a candy machine and wrote a paper on how Hershey candy bars are made of nickel, but much of our medical and biochemical literature has been just that naive as it has struggled to understand the human machine. As medical literature has developed, there has been no rigorous method to keep the definitions of each disease entity precise and consistent among all contributors to that literature; people using the same words have often been talking about different things.

While the above vocabulary and confusion have been building up over the years, anatomists, biochemists, physiologists, and so on have been trying to delineate each structure and process inside of the "black box" of the human body. This has resulted in a second elaborate literature that uses its own terms and definitions.

When all these individuals working inside and outside the human body meet over a common problem such as diabetes, difficulties in communication can arise because each defines terms from an individual point of view. To a clinician, the diabetic person may be someone with a high blood sugar and a retinopathy; to the immunologist with a new technique to measure insulin in the blood, the patient is a particular type of diabetic with a high or low blood insulin; others may think in terms of the glucagon producers, or the high levels of antibodies to insulin, or defective receptor mechanisms. The more we know, the more we realize that no two diabetic patients are exactly alike and so diagnostic tests and treatments will not have uniform effects on what we categorize as single diseases when looking on the outside of the "black box." So we arrive again at the conclusion of the uniqueness of individuals.

Regardless of the past, we can now try to define all procedures and problems in medicine in the same structure and process terms, and look for intersections among them. Old names such as "Addison's disease" can be coupled to common terms of structure and process. Indeed that very name is a link to the wisdom of the past, since it usually represents a combination of symptoms and signs realized by the patient. We cannot ignore past literature organized under old terms, because useful diagnostic, treatment, and prognostic information is there for those groupings, which were empirically derived. Digitalis helped dropsy before people understood the dynamics of heart failure. Our job is to use the computer as a tool to maintain communication between these two worlds and have definitions available at the level appropriate to the task at hand. This can best be accomplished by expressing medical entities in terms of structure-process diagrams.

When we talk about the probability of any one entity given another entity, that probability depends on how carefully, in terms of structure and process, we are defining the entities. The probability of all diabetic patients defined in one way having a given characteristic is different than the probability of just defect-ive receptor mechanism diabetics having that same characteristic. In addition, one has to talk about those probabilities in terms of propensities—and the pro-pensities relate directly to the environmental effects on structures and processes in any system. For example, two diabetics can have exactly the same derange-ment in structures and processes but be exposed to a very different set of envi-ronmental influences that affect carbohydrate metabolism, such as exercise at work, other drugs such as contraceptives, other problems such as infection, and a wholly different emotional environment.

In summary, various combinations of deranged structures and processes, combine to form the molecules or entities of clinical medicine—and the possible combinations are unlimited and each individual is a unique set. We should make every effort to define the traditional words of medicine in terms of the struc-tures and processes that present medical science considers to be the basis for the entity in question. This will obviously change as medical science develops and the definitions should be thought of in a dynamic way.

COMPLEXITY AND ILLUSIONS IN EVERYDAY PRACTICE

Since the practitioners and the investigative scientists who support them are up against a massive number of combinations and permutations of events, even among known structures and processes, to say nothing of the unknown ones, it is not surprising that detailed analysis of the performance of the average medical provider shows it to be erratic and inconsistent with the performance of many other providers. So many opportunities exist for misrepresentation of events and misapplication of knowledge that it is undoubtedly true that many of the right interpretations that we do make are obscured by less well-advised actions, and result in net harm to an individual. Fortunately, natural homeostatic mechan-isms that have evolved over millions of years are in control most of the time and dwarf most of our efforts, good and bad. It is because of all the unknowns and these homeostatic mechanisms that progress notes become the most important part of care, since every step we take must be considered as a first approxima-tion, to be modified as results appear. Not having kept rigorous progress notes (feedback loops) and not having the tools to work more precisely with our lan-guage, our options, and our results, have led most of us to live with all sorts of illusions—one of which is that other people think of entities in the same way we do. Another illusion that has been fostered with serious consequences is that thinking in medicine that is rational and logical within a small number of known, stated variables continues to be rational and defensible when applied to a unique human being who contains many more relevant variables (structures and processes) than were ever considered when the "rational" diagnosis or treatment was conceived.

It is because of these facts that seemingly irrational ideas in medicine could, from the total point of view, be more rational than the so-called "scientific rational" ones. An Indian medicine man or an acupuncturist could be setting into motion a series of complicated interactions that have evolved over millions of years, which in turn deal more effectively with a problem than the "scientific" specialist, because of the breadth of context in which actions are taken.

Indeed, we may be on the threshold of understanding many processes at the level of the mind, brain, and spirit that have heretofore escaped us. It is through this new understanding that we may well see linkages between traditional oriental medicine, western medicine, and medicine of the American Indian.

Modern communication tools, particularly the computer, can help solve these problems of complexity and context, and it is our obligation to use them and then communicate to patients exactly where the boundaries are between our knowledge and our ignorance. By getting command of these details, we can build a system in which problems can be more precisely defined. Students will not flounder so long before they begin to help us solve problems, because we will be better able to communicate to them the frontiers of our knowledge. We should go out of our way to delineate the boundaries between understanding and ignorance and clearly delineate the grey areas in between and label them as "hypotheses." The emphasis should be on methods of recordkeeping and data handling, whereby our first approximations can be either supported or rejected, and we can slowly boot-strap our way to a better understanding. Medical education got too deeply into the business of telling students and patients answers before they honestly revealed to both groups the boundaries of our knowledge and the massiveness of our ignorance. Expectations of patients as they seek help from medical providers must be shaped realistically. They, more than anyone in the system, must understand their own uniqueness, the complexity of the healing process, and the potential for manmade interventions to run the gamut from superficial and irrelevant, through perfectly focused or life-saving, to disastrously inappropriate and dangerous.

Two principles are implicit in the above:

1. Single classification systems frequently are not of universal utility. To group objects or diseases or anything on the basis of one characteristic will never create groupings that are precisely appropriate for another characteristic.

2. It has always been accepted that groupings of characteristics under a single name are necessary for practical purposes of management of common "problems" and for organizing our knowledge about specific relationships among "problems." Also, by focusing on a few variables and assuming all else to

be similar and constant, statistical studies can be done on large numbers of patients with similar problems. The price we pay for such statistical knowledge is a certain amount of fiction in our conclusions about given individuals, because the "constants" assumed are not constant and can vary a great deal in any given individual. The necessity for groupings can be greatly decreased as we more carefully delineate structures and processes.

A SYSTEM FOR PROBLEM SOLVING

We can now discuss problem solving and who should be taught what in terms of the above system and philosophy. For those derangements in structure and process that are definite and have clear-cut treatments such as a broken leg in an otherwise healthy person, we need good equipment and good technicians to correct the known derangements. There is no evidence that anything behond natural desire to help, manual dexterity, and practice with tools and procedures are necessary for the best possible results. Broad knowledge and theoretical understanding may underly the design of the tools and procedures, but they are not prerequisite to successful application.

For the medical providers who deal with defined problems in otherwise healthy people, it is pointless and perhaps even counterproductive to insist they spend long years of schooling memorizing information in the name of giving them understanding. In the first place, they usually do not really understand the issues without experience, and they do not remember what they learn anyway. What is essential is that they first have experience solving the problems in a disciplined apprenticeship system. A certain percentage will naturally seek deeper understanding and even design new approaches, but it is unlikely that sort of progress will be brought about by formal education and complicated credential requirements.

For those problems in medicine in which the derangements in structure and process are not so definite, such as abdominal pain or a sore shoulder, it is a matter of taking the symptoms and signs determined on initial examination, developing a list of possible causes, and then systematically matching the data on a given patient against each possible cause until either a diagnosis is made or more diagnostic tests are clearly indicated. In this area, the mystique of medicine has developed and flourished. It has been considered the art of medicine to elicit findings, mentally recall complete lists of possible causes, and then state a diagnosis and plan without ever having to defend one's logic in a rigorous manner. When logicians look at this process critically, they find that experts often cannot be told from nonexperts, and the variation in procedures and outcomes from one physician to another is very great indeed.

When one looks at what we have been expecting medical providers to do in their heads, it is apparent that the best possible problem solving in these complex situations exceeds the capacity of the average human mind. The mind can neither remember all of the possibilities nor extemporaneously analyze the data to choose among them. It is true that the mind is enormously capable of recognizing patterns in a second if it has seen them many times before and if the pattern is presented to the eye and mind in a highly organized state, as it is, for example, in a familiar face. But if a mind is asked to create patterns after it gets data piece by piece as a prerequisite to recognition, then it is ineffective. It is in this area that computers can help. They can be programmed to seek the appropriate data, organize it quickly, and at a minimum present it in recognizable patterns to the eye for easy recognition and matching or at a maximum do a series of computations and present an ordered list of probabilities to the provider. To be done rigorously, however, this presentation requires data on procedures we do not have and more computer time for calculating than is available.

Much of the time and money that now go into making a "physician" are expended in trying to program the mind (the human computer) to do these tasks. It is expensive to try this way. If teaching can be thought of as programming the human computer, we must remind ourselves that each student brings different hardware to the task, the software he has already developed is usually unknown to the teacher, basic computing facilities are inadequate, and his printer (the handwriting) often is completely out of order. The question is being asked more and more insistently: Why do we even try to teach some of the things we do? Why don't we start with computers in the first place?

Although more and more data are accumulating that demonstrate empirically that computers can outperform human memory and analytical capacities, an examination of the requirements of some simple problems in medicine would have proved it to us. For example, a person with a painful shoulder can have remarkably correct conclusions drawn among ten or twelve possibilities if the results of twelve carefully performed maneuvers on physical examination (looking for pain, for weakness, for limitation of movement on each) are carefully analyzed. But the mind fails at this in most instances, because it forgets some of the maneuvers or diseases, it performs the maneuvers inadequately, or it gets confused as to how to draw the proper conclusion from the large number of combinations of positive findings that suggest each disorder. Once the public understands these simple points they will be less willing to accept credentials alone as a guarantee of adequate performance, even in a minor illness. For those problems, such as a painful shoulder or abdominal pain, where evidence at first is indirect, details are numerous, and analysis complex, the patient must eventually seek help from highly organized systems of care, not single individuals.

We are at a crossroads in the development of medical practice. When physicians began to struggle to extract the right answer from the skillful handling of many variables, each of which was cheaply and simply obtained by history and physical examination, they had at least two alternatives: they could seek the help of machines to manage the many variables simply acquired on history, physical examination, and basic laboratory data; or they could abandon rigorous interpretation of those variables and go on after new and frequently more risky and expensive tests in the hope that they as individual providers would find one that would give them an absolute answer without a lot of analytical thought. Thus, to try to find the major single test, more and more x-rays, CAT scans, and complicated procedures have been done in the pursuit of everyday medical problems. Following this course for the problem "shoulder pain," the provider would abandon the twelve maneuvers on physical examination (if he ever knew them in the first place) and simply order an x-ray of the shoulder. The trouble with this course is that we endow the x-ray with a capacity to find soft tissue difficulties that it was never designed to do, but the report saying the shoulder is normal is often transmitted to the patient, who is thus made to feel that really nothing is wrong with him. He silently leaves in dismay and suffers with his symptoms and dysfunction because we couldn't manage the procurement and analysis of many simple details, but preferred to work as specialists in a limited context.

The narrower the context and the less data available, the more dependent one is on intuitive leaps or probabilities based on heterogeneous populations of people. Careful matching of all of a patient's characteristics to each patient in a study, rather than just looking at the bottom line in some journal article, can be tedious but very productive. Careful matching of many details might show that a patient is much closer to the 5% who died than to the 95% who survived when all characteristics are compared. For that individual, the use of the 5% figure in any calculation is deceptive. Up until now, careful matching has been neglected for several reasons: (1) data from patient records and from literature have not been available; (2) there has not been common language for the data that are available; (3) the data have not been in electronic form for rapid comparison; and (4) the role of the patient on his own behalf has never been emphasized. In regard to point 4, the patient, who is peculiarly well equipped by motivation, time, and detailed knowledge of many factors in his own life, can be very helpful in the matching process, if he is given the tools to be an active member of the team that cares for him. A patient's previous experience with drugs is particularly valuable, and should always take precedence over any notions we have about a drug that are based on statistical information from large populations.

We simply cannot calculate our way out of a tough position if the basis for our difficulty is paucity, disorganization, and inaccessibility of data and lack of time and motivation to extract as much as possible from that data. It is pathetic, if not scandalous, how crippled the whole field of medicine is because it will not take vigorous, global action in the management of all the data on which rational behavior in medicine depends. The humanitarian and economic consequences are enormous.

How unwise it is to blame technology in general for the increasing costs of medicine without commensurate benefit, when we can use technology to manage information to control all the specialized technology that has been applied to the diagnosing and treating of human illness.

The patient who has symptoms and signs but no diagnosis, after pursuit of a problem by either an individual provider or a whole system of care, needs above all the assurance that all the right variables were considered, all the appropriate possibilities were ruled out, and a systematic plan for observation was established. The public will realize more and more that no single human mind, no matter how dedicated, on its own in a busy office or hospital, can provide this assurance. Furthermore, no training program using present educational premises and tools can ever get the unaided mind to perform in such a fashion.

For patients with known diagnoses of chronic disease, the issue is not how much training or credentials physicians have, but when we will invest in the right guidance tools for people who are dedicated to helping others, who charge little, and who are steady over the long haul. These patients need help with the everyday unsophisticated, daily details of patient care; it is this meticulous, daily attention to details that spells the difference between success and failure far more often than any brilliant insight by a highly credentialed person at one point in the course of a twenty-year disease. The book by Fred Cook about his wife, who died after a long chronic illness and major heart surgery because a simple detail about anticoagulants was not taken care of, is testimony to this fact.

Sloppy records and verbal transmission of detail in patient management account for far more failures than the medical profession likes to admit. We do not even have the feedback loops that would make us change our misguided ways. The usual forces of economics do nothing to help us, for a physician gets paid as much for wrong decisions as for right ones—perhaps even more, since the uncured patient will return, with a second payment.

The more our knowledge of structures and processes grows and the more capable we become of monitoring them, the more organized we can become in building good guidance systems for the management of patients. We remember the kindness and compassion under adversity of old-fashioned doctors; we can still have these fine characteristics, but we should not imply that expensive training programs are necessary to develop them. To the extent that this image is that of "the physician," then it is the skillful nurse, the caring neighbor, the skilled technician, and the constantly present spouse who is the "true physician." The M.D. who appears for a moment to write an order or do a technical procedure and then leave is but a technician and should be recognized as such.

PROMIS AS A GUIDANCE SYSTEM

Having stated some of the philosophical notions that underlie PROMIS, we now must translate these notions to the real world of medical practice and medical education. I shall do that not by starting with present details of medical practice, but with an analogy. From the analogy, we can consider PROMIS in its present form and PROMIS in terms of future goals.

The Analogy: The world of travel for the average individual.

Any individual in this country is free to travel any way he pleases. He does not need to take travel courses or pay high prices to consultants who are specialists on the details for getting from one specific point on the map to the other. (There are no specialists who, for example, passed their specialty boards in Indiana by memorizing the roads, intersections, facilities, caution signs, and red lights in the state of Indiana.) Nor is it necessary for the traveler to consult a generalist in travel who helps him conceive new trips and work out the details of taking them. Nor does he, unless he is unusually compulsive, feel any need to memorize the trips of others, follow exact pathways taken by others, or travel under precisely the same conditions as others. He could not if he tried.

What does he do? He learns from a very early age that there is a system for travel that is made up of roads, places, maps, vehicles, policemen, other travelers, laws, risks, and benefits. He learns to travel within that system, setting his own goals in terms of his own values. The final details of his pathways are only known after the input stops, and most of the time those pathways are unique to him and to the conditions at the time. Even when he repeats the same overall trip, he does not try to remember the details or to repeat the details of the last trip since he cannot duplicate the conditions of the last trip.

A map can be full of detail and yet be used effectively by many people, because an individual approaches a map with a goal in mind: once he finds two points on the map—where he is and the destination—the complexity melts away; all the details not involved with his options for that trip are ignored. He is relaxed because he knows he does not have to memorize the map; he can look as often as he wants and when he needs to. He does not pay for each look—just 50 cents for the map and an infinite number of looks. What he expects from society are good roads and good maps, for which he pays taxes and a willingness to function within the traffic rules and other laws that allow the system to accommodate many individuals for unique trips and goals.

Highway engineers and mapmakers provide good maps and roads without ever dictating the full details of any single user's trips or goals. They do watch the use of various options by large numbers of people and fix them when observations suggest it to be appropriate. They can widen a bridge and improve everyone's travel across that bridge regardless of where each crosser of the bridge came from or where he is going. Depending on the sophistication of their information system and traffic analyses, they can harvest an enormous amount of information on how options and sequences of options are used. This information is then available to the highway department to devise better options, facilitate the more efficient sequences and inform travelers. Travelers then can integrate the overall information with their unique personal desire and goals.

Not only would it be expensive to try to provide every traveler with a paid travel agent for all travel eventualities, with the traveler in a passive mode much of the time, but it would be impossible to reach the standards of travel that could be achieved by the traveler alone once he is given the right tools, information, and responsibility. This has to be true, because not only is the traveler himself aware at all times of conditions for decision making, but he is also the only one who can determine his goals and meet his own desires in the long run. If he is willing to turn even his goals and desires over to someone else, he has degenerated into severe dependency. Those who created that dependency with the motive of helping him have in the long run destroyed him as an effective individual in society. Society itself suffers when it is made up of large numbers of such dependent individuals.

PROMIS AND GUIDANCE

With the foregoing principles and analogy in mind, what has PROMIS built and what are its goals? PROMIS is the computerized problem-oriented medical information system that allows one to monitor the structures and processes of individuals and then intervene in a defined manner. It also allows individuals to convert their own perceptions of problems into the language of the system so that the various options for dealing with the problem are available; users can then make choices in the context of their own unique lives. It is in effect an electronic medical map for all travelers through the medical landscape. But it is even more than that, because by coding choices and making all the electronic data available for population studies in a continuous dynamic way, the system can improve through usage. This is a merging, electronically, of patient care data, a library system of medical options, and a population study system that makes the patient care data evolve over time, to become the principal source of the library system itself. It is impossible to convey the technology and philosophy of PROMIS in a brief prose description. All those who have interacted with PROMIS in its present form have stated that merely reading about it and discussing it are inadequate. The closest one can come on paper is to print representative sequences of displays, as we have done in at least two detailed articles.[4,5] What follows here is a limited introduction; the reader who has greater interest should visit the PROMIS Laboratory.

Figures 1 and 2 show the beginning of the system for getting the initial data base from which problem statements can be written. One touches "Data Base" on the "Add To" side of the screen in Figure 1 and proceeds through the choices on the display that immediately appears in Figure 2. As one gets into the specific content of the displays, such as descriptors of a cough or details of a heart examination, no two patients elicit the same sequence of choices through the displays because no two patients have the same combination of derangements of structures and processes. Medical providers are available to help the patients with those steps they cannot do for themselves. As computerized guidance and problem solving systems are developed and integrated into our work and early education, more and more patients will be able to negotiate many of the

```
B    , Oren    . . . .
                      IIIB    , Oren    . . . . . . . . . .  M 63 000-000-0...
-- ------------------------------4 Phases of Medical Action----------------------
         --------- RETRIEVE:  ----------          ---------- ADD TO:  ------------

         -Data Base    -Exp-                      -Data Base    -Exp-

         -Problem List                            -Problem List    -Exp-

         -Initial Plans                           -Initial Plans    -Exp-

         -Progress Notes    -Exp-                 -Progress Notes
         -----------------------------            ------------------------------
         -Other retrievals                        -Other Actions

         -Flowsheets          -Graphs            -Emergency Management    -Exp-

         -Retrieve from past admissions           -Consult reply     -Attending note

         -To printer                              -Audit
------------------------------------------------------------------------------
-Choose other ward / other functions     -Choose other patient on this ward
Lawrence L. Weed----------------------------------------------------------64.101----
Eras Sen          Review Erase 1  -Opts- Confirm -Help-                Retriev
- -- - - - - - - - - - - - - - - - <END> - - - - - - - - - - - - - - - - - -
```

Figure 1

```
B    , Oren    . . . .
                      B    , Oren  . . . . . . . . . .  M 63 000-000-0...
----------------------------------------Data Base----------------------------------

-Data to collect on admission

-Patient's sickness ("major complaints")    -Exp-

-Health care profile    -Exp-

-Social profile    -Exp-

History data base:    -Exp-    -questionnaire          -other additions

-Physical exam data base    -Exp-

-Laboratory data base    -Exp-

Present illness:    -Exp-      -begin new PI    -Exp-    -add to existing PI

                                                            -Next Frame-
Lawrence L. Weed------------------------------------------------------------64.131----
Eras Sen Ret/Add Review Erase 1  -Opts- Confirm -Help-                Retriev
- - - - - - - - - - - - - - - - - <END> - - - - - - - - - - - - - - - - - -
```

Figure 2

steps on their own; not because they learned medicine; but because the system can lead them step by step to very high levels of sophistication in the problem-solving process. The user is the needed expert on the "conditions at the time" (he or she is living under them) and on his or her own goals. The system is the expert on the choices available at each step; and the system through analysis of its own usage can keep updating these choices—removing bad ones and introducing new ones. The number of people maintaining and building such a guidance system needs to be only a small fraction of all those using it with or without theoretical understanding of it. For each cartographer, there are literally millions of travelers.

```
B     Oren  . . . .
                              B   , Oren  . . . . . . . . . .  M 63 000-000-0...
----------------------------------4 Phases of Medical Action----------------------------
       --------- RETRIEVE: ---------              ---------- ADD TO: -----------

       -Data Base   -Exp-                         -Data Base    -Exp-

       -Problem List                              -Problem List    -Exp-

       -Initial Plans                             -Initial Plans   -Exp-

       -Progress Notes   -Exp-                    -Progress Notes
       --------------------------------          --------------------------------
       -Other retrievals                          -Other Actions

       -Flowsheets          -Graphs               -Emergency Management   -Exp-

       -Retrieve from past admissions             -Consult reply    -Attending note

       -To printer                                -Audit
----------------------------------------------------------------------------------------
-Choose other ward / other functions    -Choose other patient on this ward
Lawrence L. Weed----------------------------------------------------------64.101----
Eras Sen         Review Erase 1  -Opts- Confirm -Help-                   Retriev
- - - - - - - - - - - - - - - - - - - <END> - - - - - - - - - - - - - - - - - -
```

Figure 3

```
Blow, Oren  . . . .
                              |||Blow, Oren  . . . . . . . . .  M 63 000-000-0...
------------------------------------------Problem List----------------------------------

-- Formulate Problem List --            -- Change Problem List --
   Identify abnormalities:  -Exp-          -restate active problem    -Exp-

      -from Data Base                       -change temp to major    -Exp-

   Synthesize abnormalities   -Exp-        -combine problems    -Exp-
      and add to Problem List:
      -major problem    -Def-              -discard problem    -Exp-

      -temporary problem  -Def-            -inactivate problem   -Exp-

      -inactive problem  -Def-             -activate problem    -Exp-

      -add present illness to Problem List


-Prob List-                                                  -Next Frame-
------------------------------------Level of Major Problem-------------------------------

-- A Primary Finding --                  -- A Primary Finding (cont.) --
   -Symptom                                 -Drug/surgery/other procedure   -Def-

   -Habit/life style finding               -S/P surgery/other procedure    -Def-

   -Social problem                          -Health maintenance,

   -Environmental problem                   -Incomplete Data Base,

   -Physical exam finding
                                         -- A Synthesis of Findings --
   -Lab/x-ray/other test finding            -Psychiatric/behavioral problem

   -Family history of   -Def-               -Physiological abnormality

   -H/O problem   -Def-                     -Medical/surgical diagnosis


Lawrence L. Weed-------------------------------------------------------73.3100---
Eras Sen          Review Erase 1  -Opts-            -Help-  -Info-       Retriev
- - - - - - - - - - - - - - - - - - - <END> - - - - - - - - - - - - - - - - -
```

Figure 4

Having developed a data base, the users (usually a patient together with a medical provider) are confronted with Figure 3 on a computer screen. They make the choice "Add To the Problem List" and then immediately see Figure 4. This display accommodates almost any level of sophistication, allowing one to state a problem to be solved at a very low level of abstraction, or at a very high level. Whatever level is chosen, the system will then provide guidance for solving the problem from that level on.

As stated above, it is not possible to put on paper all the possible sequences that follow the various choices on Figure 4 (there are literally thousands of displays in the computer); suffice it to say that options are available and the problem list can be quickly generated and stored, itself becoming available on the screen.

These initial steps in establishing a data base and forming the problem list require that all providers within the system use the same data structures so that their efforts will be cumulative. The defined data base from which the initial problem set will be derived emphasizes the issue of "problem stating" as opposed to "problem solving." As Bernanos has said: "The worst, the most corrupting, of all lies is to misstate the problem." Or looked at in a more positive way, as Max Planck said: "You are 95% of the way to a solution when you precisely state the problem." Asking a provider for the defined data base is equivalent to asking her for the universe of data from which she pieces out her first problem statements, and for the context in which any single one of the problems is going to be solved. A solution that looks good in one context can look very bad in another. The decision to pin a broken hip can look good if that is the only problem on the list. If we broaden the context and add severe heart failure to the list, then the solution of an operative procedure looks very bad. In a world of specialists and many medical encounters, too many people are either acting in too narrow a context or wasting time starting from scratch in getting a broad data base. There should be a single, complete data base available at all times to everyone. At present individual providers work alone using different terms and different records and their efforts are not cumulative either for the patient or for medical science. Many of the most difficult problems now facing medicine, such as carcinogenesis, cancer cures, and degenerative diseases, require cumulative information in a broad context over a long period of time and problem solving by coordinated groups of people of different skills using the most sophisticated information tools available. Tough problems in contemporary medicine will not be easily solved by the brilliant insights and efforts of a single unaided mind in a short period of time. Even in short-term problems and in episodic care there is no greater source of confusion in the practice of medicine than allowing providers of all sorts to define and state problems in any context and subject to practically no discipline whatsoever. In addition to the varied personnel and no rules, the environment itself has an extraordinary effect. The same patient seen in a generalist's office, a specialist's office, an emergency room, or on a hospital ward (after being admitted over the low threshold of a particular provider) will have four different problem lists, perhaps so different that they suggest that four different patients were seen. In hospitals, doctors, particularly those in training, define problems in terms of what they think that particular environment requires and expects rather than in terms of what the patient's disorder actually is. An almost off-hand five-minute discussion in a hallway as to whether to admit a patient has a profound effect on not only what the problem list will look like but how each problem will be pursued. The system should be far more uniform, less provincial in time and space, and less at the whim of individual problem solvers operating off the tops of their heads.

Returning to our computerized guidance system and the patient's problem list, which is immediately available on a touch sensitive screen, planning for each problem can now be discussed. After a problem is picked, Figure 5 appears on the screen. The details of how to negotiate this set of options for planning and the explanation of each of the choices will not be discussed here (see reference 4). Also, as readers pursue the examples below, they should be reminded that although the structures of PROMIS are elucidated using specific content, I do not mean to imply that PROMIS now contains content to this level of detail in all problems. However, the structures are there and the capacity to be cumulative has been developed. We shall focus on the choice "Investigate for causes of the problem." Depending on the problem, different strategies can appear after making this choice. Regardless of the strategy chosen, a list of causes for that particular problem is always available to the user. Some of the causes are expressed in clinical terms that have grown up over the years—such as diabetes causing the polyuria. Others are expressed in structure-process terms familiar to basic biological science—hyperaldosteronism causing the hypokalemia. Figure 6 is a typical causes list for epigastric pain. Figure 7 is a branch from one of the choices

```
   B    , Oren
B . . . . . M 63 000-000-0...   |Initial Plan  |  1. Heart failure, compensated.
----------------Initial Plan for Diagnosis, Physiologic abnormality--------------
                                                          -Exp for Plans

-Aims for problem management            -Emergency management

-Assess function of related body systems

 Assess and follow:      -sickness     -disabilities      -course of problem

-Investigate problem and etiology

-Watch for/prevent complications of problem

 Treat & monitor Rx:     -sickness     -disabilities      -disease process


                          -Choose another problem

                                               -Next Frame-
Lawrence L. Weed-----------------------------------------------------64.171----
Eras Sen Ret/Add Review Erase 1   -Opts- Confirm -Help-  -Info-      Retriev
- - - - - - - - - - - - - - - - - <END> - - - - - - - - - - - - - - - - - -
```

Figure 5

```
---------------Epigastric pain: causes-------------------------------
-- Urgent or common --            -- By body system --
  -myocardial infarction (1,2)      -general/systemic

  -angina pectoris (1,2)            -respiratory

  -aortic dissection (1,2)          -cardiovascular

  -ectopic pregnancy (1,1)          -gastrointestinal

  -botulism (1,2)                   -renal/urinary

  -acute pancreatitis (2,4)         -musculoskeletal

  -peptic ulcer (3,4)               -hematological

  -functional dyspepsia (3,4)       -endocrine/metabolic

                                   -Next Frame- -More chcs-
Lawrence L. Weed-------------------- Lookup mode --------------------85.263----
Eras Sen    Pop    Review Erase 1  -Opts- -Exit-  -Help-  -Info-  -Refs-  Retriev
- - - - - - - - - - - - - - - - - <END> - - - - - - - - - - - - - - - - - -
```

Figure 6

```
                      Problem name: epigastric pain...
              --------Epigastric pain: cardiovascular causes----------

-hepatic artery aneurysm (1,3)        -portal vein obstruction (1,1)

-acute pericarditis (1,3)             -acute rheumatic carditis (1,1)

-hepatic vein obstruction (1,3)

-myocardial infarction (1,2)

-pericardial effusion (1,2)

-aortic dissection (1,2)

-angina pectoris (1,2)

-Type in cause

                                   -Next Frame-
Lawrence L. Weed-------------------- Lookup mode --------------------85.273----
Eras Sen    Pop    Review Erase 1  -Opts- -Exit-  -Help-  -Info-  -Refs-  Retriev
- - - - - - - - - - - - - - - - - <END> - - - - - - - - - - - - - - - - - -
```

Figure 7

(cardiovascular causes) on Figure 6. Figures 8 and 9 are structure-process definitions on the problems allergic asthma and myasthenia gravis. The upper part of the structure-process definitions merge into the clinical definition of disease and one can have the clinical world and the basic science world beginning to communicate with one another in rather precise ways.

One can systematically go through the causes list, touching each cause and getting an array for guidance for ruling out that cause, as seen in Figure 10 (an array for investigating iron deficiency). Or instead of going down through a long list of causes step by step, one can be directed to one or two causes by cues from the patient's unique problem list or data base or by one's own intuition based on

```
                        Problem name: allergic asthma
              ----Allergic asthma: structure-process definition-----

-- Level --           -- Structure --               -- Process --

Body system       Respiratory system           Airways obstruction

Organ             Bronchi                       Spasmodic narrowing
                                                Mucus plugging
                                                Edema of mucosa

Cell              Mast cell                     Release of mediators
                  Smooth muscle cell            Contraction
                  Capillary endothelium         Incr. permeability
                  Mucus glands                  Incr. secretion
                  Irritant receptors            Stimulation -> vagal reflex response
                  Eosinophils                   (h)Release of inhibitors
                                                (h)Phagocytosis of free mast cell
                                                    granules
Subcellular

Molecule          IgE                           Binding to mast cell in combination
                                                    with allergen
                  Histamine, SRS-S,             Stimulation of bronchial smooth mus-
                   (h)bradykinin                    cle, mucosa, and irritant receptors
                  (h)Prostaglandins             Potentiation of action of histamine,
                                                    SRS-A
                  ECF-A                          Stimulation of migration of eosino-
                                                    phils
                  (h)Arysulfatase B             Inactivation of SRS-A
                  (h)Histaminase                Inactivation of histamine



                                                -Prev chcs-  -Next Frame-
Lawrence L. Weed-------------------- Lookup mode --------------------81.1523-2-
Eras Sen   Pop   Review Erase 1  -Opts-  -Exit-   -Help-   -Info-   -Refs-   Retriev
- - - - - - - - - - - - - - - - - - <END> - - - - - - - - - - - - - - - - - - -
```

Figure 8


```
              -----Myasthenia gravis: structure-process definition----

-- Level --           -- Structure --               -- Process --

Body system       Neuromuscular

Organ             Voluntary muscles             Weakness and fatigability

Cell              Neuromuscular junction        Failure of transmission of nerve
                                                impulse

Subcellular       Muscle cell end-plate         Reduction in amplitude of end-plate
entity                                          potentials

Molecule          Acetylcholine receptor        Reduction in available receptors on
                   glycoprotein                     post-synaptic membrane
                  Antibody to acetyl-           (h)Incr. degradation of receptors
                   choline receptor             (h)Blockade of active site

                                                -Next Frame-
Lawrence L. Weed-------------------- Lookup mode --------------------81.1648---
Eras Sen   Pop   Review Erase 1  -Opts-  -Exit-   -Help-   -Info-   -Refs-   Retriev
- - - - - - - - - - - - - - - - - - <END> - - - - - - - - - - - - - - - - - - -
```

Figure 9

FIG. 10a

```
---------Iron deficiency: investigation---------
      Data        Utility      -Exp      Price      Time      Side effects
-----------------|----- Rules for:------|--------|------------|----------------
 -Hx             | -likely present    |    -    |    -       |    -
                 |                    |         |            |
 -hemoglobin or  | -likely absent     | $4.00   | 10 minutes | minimal
    hematocrit   |                    |         |            |
 -rbc smear      | -absence           | $4.00   | 10 minutes | minimal
                 |                    |         |            |
  rbc indices    | -absence, likely   | $4.00   |  1 day     | minimal
                 |    present         |         |            |
  stool occult   | -likely present    | $3.00   | 10 minutes | none
    blood        |                    |         |            |
 -serum iron     | -absent, likely    | $5.00   | 2-5 days   | minimal
                 |    present         |         |            |
 -transferrin    | -absent, likely    |$10.00   | 2-5 days   | minimal
    saturation   |    present         |         |            |
                 |                    |         |       -Flowsheet    -Def-
  iron therapy   | -likely absent,    | $5.00   | 10 days    | minimal
                 |    present         |         |            |
 -cobalt         | -absence           |     Not available at MCHV
    excretion    |                    |         |            |
  bone marrow    | -absence, presence |$40.00   |  2 days    | moderate
                 |                    |         |            |
  liver biopsy   | -absence, presence |   Not orderable for this work-up
                 |                    |         |            |
```

FIG. 10b   Investigate for Iron deficiency: transferrin saturation

1. Obtain a   serum iron   and   total iron binding capacity.

   transferrin saturation (%) = serum iron X 100/TIBC

-2. Interpret results

FIG. 10c
```
Doc:  307              Supporting documentation                    Page  1
Fact 135.00355
    IF transferrin saturation is > 16 % THEN
       Iron deficiency is absent.
    OTHERWISE IF < 5 % THEN
       The likelihood of iron deficiency is very high.
    OTHERWISE
       The findings are consistent with but not diagnostic of iron deficiency.
    Refs:
 Fact 135.00303
    A transferrin saturation of less than 16% (with an average of 7%) is
    a manifestation of iron deficiency that is always present.

 Fact 135.00333
    Dx: iron deficiency
    Mf: transferrin saturation less than 5%
    P[Dx|Mf] = high
- - - - - - - - - - - - - - - <END> - - - - - - - - - - - - - - - - - - - - -
```

Guidance in investigating the possible cause of a problem is displayed to the user in an array as in (a). The array presents ways in which iron deficiency can be "ruled out" or "ruled in." Frame (b) is one such way, using transferrin saturation whose interpretation is presented in (c).

Figure 10

vast experience in an area. For those who do not want to go through all the causes and who do not trust their memories and intuition, there is help for ordering causes. One is guided through a series of choices of basic data base facts pertaining to the problem. The system immediately does two things with each selection: it first records the positive finding, so we have the history for further management and statistical studies on populations; and it shows immediately the diseases that should cross one's mind as the positive finding appears. The system then creates patterns from these potential causes that pile up as one proceeds through the choices appropriate to that problem. By glancing at the pattern one can zero in on the few arrays that deserve detailed consideration, so that precise matching can occur for this unique patient. The time required for precise matching is nothing compared with the time, expense, and risk of x-rays and surgical procedures that are carelessly begun because of probabilities based on a few parameters, when one could have had far more certainty based on detailed matching.

CONCLUSION

Going back to our original question: "Can you teach problem solving?" it should be clear that more and more problem solving will be the result of disciplined use of problem-solving guidance systems. We cannot expect professors at MIT to run all the Three Mile Island type nuclear plants, but we can expect them to build guidance systems that guarantee that the actions of those who do run it conform to the logical analysis they would provide if they were there and had the time to do and analyze everything themselves. Since we all have to live with the actions of all of us, not just the actions of the sophisticated and the educated, it is imperative that problem solvers at all levels be coupled to the best thinking available for that problem. Teaching and education as we have known them are not up to that task and have obviously failed because they did not recognize the limitations of the human mind in the face of rising complexity at the time action is required. We got to the moon because computers and guidance systems were preprogrammed, not because bright people tried problem solving as the rocket was on its way.

Figure 11 gives the reader a glimpse of what is immediately available in the system. Figure 12 shows the sequence of choices one can go through for population studies. One can then use the statistical package in the system to analyze the data and modify options within the system as the data indicate.

After reading the above and some of the bibliography[5-8] one gets at least some feeling for how we have tried, through structured input, definitions of terms, and referenced options, to make explicit the present state of medicine and medical practice as it straddles the clinical world, which deduces much from the outside of "the black box," and the scientific world of medicine, which speaks in terms of defined structures and processes. Some disorders or entities in the PROMIS system are still defined in very old-fashioned terms and their treatments are based on statistical analyses of clinical results using drugs and procedures whose mechanism of action are unknown at the basic level of structures and processes. Other entities are at the other end of the spectrum, where both they and their treatments are related and pinpointed in specific biochemical and physiological terms. It will be a long, long time before we can scan the body at regular intervals and immediately print out a list of the precise structures and

```
------------------Other retrievals------------------
                                -- Administrative retrievals --
-emergency room problem abstract    -Patient charges    -Int-

-emergency room recycled record     -Pharmacy charges    -Int-

                                    -Encounters

-all procedures, cycled by order    -on-line administrative data

-reports without orders, chronologically    -all administrative data


-HLA match

-Determine metabolic requirements    -Ref-

                                    -Begn chcs-  -Next Frame-  -More chcs-
Lawrence L. Weed------------------------ Lookup mode ----------------------64.507-3--
Eras Sen   Pop    Review Erase 1  -Opts-  -Exit-  -Help-              Retriev
- - - - - - - - - - - - - - - - - - - <END> - - - - - - - - - - - - - - - - - - -
                 ------------------Other retrievals------------------
                                    -reason for admission

-orders and reports                 -abstract for a problem:    -Exp-

-Calculate body surface area    -Exp-    -lab data base & obj for all probs

-current aims for active prob    -Exp-   -vital signs

-current condition of active prob        -consult notes    -Exp-

-total problem list                 -attending notes

                                    -present illnesses assoc w/ problem
 All parts of the record
-arranged in standard fashion    -Exp-    -Status of investigations

-arranged in chronologic order       -audit notes
------------------Other retrievals------------------
    -pharmacy billing

    -pharmacy billing, orders only    -countersigned orders

    -drugs given with charge code    -all contingency plans    -Exp-

    -discharge summary    -Exp-        -all recommendations

    -Objectives during Hosp., all active probs

    -person coord. mgmt., all active probs    -valuables list

    -current goal, all active probs        -data base cycled, prog notes chron

    -mgmt limits, all active problems     -Hosp record with PN/IP chron

    -patient education given            -problem specific data chron

                                    -Prev chcs-  -Next Frame-  -More chcs-
Lawrence L. Weed------------------------ Lookup mode ----------------------64.507-2--
Eras Sen   Pop    Review Erase 1  -Opts-  -Exit-  -Help-              Retriev
- - - - - - - - - - - - - - - - - - - <END> - - - - - - - - - - - - - - - - - - -
```

Figure 11

processes that are out of adjustment, along with the recommended means of fixing them—much time is spent now trying to deduce basic derangements indirectly through the sophisticated analysis of all sorts of combinations of symptoms and signs that are far removed from the original difficulty. And it will certainly

```
------------------Population Studies: Index of Functions-----------------
Patient Set Operations:              Extraction of data from patient records:
  -Form patient set *  -Exp-            -Define numeric data to collect    -Exp-

  -Display patient set   -Exp-          -Collect numeric data for pt. set

  -Store criteria used to form a set


                                     Problem list studies:
                                       -Determine problem frequencies    -Exp-


-Miscellaneous functions

-Waiting time for population study requests

                                                         -Next Frame-
-------------------Population Studies: Form Patient Set-----------------------


    -Specify criteria for set membership


    -Set consists of a single patient: type in id number


    -Form set from stored criteria




                                                         -Next Frame-
Lawrence L. Weed-------------------------------------------------65.497----
Eras Sen          Review         -Opts-          -Help-
- - - - - - - - - - - - - - - - - <END> - - - - - - - - - - - - - - - -

-------------------------Population study: add to request-------------------
                          Attribute is a:
    -Problem, alpha lookup       -Problem, access by code

    -Procedure, alpha lookup     -Procedure, access by code

    -Set        -Exp-

    -Ward                        -Left parenthesis (start subexpression)

    -Record usage attribute   -Exp-

    -Order, problem condition status    -Exp-


-Review request specifying frames in lookup mode

Lawrence L. Weed-------------------------------------------------65.319----
----------------------Population study: add conjunction------------------


    -none                        -AND

                                 -OR

Lawrence L. Weed-------------------------------------------------65.321----
Eras Sen          Review Erase 1  -Opts-          -Help-
- - - - - - - - - - - - - - - - - <END> - - - - - - - - - - - - - - - -
```

Figure 12

```
-------------------Population Studies : Display Patient Set--------------------

Display:

   -Criteria used to form the set and number of patients in set

   -Names of patients in set, selectable
      [This provides access to records of patients in the set. Selection of
      a patient from this list immediately generates a retrieval of data in
      the record.]


   -Names of patients, to be printed, including names of patients whose
      records are off-line, and optionally including procedure values
      from the procedure value entity file.



                                                              -Next Frame-
Lawrence L. Weed------------------------------------------------------65.463----
Eras Sen              Review Erase 1   -Opts-          --Help--
- - - - - - - - - - - - - - - - - - - <END> - - - - - - - - - - - - - - - - - -
```

Figure 12 (continued)

be a long time before our scans are so complete and precise that we will be tell-ing the patient what symptoms and signs they might expect and how to manage them, instead of hearing the symptom first from the patient and then trying to figure out what is wrong. But patients and new students particularly should un-derstand what is happening to medical science and practice, and with their help we can gain a firmer grip on the information problem and accelerate the whole process of improving the science and practice of medicine. Once every structure and process is coded and every drug and treatment has its mechanism of action coded in terms of those same structures and processes, the correlations possible will be far beyond anything the unaided mind could ever do.

As logic dictates new options, population studies on the data generated can validate or suggest removal of those same options. The system will grow in depth and rigor with use. We shall be able to accommodate to each patient's uniqueness as we slowly gain command over the details of structure and func-tion that determine that uniqueness.

And, finally, if we can develop tools that help us deal successfully with complexity in the field of medicine, those same tools can become the basis of education and problem solving in many areas of our society. If we ever expect to couple the best thinking to the everyday actions of us all, we must abandon many of the previous premises and tools of education, for it is in those false premises and inadequate tools that our real world failures have their deepest roots.

References

1. Castle M, Wilfert CM, Cate TR, Osterhout S. Antibiotic use at Duke University Medical Center. JAMA 1977;237:2819-22.
2. Casscells W, Schoenberger A, Graboys T. Interpretation by physicians of clinical labor-atory results. N Engl J Med 1978;299:999-1000.

3. Elstein AS, Schulman LS, Sprasks SA, et al. Medical problem solving and analysis of clinical reasoning. Cambridge: Harvard University Press, 1978.

4. Weed LL. Appendix 4, an organized approach for dealing with a well defined problem. In: Your health care and how to manage it. Essex Junction, VT: Essex Publishing Company, 1978:200-209.

5. Weed LL and The PROMIS Laboratory Staff. 'Representations of medical knowledge' and PROMIS. In: Orthner FH, ed. Proceedings of The Second Annual Symposium on Computer Application in Medical Care. New York: Institute of Electrical and Electronics Engineers, Inc. (IEEE), 1978:368-400.

6. Schultz JR, Davis LW. The technology of PROMIS. Proceedings of IEEE 1979;67:1237-44.

7. Walton PL, Holland RR, Wolf LI. Medical guidance and PROMIS. COMPUTER Magazine (ISSN 0018-9162). Long Beach, CA: IEEE Computer Society 1979;12:19-27.

8. Wanner JF. Wideband communication system improves response time. Computer Design, December 1978:85-91.

Section V. Tools for Supporting the Decision-Making Process

CHAPTER NINETEEN

Decision Making in Radiology: ROC Curves

Barbara J. McNeil, MD, PhD

The evaluation of new diagnostic procedures is becoming as commonplace as is the evaluation of new therapeutic procedures. And, just as the need to evaluate therapies led to the generation of a variety of new methodologic techniques, the randomized clinical trial being the most common, so too has the need to evaluate diagnostic procedures led to the introduction of a variety of other methodological techniques.[1-3] Some of these are quite familiar to most physicians by now. For example, there has been a flurry of articles recently on Bayes' theorem, decision matrices, and predictive values. Other techniques, borrowed heavily from signal detection theory and cognitive psychology, are just being recognized for their potential. In this chapter we shall spend time on one of these unfamiliar techniques for evaluating new diagnostic technologies; we shall emphasize the use of receiver operating characteristic (ROC) curves in radiology.

BASIC DEFINITIONS

When tests do not have binary outcomes (normal, abnormal) of the type described by a decision matrix but instead have a continuum of values (any one of which can be selected as the boundary between normal and abnormal), the true and false positive ratios vary with the value selected as the cutoff point. Schematically this can be seen by plotting the frequency of a particular test outcome measured along a continuum scale for the normal and diseased individuals. In general, there is almost always considerable overlap between these two distributions. For example, consider the situation in Figure 1. Here, four possible outcomes—true positive (TP) events, false positive (FP) events, true negative (TN) events, and false negative (FN) events—can be graphically depicted as four areas produced by the selection of a cutoff point between the two frequency distributions. For example, if the cutoff point is 50, the sensitivity and the specificity of

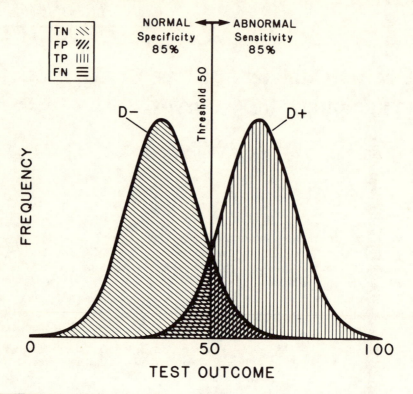

Figure 1. Hypothetical distribution for laboratory tests performed in diseased and normal individuals. On the ordinate is the proportion of patients having a particular laboratory value; the abscissa represents values on a scale from 0 to 100. The left-hand bell-shaped curve describes the distribution of test results in a healthy population whereas the right-hand distribution describes results in a diseased population. The vertical line placed at a test value of 50 indicates the cutoff point used to separate normal from diseased individuals. At that level, the proportion of normal patients with "abnormal" test results is 15% and the proportion of abnormal patients with abnormal test results is 85%.

the test are 85%. If a test result of 55 or more were needed to be considered abnormal, the sensitivity would drop to 65% and the specificity would rise to 95%. In other words, a stricter threshold would allow more of the normal patients to be classified correctly, but would lead to the identification of fewer of the abnormal patients, i.e., a higher specificity but a lower sensitivity.

By plotting different TP and FP ratios as a function of the cutoff point selected it is possible to generate a receiver operating characteristic curve (Figure 2) and display explicitly the tradeoffs involved in the selection of a cutoff point for the separation of normal from diseased patients. Generally cutoff points corresponding to the region in the lower left part of the curve are used with screen-

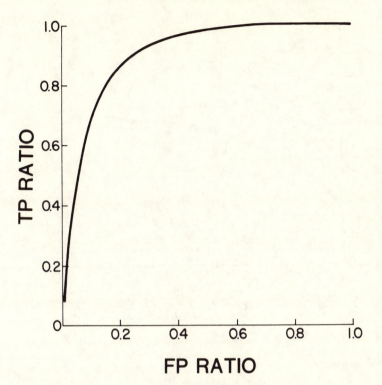

FP RATIO

Figure 2. ROC curve for data in Figure 1. On the ordinate is the true positive ratio and on the abscissa the false positive ratio. As the cutoff point separating normal from abnormal patients rises, the proportion of diseased patients detected drops (true positive ratio); the false positive ratio also drops.

ing tests, where the presence of a large number of false positive tests would lead to a large number of unnecessary secondary confirmatory tests. On the other hand, cutoff points corresponding to the region in the upper right part of the curve are used when a high morbidity is associated with failing to diagnose and treat disease and a low morbidity associated with treating unnecessarily.

Although ROC curves as described above have been used extensively in radiology, as will be described below, they can be used for virtually any test with nonbinary outcomes. For example, stress electrocardiograms can be evaluated in this fashion.[4,5] In this case, correlating ST segment depressions with the presence or absence of coronary artery disease at angiography leads to the ROC curve shown in Figure 3. It was created by considering abnormal only ST segment depressions corresponding first to 2.5 mm or more, then 2.0 mm or more, then 1.5 mm or more, and, finally, all depressions greater than or equal to 1.0 mm. With this format, we can clearly see that even with the most liberal of interpretive

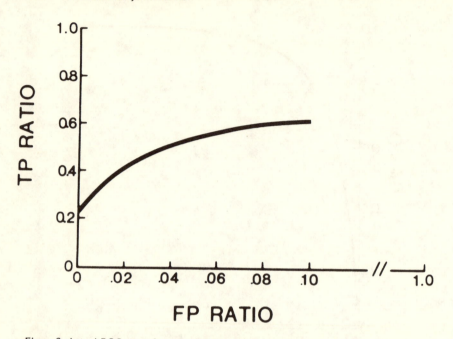

Figure 3. Actual ROC curve for data on ECG stress testing (reference 4). The ordinate is the true positive ratio and the abscissa is the false positive ratio. At the extreme left when only strict criteria for abnormality were used (that is, depressions greater than or equal to 2.5 mm), the false positive ratio is virtually 0, but the sensitivity is similarly low (21%). At the right, with more liberal criteria involving test results called abnormal with smaller depressions, both the true positive and false positive ratios rise. (Reprinted with permission from Parisi, A. F., and Tow, D. E., Noninvasive approaches to cardiovascular diagnosis, New York: Appleton-Century-Crofts, 1978:226.

criteria (rightmost part of the curve), only 62 percent of patients with coronary artery disease are detected by this test; at the same time about 10 percent of patients without coronary artery disease will also have abnormal tests results. If we use the most strict criteria available (only depressions > 2.5 mm are abnormal), represented at the leftmost part of the curve, the false positive rate drops practically to zero, but so does the sensitivity; only 21 percent of patients with coronary artery disease are detected.

ROC CURVES AND IMAGE EVALUATION

By far and away the most common and probably the most important use of ROC curves has been in the evaluation of tests involving image interpretation. Radiographic images are the prime example of their use in this regard, and although ROC curves were suggested over 15 years ago for the evaluation of imaging systems, their use has only recently been popularized (see for example references 3, 6, 7). This greater use is probably due to the increased awareness by researchers and practicing physicians of the need for *unbiased* estimates of image performance; this awareness has come as a result of a large number of new and potentially competitive imaging modalities.

In clinical medicine the key question to be asked of any new test is, "How much more information do I get from the new test as compared with the old?" For imaging modalities the answer is considerably more complicated than for other tests because of the possibility of interpreter bias in the recognition of a potential lesion. A reader tends to overcall or undercall lesions, depending on his or her perception of the consequences of mistakes. Such biases are in part responsible for radiographic interpretations taking such forms as "definitely abnormal," "probably abnormal," "probably normal," etc. These same categories can be used in an experimental situation to quantitate the inherent ability of one imaging modality to detect lesions compared with that of another modality.

Consider a new imaging modality that is used on 200 patients, 100 of whom have the disease being sought and the other 100 of whom do not. Give a radiologist all 200 images and ask him or her to read them and place them in one of five categories: definitely abnormal for the disease in question, probably abnormal, possibly abnormal, probably normal and definitely normal. Then, by *independent* means (e.g., biopsy) determine whether the disease was present or absent in each of the 200 patients. With this information it is possible to construct Table 1. For example, the radiologist indicated that 50 of the 200 examinations were "definitely abnormal," and by independent means we ascertained that 45 of them actually had disease and 5 did not. He said that 35 of the 200 examinations were "probably abnormal" and of these 25 were in patients who truly had the disease and 10 were in patients who did not. If we take the position that only examinations read as definitely abnormal should be called abnormal, then only 45 of the 100 patients with disease would be identified (TP ratio = 45%) and only 5 of the 100 patients would be misclassified (FP ratio = 5%). Similarly, if we think that in a clinical situation it is reasonable to call abnormal

Table 1. Creation of ROC Curve for an Imaging Modality

Reading	Present	(TP ratio)	Absent	(FP ratio)
		Disease State		
Definitely abnormal	45	(0.45)	5	(0.05)
Probably abnormal	25	(0.70)	10	(0.15)
Possibly abnormal	16	(0.86)	15	(0.30)
Probably normal	9	(0.95)	20	(0.50)
Probably normal	5	(1.00)	50	(1.00)
	100		100	

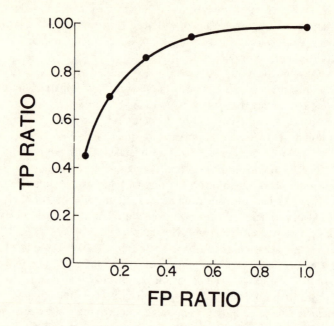

Figure 4. ROC curve for the hypothetical data in Table 1. The ordinate again represents the true positive ratio and the abscissa represents the false positive ratio. For images called abnormal, only if the reading was called "definitely abnormal" the true positive ratio is 45% and the false positive ratio is 5%. As the criterion becomes less strict and images are called abnormal for readings "definitely abnormal," "probably abnormal," or "possibly abnormal," the true positive ratio rises to 86% and the false positive ratio rises to 30%.

those patients whose studies are said to be *either* "definitely abnormal" *or* "probably abnormal," the TP ratio rises to 70% and the FP ratio to 15%. By altering the cutoff point a series of TP and FP pairs can be created. If these are plotted on linear paper, then the ROC curve shown in Figure 4 results. It should be apparent that the higher and the farther to the left of the graph an ROC curve is, the better the imaging modality (see Curves A and B, Figure 5). For example, of two imaging modalities generated on the ROC curves shown on Figure 5, it is immediately apparent that technique A is better than technique B.[6] For any TP ratio the FP ratio for curve A is lower than that for curve B. Its likelihood ratio is thus higher, and imaging modality A is better at distinguishing regions representing disease from regions representing no disease. It is also apparent that the area under curve A is larger than that under curve B, suggesting another means of comparing two modalities and their corresponding ROC curves; this approach will be discussed in greater detail below.

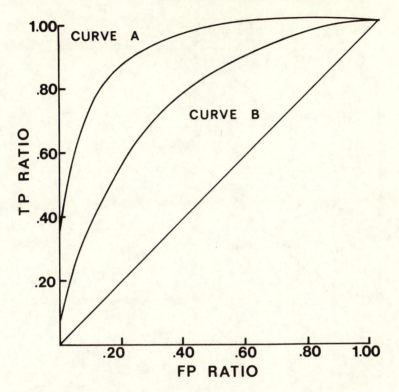

Figure 5. Hypothetical ROC curves for two competitive imaging modalities. Although both curves are concave downward, curve A represents a significantly better imaging modality than curve B because for any given true positive ratio the false positive ratio on curve A is considerably less than for curve B. The diagonal line indicated in this figure represents chance performance, that is, an imaging modality whose true positive ratio would exactly equal its false positive ratio. (Reprinted with permission from Radiology 1977;123:614.)

STATISTICAL TECHNIQUES FOR THE ROC

One question at this point should be "How have we drawn the curves in Figures 4 and 5?" Free hand? Least squares fit? It is clear that the answer to this question is important, because if we are to compare two ROC curves that are close together, we need good statistical techniques to determine whether or not they are statistically different. These techniques have been developed using a transformation of the data leading to ROC curves that are straight lines (e.g., see Figure 6 as a transformation of Figure 5). The rationale for this transformation follows.

ROC curves were originally used in psychophysical experiments involving the identification of visual or auditory stimuli in the midst of appropriate

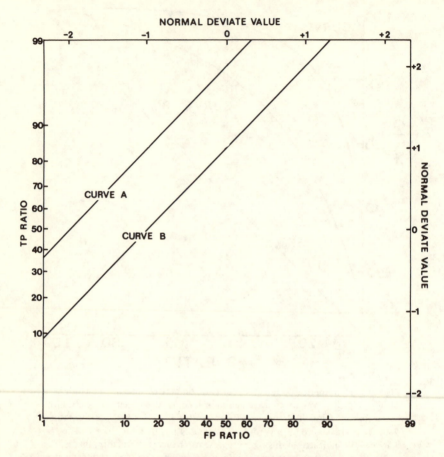

Figure 6. ROC curves for data in Figure 5 plotted on double probability paper. When the data in Figure 5 are plotted on double probability paper, the ROC curves become linear as shown here. As described in the test, this transformation provides a convenient way of fitting ROC data by a maximum likelihood estimation (reference 8).

background. In these circumstances the stimuli (called the "signal") and the background (called the "noise") are generally both normally distributed, just as are the hypothetical data for the diseases and nondiseased patients shown in Figure 1. It is known that if resulting TP and FP ratios are obtained in such circumstances, and if the normal deviate values of these ratios are obtained and plotted, a *straight line* results. (In other words we must determine how many standard deviations of the normal curve are represented by particular TP and FP ratios.) This entire process can be performed using binormal graph paper, also called double probability paper. Depending on the relative standard deviation of the two distributions, the slopes of these lines may be greater than, equal to, or less than 1.00.

A line can be drawn through a series of points on an ROC graph by eye or by use of a maximum likelihood estimation technique. It *cannot* be obtained by a straightforward linear regression of the normal deviate values; such regressions assume *independence* among all TP-FP pairs, and as shown in Table 1, consecutive TP, FP pairs are not independent. The second ratio depends, for example, on observations that were part of the first and second ratios. The most common maximum likelihood technique used for this purpose is called the Dorfman and Alf technique; it uses as input data four TP-FP pairs, and it provides, among other things, fitted TP and FP values and the area under the curve and standard deviations around all these parameters.[8] The area ranges from a low value of 0.50, indicating that each TP ratio is the same as its FP ratio (i.e., chance performance), to 1.00 for perfect detection.

JOINT ROC CURVES

So far we have talked only about the use of ROC curves to evaluate imaging modalities and their ability to differentiate diseased areas from nondiseased areas. This is clearly the first step in evaluating new imaging modalities. In fact, though, as techniques become more sophisticated in their ability not only to detect diseases but also to classify or localize them, additional analyses are often desirable. This also can be done with ROC curves. The question in this case becomes "Of all positive responses as to disease presence, how many of them are also correct as to disease classification?" Thus, the ordinate of a resulting ROC curve becomes true positive responses reflecting both detection *and* classification and the abscissa reflects false positive responses for detection. Thus, only the ordinate is changed; no subdivisions are made on the abscissa.

To illustrate the differences between single and joint ROC curves, let us consider a recent analysis comparing computed tomography (CT) and radionuclide (RN) imaging in the brain.[7,9] For the lesion detection part of the study, the resulting ROC curves are shown in Figure 7; for detection, the curve for CT is everywhere above that for RN, thus indicating CT's superiority over RN. Creation of joint ROCs requires more information. In fact, when the comparative study was originally performed, the radiologists were asked in their reading of images to specify, for the definitely, probably, or possibly abnormal cases, the anatomic location of the disease responsible for the CT or RN image. They were also asked for their most likely diagnosis. The ROC curves for detection and localization generated in this fashion for CT and RN are shown in Figure 8. Note that each one is below the corresponding single ROC curve repeated in the left panel in Figure 8. This must happen because data reflecting disease detection plus localization are a subset of those reflecting only disease detection. In fact, it could even happen that a joint ROC curve would be below the diagonal even if the single ROC curve was everywhere above it.

The above example has related to disease detection plus disease classification. You might imagine that for some modalities the ability of a modality to

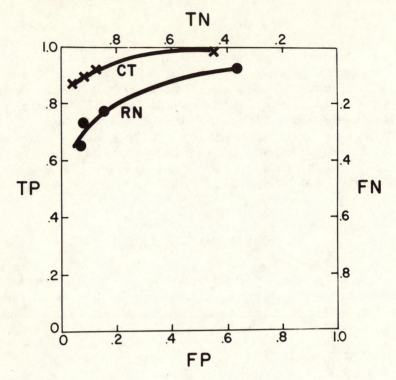

Figure 7. ROC curves for computed tomography and radionuclide scanning of the head. The data for computed tomography are on an ROC curve everywhere above the curve for radionuclide imaging, thus indicating the superiority of the former technique. For example, at a true positive ratio of 85%, the false positive ratio of computed tomography is only about 4% whereas that for radionuclide scanning is about 35%.

detect and localize might be more important than its ability to detect and classify (e.g., comparison of computed tomography and ultrasound in their ability to localize disease for closed biopsy). An analogous approach to that just described would be used and is shown in the remaining panels of Figure 8 for CT and RN of the head.

STATISTICAL ANALYSES

The general problem here is the identification of statistically significant differences between or among ROC curves. Although the psychophysical literature suggests a number of different criteria by which ROC curves may be computed, so far we have mentioned only one quantitative criterion, i.e., the area under the curve. This limited discussion of criteria appears in order because, operationally,

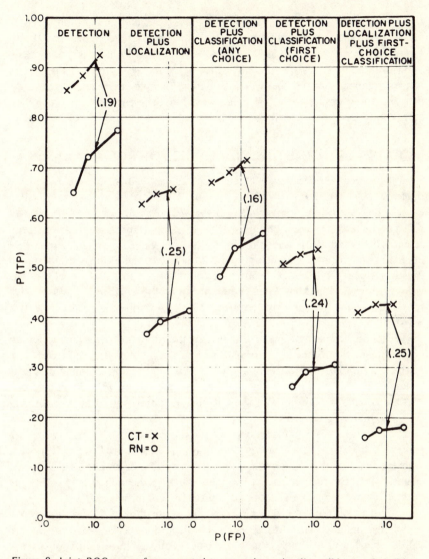

Figure 8. Joint ROC curves for computed tomography and radionuclide scanning with detection ROC curves plotted for comparison on the left. These data show that for each of the five tasks the ROC curves for computed tomography lie above those for radionuclide scanning. For all tasks involving detection plus something else (panels 2, 3, 4, 5) the ROC curves are depressed relative to those for detection alone. This phenomenon occurs because these combined tasks are a subset of the detection task alone. (Reprinted with permission from Science 1979;205:754. Copyright 1979 by the American Association for the Advancement of Science.)

the rationale for the area measure is the most clear, and, in addition, the area measure has been found applicable to most imaging systems studied to data. As stated earlier, the area and its variations are obtained from a maximum likelihood estimation. A test for this difference between two proportions is used to test for significant differences when the data in the two or more curves are independent (for example, when they are derived from different patients). Otherwise, more complicated analyses are required.[10]

CAVEATS IN THE DESIGN AND USE OF ROC ANALYSES

Several problems in the design of experiments can lead to subtle biases in the final results.[9] First, in comparing two or more modalities, the health care system is such that it is often impossible to obtain *all* images with *all* modalities on *all* patients. Instead, there may be a disparity. It is important to determine that differences (or lack thereof) among the modalities ascertained by studying the whole population are maintained when only the subset having all of the relevant modalities is included in the ROC analysis. It could happen that a group of patients with "easy-to-find" lesions would be examined by the worst of the three modalities and not by the other two, thus artificially inflating the sensitivity of the worst modality.

Second, it is important to ensure that the results of one examination do not influence the technical performance of another. Otherwise, the ROC curve of the second modality reflects the second *plus* information from the first. The easiest place for this kind of bias to creep in occurs when tomographic modalities are compared with nontomographic and the latter is used to guide the *site* for tomagraphic sectioning.

Third, technically unsatisfactory examinations have to be dealt with in a consistent manner. If their being "technically unsatisfactory" is a reflection of inherent limitations of the technique, then they cannot be excluded from the analysis. Instead, they must be included—putting them in the "possibly abnormal" category may be one type of appropriate compromise.

A different kind of problem can arise in the analysis of ROC results from a well-designed study. This difficulty relates to appropriate evaluation of two modalities that have ROC curves that cross (as in Figure 9). In this situation a single area under the curve measure is inappropriate because significant differences in sensitivity or specifity for one modality might occur in one region of the curve but not in another.[11] For example, curve B in Figure 9 appears better than that for curve A at FP ratios of less than 20%, the usual operating region for imaging modalities. However, A is better for FP ratios of more than 20% and the resulting areas are virtually identical.

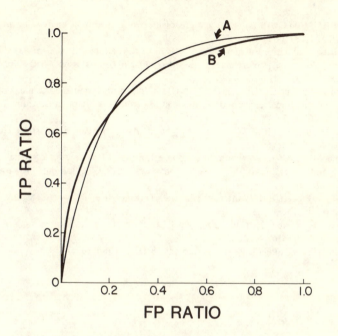

Figure 9. Crossing ROC curves. These hypothetical curves A and B indicate the complexity arising when at a low false positive ratio the sensitivity of one imaging modality (B) is greater than that for the other imaging modality (A), where at high false positive ratios the converse holds.

CONCLUSIONS

This brief review was intended as a simple introduction to receiver operating characteristic curves and their use in diagnostic medicine, particularly radiology. In brief, this technique is an ideal one for comparing competitive imaging modalities because of its ability, in a carefully designed study, to produce unbiased estimates of lesion detectability and, in addition, of lesion detectability *plus* other relevant indexes (e.g., disease location, disease classification).

References

1. Swets JA, ed. Signal Detection and Recognition by Human Observer. New York, John Wiley and Sons, 1964.
2. McNeil BJ, Keeler E, Adelstein SJ. Primer on certain elements of medical decision making. N Engl J Med 1975;293:211-15.
3. Swets JA. ROC analysis applied to the evaluation of medical imaging techniques. Investigative Radiology 1979;14:109-21.

4. Rifkin RD, Hood WB. Bayesian analysis of electrocardiographic exercise testing. N Engl J Med 1977;297:681-6.
5. McNeil BJ. Validation of noninvasive tests in cardiovascular disease. In: Parisi AF, Tow DE, eds. Noninvasive approaches to cardiovascular diagnosis. New York: Appleton-Century-Crofts, 1978:211-28.
6. McNeil BJ, Weber E, Harrison D, et al. Use of signal detection theory in examining the results of a contrast examination: a case study using the lymphoangiogram. Radiology 1977;123:613-17.
7. Swets JA, Pickett RM, Whitehead AF, et al. Assessment of diagnostic technologies. Science 1979;205:753-9.
8. Dorfman DD, Alf E. Maximum likelihood estimation of parameters of signal detection theory and determination of confidence intervals—rating method data. J Math Psychol 1969;6:487-96.
9. .Swets JA, Pickett RM, Whitehead JF, et al. Technical Report No. 3818. Bolt, Beranek and Newman, Inc., 1979.
10. Hanley JA, McNeil BJ. Comparing two ROC curves from the same sample of subjects. Radiology 1982 (In Press).
11. Habicht JP. Assessing diagnostic technology. Science 1980;207:1414.

CHAPTER TWENTY

The Timing of Surgery for Resection of an Abdominal Aortic Aneurysm: Decision Analysis in Clinical Practice

Stephen G. Pauker, MD

INTRODUCTION

Clinical decision analysis is a relatively new discipline that is increasingly infiltrating the medical literature and beginning to form the basis for health policy decisions.[1-12] It applies the established tools of decision analysis[13] to a new domain, medicine. Even more recently, decision analysis has begun to be applied to patient care, and the technique is being slowly adapted for bedside use.[14-17] This paper presents the clinical decision analysis of an actual clinical case seen in consultation at the New England Medical Center Hospital and demonstrates the feasibility of applying these tools to selected clinical cases. Since this analysis was developed "at the bedside," much of the data utilized were the subjective "rough and ready" estimates of experienced clinicians. To retain the flavor of this setting, no attempt is made in this paper to provide references to the literature to document these data. Our purpose here is to demonstrate how logical thought can be applied "in real time" to actual clinical decisions. Certainly, some of the data will be shown to be erroneous, but mistakes are the burden of any clinician. Indeed, as will be suggested later, one of the advantages of this approach is the documentation of the reasoning process and the data base from which the decision

This research was supported, in part, by Research Career Development Award 1 K04 GM 00349 from the National Institute of General Medical Sciences, by research grant 1 P04 LM 03374 and training grant 1 T15 LM 07027 from the National Library of Medicine, and by grant 1 P41 RR 01096 from the Division of Research Resources, National Institutes of Health, Bethesda, Maryland.

I am indebted to several of the surgeons of the New England Medical Center Hospital for referring this patient for consultation and for being bold enough to attempt to quantify their expertise by making subjective probability estimates. Any erroneous data found in this manuscript undoubtedly relate to my inadequacies in understanding their clinical knowledge and translating that understanding into the decision analytic framework.

was made, and one of the great sources of resistance to this approach is this explicit documentation wherein many of one's errors are laid bare for all to see.

PRESENTATION OF THE CASE

Mr. CMK is a 51-year-old man with ankylosing spondylitis and long-standing hypertension. He has a known abdominal aortic aneurysm that, in the past two years, has increased in diameter from 6 cm to 8 cm. Recently, he has had some nondescript epigastric and back pain. Five months ago, a silent myocardial infarction was detected on a routine electrocardiogram. He is now admitted to the hospital for elective aneurysm repair. Aortogram again shows the aneurysm. After the aortogram, the patient developed crushing anterior chest pain. Electrocardiogram demonstrated an evolving anterior myocardial infarction, a diagnosis confirmed by serum enzyme studies and a technetium pyrophosphate scan. The patient's course is otherwise uncomplicated, without congestive heart failure, hypotension, or arrhythmia; however, his back pain continues.

It is generally agreed that an abdominal aortic aneurysm of this size should be resected, but the proper timing of such surgery is unclear. Since the "anesthesia risk" of patients who suffer a myocardial infarction is high in the immediate peri-infarction period and declines with increasing delay after infarction, it is often recommended that elective surgery be delayed at least six months. Unfortunately, aneurysm resection in this man can hardly be considered elective. With increasing delay before resection, the likelihood of preoperative rupture of the aneurysm increases, and the consequences of such rupture would be dire indeed. Thus, the patient is referred for clinical decision analysis in an attempt to discover when surgery might best be performed.

THE CLINICAL DECISION ANALYTIC APPROACH

The basic philosophy of decision analysis is to break a complex problem into a series of equivalent more limited problems and to attack each of those problems separately. The formalism of decision theory (i.e., the principle of averaging out or folding back) is then used to combine the smaller solutions into an overall approach. The underlying assumptions are that the smaller problems are more manageable and that the formal process of combination is more reliable and less subject to error than intuitive informal reasoning.

The process of clinical decision analysis can be separated into five steps. First, the problem must be structured, that is, the set of available strategies and outcomes to be considered must be explicitly specified. The notation of the decision tree is used in providing this structure. As will be demonstrated below, a square node is used to denote a decision point or choice fork that is under the control of the physician; a circular node is used to denote a chance event or chance fork not under the physician's control. It is assumed that the set of branches of each chance node constitute a set of mutually exclusive and exhaustive events, that is, it is assumed that the likelihood of each outcome branch of a chance node can be denoted as a probability and that the sum of all such branch probabilities is unity at each chance node. The process of creating a decision tree to represent a clinical problem always involves a dynamic tension between detail and manageability. The notation can represent problems of arbitrary complexity, but the resulting decision trees become far too "bushy" to be useful or comprehended. The guiding principle should be to provide as much detail as would be *used* in informal decision making. As will be explained below, the process of sensitivity analysis allows the physician to modify the structure and examine the effect of such modifications on the decision.

The second step in the decision analytic process is to specify the likelihood of each outcome's occurring. The language used for such specifications is the language of probabilities, i.e., a number between zero and one, where zero indicates that the event will not occur and one indicates it surely will. The probability of two events both occurring is equal to the product of their probabilities (conjunction), whereas the probability of either of two events occurring is equal to the sum of their probabilities (disjunction). Finally, the likelihood of an event not occurring is equal to one minus the probability of the event occurring. The source of these probabilities can be problematic, since such data are often not clearly available in the literature. However, if the medical literature is viewed merely as a description of past events that are useful in predicting future events, then the probabilities used in the analysis can be viewed as predictions of future events in a particular patient. In this context, the literature, or any other source of experience, can serve as anchor points for the predictive probabilities used in this analysis. Of course, since the details of every patient's presentation are unique, these experience-based estimates must often be adjusted to reflect the individual characteristics of each patient. When the requisite data are not available in the literature, one turns to the expert judgment of experienced clinicians (just as one does in informal clinical judgment) — now in the form of subjective probability estimates. Since much of the physician's training is devoted to the issues of examining and estimating prognosis, subjective probability estimates only represent the formalization of such prognostication in a relatively standard language. It must, of course, be noted that the various probabilities used in a particular analysis often are derived from diverse sources, including the literature and a variety of expert consultants. Indeed, one of the beauties of this approach is the ability to combine, in a thoughtful fashion, the diverse opinions of several physicians, often each focused on a different aspect of the patient's presentation.

The third step in the process is the assignment of relative values, or utilities, to each potential outcome of the decision. Comparison of the many potential outcomes may involve one or several different attributes (e.g., survival, quality of life) and may involve discrete (e.g., alive or dead after five years) or continuous (e.g., life expectancy) scales. Ultimately, however, a single scale that ranks all potential outcomes must be created. In ordering the various outcomes, the physician must first decide whose utilities are to be optimized by the decision-making process (the patient's, the physician's, society's). If the patient's utilities are to serve as the basis for the analysis, then the physician must decide how that individual's attitudes will be assessed and incorporated into the analysis. Will the physician's own attitudes be used as a proxy? Will the physician try to imagine himself in the patient's place? Will the patient be asked—directly or indirectly? Will the average attitudes of a previously interviewed segment of society be used? Will financial consideration be used as a proxy for society's attitudes? These thorny questions have no simple solutions, but it is well to remember that, implicitly or explicitly, they must be addressed.

The fourth step is to choose the best action—by the process of averaging out or folding back. The assumption here is that the best management strategy is the one that on average, would yield the best outcome, where best outcome is meant to imply the highest average utility on the single unified utility scale previously developed. The expected utility of a chance node is calculated by multiplying each branch probability by the associated branch utility and then summing these products. The process is begun at the right-hand outcome branches of the tree and continued leftward into the trunk of the tree. Decision nodes are treated somewhat differently. Here, it is assumed that the rational decision maker will choose the alternative with the highest expected utility, so suboptimal branches are discarded and the entire decision node is assigned the utility of the branch with the highest expected utility. In the process of folding back, certain probabilities and utilities may not be assigned specific numerical values but, rather, may be carried as algebraic symbols, resulting in expected utilities that are algebraic expressions. When the root decision is reached, the strategy with the highest expected utility is chosen. Examining the folded tree (with all suboptimal choices discarded) provides the physician with a relatively complete strategy for managing his patient.

The final, and perhaps the most important, step in the clinical decision analytic process is the sensitivity analysis. The first three phases of the analysis (creating structure, estimating probabilities, and assigning utilities) involve many assumptions and the use of much soft data. It is through sensitivity analysis that the impact of the assumptions is examined. The range of possible values for each probability is specified, and the tree is again folded back for various values (most often the extremes) of the range. If the decision is not changed, it is said to be insensitive to such variations and can be considered quite robust. If the decision is changed, then it is said to be sensitive to such variations, and an attempt should be made to better define the range of that parameter. Such sensitivity analyses are, at first, carried out one at a time. Eventually, several parameters may be varied together, especially if those parameters are in some way linked. Similar sensitivity analyses are carried out on the utilities used in the model. Finally, the structure of the tree, involving considerations such as changes in the time horizon and either adding or subtracting branches at various places in the tree can be examined. In the final type of sensitivity analyses, it is important to take the view that each assigned utility merely represents a summarization of a (potentially) expanded tree. Thus, at any point where the physician finds it difficult to assess a utility to an outcome, that outcome can be expanded to a detailed tree segment involving more narrowly defined outcome states. This process can be continued, at the expense of expanding the tree and increasing the calculational burden of the averaging out process, until the physician finds the outcome states sufficiently constrained to allow him to comfortably assign utilities.

ANALYSIS OF THE CASE

Having presented the difficult case of a patient with a large aortic aneurysm and a recent myocardial infarction, and having outlined the general decision analytic approach, let us now combine these two themes into a clinical decision analysis. In its most simple form, the decision could be structured as shown in Figure 1, where the physician must decide whether to operate now or to delay from one to six months. If a utility could be assigned to each strategy, the physician could simply choose the strategy with the highest utility.

First, one must decide the time horizon for the analysis and the basis for utility assignment. In this particular case, a time horizon of six months was chosen since the surgeons caring for the patient felt that elective surgery would be performed within that time frame in any case. Death from either aneurysm rupture or perioperative complications was defined as a bad outcome and survival after aneurysm resection was defined as a good outcome. On that utility scale,

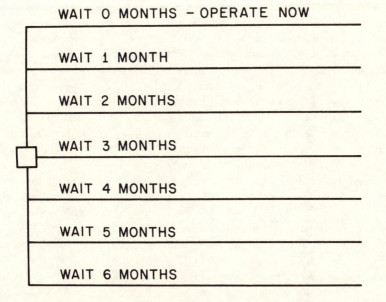

Figure 1. A simple decision tree for selecting the optimal surgical delay. The square node denotes the decision that the physician faces.

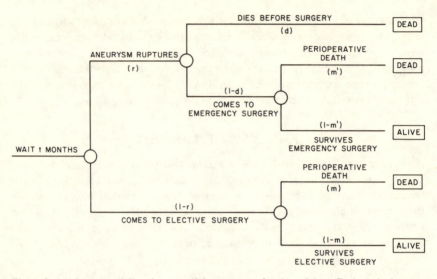

Figure 2. A sub-tree modeling the potential outcomes of various delays. Each circle denotes a chance node. Each rectangle encloses an outcome state. The symbols in parentheses denote the probabilities of various chance events.

the assignment of utilities to each outcome in Figure 1 was felt to be too difficult, so each outcome was expanded into a partial decision tree. The general form of each of those trees is shown in Figure 2. If such an expansion were physically made in Figure 1, the resulting tree would have 35 end branches and would be difficult to conceptualize. Furthermore, such a 35-branch tree would deal only with options of operating at monthly intervals. If the physician wanted to consider intervals of two weeks (e.g., two weeks, one month, six weeks, etc.), then the resulting tree would have 61 branches and be quite unmanageable. Thus, the choice was made to represent the problem by the tree shown in Figure 2, with the delay before surgery being represented by a parameter "t." The optimization problem can now be restated as "select the value of t for which the expected utility is highest." Note that Figure 2 involves four probabilities, some of which are a function of t, and only two utilities; we have quietly, but explicitly, made the assumption that death before surgery from aneurysm rupture and perioperative death are both equally bad outcomes and that, in the time frame of the analysis relative to this man's life expectancy, both would be equally bad whenever in the next six months they were to occur. If we assign the outcome alive a utility of one and the outcome dead a utility of zero, then the expected utility calculated from folding back the tree will be precisely the probability of being alive at the end of the time horizon for analysis. The probability and utility of each outcome are shown in Table 1, as is the expected utility of the tree in Figure 2.

Table 1. Calculation of Expected Utility

Outcome	Probability	Utility	Product
Aneurysm ruptures Dies before surgery	$r \times d$	0	0
Aneurysm ruptures Dies at surgery	$r \times (1-d) \times m'$	0	0
Aneurysm ruptures Survives surgery	$r \times (1-d) \times (1-m')$	1	$r \times (1-d) \times (1-m')$
Elective surgery Perioperative death	$(1-r) \times m$	0	0
Elective surgery Survives	$(1-r) \times (1-m)$	1	$(1-r) \times (1-m)$
Expected utility (sum of products)			$r \times (1-d) \times (1-m') + (1-r) \times (1-m)$

Now let us make some more detailed assumptions about the relations between the delay before surgery (t) and the various probabilities $(r, d, m',$ and $m)$. For an 8-cm aneurysm, we assume the likelihood of rupture is 80% in the next year. Since the aneurysm can only rupture once, we can define the relation between the probability of rupture (r) after t months to be $1 - \exp(-kt)$, where k is the monthly rupture rate and equals 0.134. (This corresponds to the assumption of a constant monthly rupture rate and, thus, simple exponential decay of the likelihood of the aneurysm remaining intact. After one year, we would have $r = 1 - \exp(-12k) = 80\% = 0.8$. Thus, $\exp(-12k) = 0.2$, and we can solve for k.) The relation between the probability of rupture and delay before surgery is shown in Figure 3. For example, after six months, there is a 55% chance of the aneurysm's having ruptured, whereas after three months that chance is only 33%. In a man with a recent myocardial infarction, we assume that, if the aneurysm ruptures, the chance of his dying before emergency surgery (d) is 80%, significantly increased from the usually quoted likelihood of 50%. Finally, we assume that the perioperative mortality rates for both elective (m) and emergency (m') surgery decline with increasing delay before surgery, but that at all times within the next six months, the perioperative mortality rate for emergency surgery is twice that of elective surgery $(m' = 2m)$. Figure 4 shows the decline in the perioperative mortality rate for elective aneurysm resection (m). The probability of perioperative death is assumed to be 0.45 in the peri-infarction period, to fall to 0.25 after two months, to 0.15 after four months, and to 0.10 after six months. (Over the time frame of this analysis, the relation between mortality rate and delay before surgery can be viewed as a modified declining exponential of the form $b + (c \times \exp(-dt))$ where b is the baseline operative mortality rate of 5% and where c is the correctable or excess risk due to recent myocardial infarction

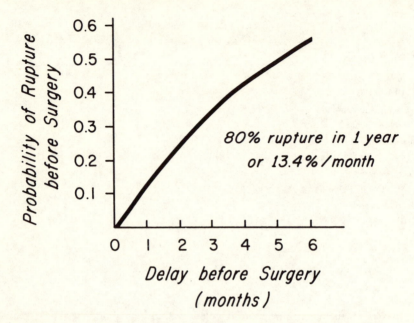

Figure 3. The relation between the delay before surgery and the probability that the aneurysm will rupture (*r*). The data assume a constant monthly rupture rate of 0.134/month, or a probability of 0.8 of rupture in one year.

(40%). The contribution of the excess risk declines exponentially with time, with a half-time of two months.)

Having specified the structure of the problem, estimated the probability of each potential outcome, and assigned a utility (in this case, either zero or one) to each outcome, we are now in a position to calculate the expected utility of each management strategy, i.e., for each potential period of delay before surgery. For example, if *t* equals zero (i.e., for the strategy "operate now"), we have $r = 0$, $d = 0.8$, $m = 0.45$, and $m' = 0.90$; thus, the probability of survival at the six-month point would be 0.55. Similarly, for the strategy "wait for six months" ($t = 6$), we have $r = 0.55$, $d = 0.8$, $m = 0.10$, and $m' = 0.20$; the probability of survival at the six-month point would be 0.49. Clearly, it would be worse to delay six months than to operate in the peri-infarction period. Nonetheless, there remains the question whether some other strategy of delay might be even better. Figure 5 shows the relation between the probability of being alive after six months and the delay before surgery. Indeed, there is an optimal period of delay, which is shown to be approximately 1.6 months. Returning to Figure 1, we see that the optimal strategy was not one of the seven rough management plans outlined there but, if one had to choose among the plans shown there, the choice should be for a two-month delay.

Having selected the best management strategy under our baseline assumptions, we can now proceed with sensitivity analyses that address some of the

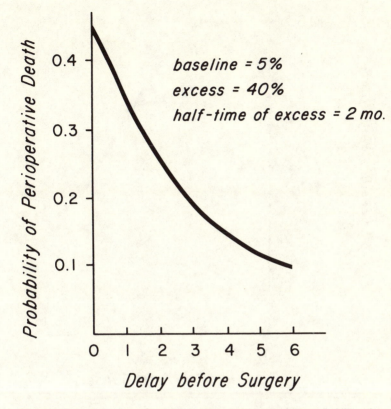

Figure 4. The relation between the delay before surgery and the probability of perioperative death after elective surgery (*m*). The data assume a baseline risk of 5% plus an excess correctable component of 40% with the excess decaying exponentialy with a half-time of two months.

"soft" assumptions that we were forced to make in this bedside analysis. Let us first consider the likelihood of death before emergency surgery (*d*) if the aneurysm were to rupture. We had assumed a baseline value of 80%, but made that assessment deliberately higher than the commonly quoted figure of 50%. In Figure 6, the entire analysis is repeated for preoperative death rates ranging from 30% to 100%. As the preoperative death rate declines, the likelihood of survival increases for all management strategies involving delay before surgery, but more important, as the preoperative death rate declines, the optimal delay increases, reaching 2.6 months for *d* = 0.6 and 4.6 months for *d* = 0.4. For *d* = 0.3, the likelihood of sudden death has become low enough that surgery should be delayed at least for the full six-month time frame of the analysis.

Next consider the probability that the aneurysm will rupture (*r*) prior to elective surgery. That likelihood was translated into a monthly rupture rate— 0.134/month under our baseline assumption. If the same problem were faced in

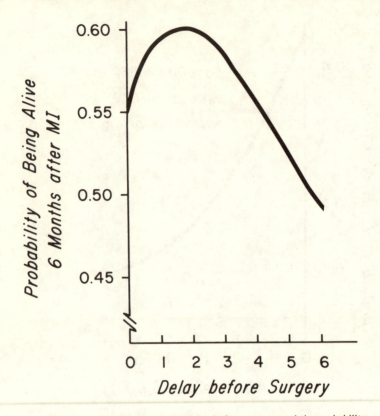

Figure 5. The relation between the delay before surgery and the probability of being alive after six months. The optimal delay is 1.6 months.

a patient with an aneurysm of different size, then the rupture rate and, presumably, the optimal delay before surgery would be different. Figure 7 depicts the rough relation between aneurysm size and the annual rupture rate. For example, if the aneurysm were 10 cm in diameter, then there would be roughly a 95% chance of rupture in one year, or a rupture rate (k) of 0.25/month, again, found by constructing the relation $1 - 0.95 = 0.05 = \exp(-12k)$ and by solving for k. Similarly, if the aneurysm were only 6 cm in diameter, then the likelihood of rupture after a year's delay would be 20%, or a rate of only 0.0186/month. The effect of these changes in aneurysm size on the optimal surgical delay can be seen in Figure 8. If the chance of preoperative death after rupture is 80% (baseline assumption), then one should delay the full six months for a 6 cm aneurysm but operate immediately on a 10-cm aneurysm. However, if the chance of sudden death with rupture fell to 40%, then a patient with a 7-cm aneurysm should have surgery delayed the full six months (compared with 3.8 months under the baseline assumption), whereas even a patient with a 10-cm aneurysm should have surgery delayed 3.8 months.

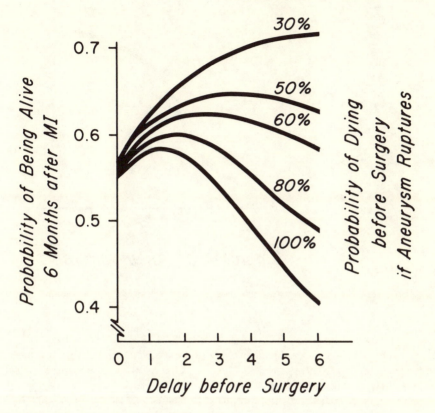

Figure 6. The effect of the probability of sudden death after rupture on the probability of being alive after six months.

Next, let us consider the general relation between perioperative risk and the optimal delay before surgery. In this analysis we have separated that risk into two components—a baseline risk (5% in this case) and an excess risk (40% in this case), which declines exponentially with increasing delay after the myocardial infarction. Changes in the baseline risk of even moderate extent (e.g., doubling it to 10% or removing it entirely) resulted in only minor changes in the optimal delay before surgery (e.g., changes of less than one week). In contrast, even small changes in the correctable portion of the risk (i.e., the excess risk) or the rate of decay of that excess risk had a major impact on the optimal delay. The reason for this extreme sensitivity should be obvious—in delaying surgery, the physician is trading the risk of aneurysm rupture against a decline in operative risk and that decline (over time) is, in this model, totally dependent on the magnitude of the excess risk. Note that this conclusion does not deny the importance of the baseline risk—that parameter will have a major influence on the decision of whether or not to attempt aneurysm resection but has relatively little effect on the choice of *when* to perform the surgery.

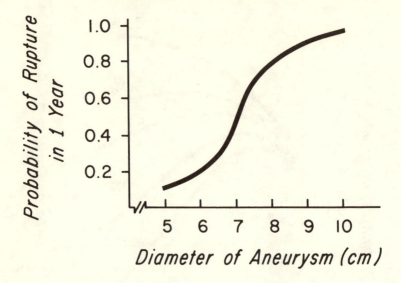

Figure 7. The relation between aneurysm size and the probability of rupture in one year.

This analysis also assumed that the perioperative mortality rate for emergency surgery (m') was twice that of elective surgery (m). Under the baseline assumptions, varying the factor used to adjust the mortality rate for emergency surgery had little effect on the optimal delay. When the chance of preoperative death after rupture (d) became low, however, then a more pronounced relation between that factor and optimal delay was seen.

All the sensitivity analyses performed thus far have dealt with changes in the probabilities of various events. Changes in utility might also be investigated. For any decision in which only two outcome states are defined (e.g., dead and alive), all utility scales will provide identical decisions. On the other hand, if one chose to consider the time alive before death to be a significant measure of worth (e.g., that death after four months was a better outcome than death after one month), then the utility scale would be more detailed, and a sensitivity analysis of the utilities might be performed.

Finally, one might consider changes in the structure of the problem. We have thus far assumed that the only causes of death in the time frame of this analysis are either surgery or aneurysm rupture. However, this man has recently suffered a myocardial infarction—what would be the effect of considering the possibility of his dying from his heart disease within the next six months? Sensitivity analysis of this structural change showed almost no effect on the optimal delay before surgery! Of course, if the decision under consideration were whether or not to perform surgery, a greater effect might have been seen, but recall the utility structure used for this analysis. Being alive after six months was the

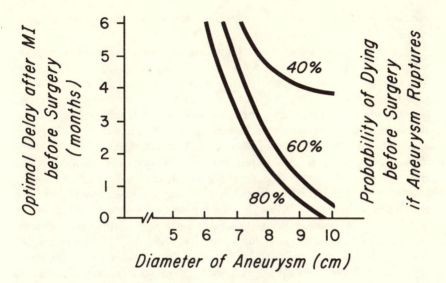

Figure 8. The relation between aneurysm size and the optimal delay before surgery. As the likelihood of sudden death after rupture falls, the optimal delay increases and the relation between aneurysm size and delay becomes less marked.

best outcome, and dying was the worst. Since the patient can only die once, the outcome of successful surgery followed by death from heart disease (in the six-month time frame) was no worse than any other death in that time frame. Of course, such "bad luck" would constitute an unfortunate drain on society's or the patient's family's resources but, if such resource considerations should have an influence on the decision-making process, then they must be considered explicitly in the utility structure from the outset, and some "trade-off" between resources and survival must be established. Indeed, if physicians consider such factors in their implicit clinical decisions now, then they must be making some of these trade-offs themselves. One might argue convincingly that it would be better if such trade-offs between lives and resources were made explicitly, where they could be examined and where the input of other concerned individuals—like the patient or his family—might be sought.

DISCUSSION

This brief example of the use of decision analysis in clinical medicine has addressed a difficult clinical problem recently faced at the New England Medical Center Hospital. The clinical decision analysis presented here involved structuring the problem domain, estimating the likelihood of a variety of events, creating a quantitative ranking of the relative worth of the various potential outcomes, calculating which management strategy would, on average, provide the best outcome, and finally examining the impact of the explicit assumptions that were made.

The process is straightforward, but can certainly be time-consuming. The actual analysis was performed on the ward with only pencil, paper, and a hand-held calculator, and took approximately three hours to complete, including the data acquisition phase, which involved discussion with several vascular surgeons. In the preparation of this paper, the calculations were repeated, and several additional sensitivity analyses were performed, using a mini-computer[18] and requiring approximately 30 minutes to complete. Certainly this time-intensive approach to medical decision making must be reserved for the minority of clinical decisions—situations that involve unusual risks or particularly uncertain data. It is probably unreasonable to expect every physician to develop and maintain an expertise in performing such analyses, although some exposure to these techniques might affect his general problem-solving skills in a positive way. Rather, one might expect a cadre of specialists to develop—physicians, well-versed in these techniques, who are willing to share their expertise, in the form of consultations, with others. Even then, these analyses must be reserved for those situations in which the time investment is likely to be clinically helpful. Of course, it may be well to perform "one-time" generic analyses of a variety of clinical situations that commonly occur and then publish the results of those analyses in a form that might be efficiently used by other clinicians.

In the end, each physician and the medical community as a whole must decide whether this type of explicit, logical approach to clinical decision making offers sufficient advantages to the patient, to the physician, and to society to justify the resource investment required to perfect, disseminate, and utilize it. Table 2 provides a limited and somewhat lighthearted comparison of some of the advantages and disadvantages of the approach. The juxtaposition of certain items in that table has been quite deliberate. The first and last items—the explicitness of clinical decision analysis and its ability to document clinical reasoning—can be viewed as either advantages or disadvantages, depending on the quality of the reasoning involved.

Table 2. A Balance Sheet Concerning Clinical Decision Analysis

Advantages	Disadvantages
Explicit	Explicit
Provides structure	Encourages oversimplification
Allows diverse data to be combined	Requires data
Allows explicit consideration of utilities and patient input	Unfamiliar
Allows examination of impact of soft data	Time consuming
Separates large problem into smaller, more manageable ones	Demystifies medicine
Provides documentation of reasoning	Provides documentation of reasoning

To the extent that clinical decision analysis improves the general level of clinical reasoning, helps limit the use of scarce resources, and provides better patient outcomes, it will be a positive force in medicine. In doing so, however, it will undoubtedly precipitate changes in medical education and in the very style of medical practice. Our ability to meet these challenges and make whatever changes are necessary to incorporate these developing technologies into our rituals of practice constitute one of the great strengths of medicine. Surely we shall succeed!

References

1. Lusted LB. Introduction to medical decision making. Springfield, IL: Charles C Thomas, 1968.
2. Schwartz WB, Gorry GA, Kassirer JP, EssignA. Decision analysis and clinical judgment. Am J Med 1973;55:459-72.
3. McNeil BJ, Keeler E, Adelstein SJ. Primer on certain elements of medical decision making. N Engl J Med 1975;293:211-15.
4. Pauker SG, Kassirer JP. Therapeutic decision making: a cost-benefit analysis. N Engl J Med 1975;293:229-34.
5. Kassirer JP. The principles of clinical decision making: an introduction to decision analysis. Yale J Biol Med 1976;49:149-64.
6. Pauker SG. Coronary artery surgery: the use of decision analysis. Ann Intern Med 1976; 85:8-18.
7. Weinstein MC, Stason WB. Hypertension: a policy perspective. Cambridge, MA: Harvard University Press, 1976.
8. Bunker JP, Barnes BA, Mosteller F, eds. Costs, risks, and benefits of surgery. New York: Oxford University Press, 1977.
9. Pauker SG, Kassirer JP. Clinical application of decision analysis: a detailed illustration. Semin Nucl Med 1978;8:-324-35.
10. Pauker SG, Pauker SP. Decision making in the practice of medicine. In: Hill P, ed. Making decisions. Reading, MA: Addison-Wesley, 1979;152-76.
11. Weinstein MC, Fineberg HV. Clinical decision analysis. Philadelphia: W.B. Saunders Co, 1980.
12. Pauker SG, Kassirer JP. The threshold approach to clinical decision making. N Engl J Med 1980;302:1109-17.
13. Raiffa H. Decision analysis. Reading, MA: Addison-Wesley, 1968.
14. McNeil BJ, Weichselbaum R, Pauker SG. The fallacy of the five-year survival in lung cancer. N Engl J Med 1978;299:1397-1401.
15. Pauker SP, Pauker SG. The amniocentesis decision: an explicit guide for parents. In: Epstein CJ, Curry CJR, Packman S, Sherman S, Hall BD, eds. Risk, communication, and decision making in genetic counseling, Part C of Ann Review of Birth Defects, 1978. National Foundation-March of Dimes. Birth Defects Original Article Series XV:5C, New York: Alan R. Liss, 1979;289-324.
16. McNeil BJ, Pauker SG. The patient's role in assessing the value of diagnostic tests. Radiology 1979;132:605-10.
17. Barza M, Pauker SG. The decision to biopsy, treat, or wait in suspected herpes encephalitis. Ann Intern Med 1980;92:641-9.
18. Pauker SG, Kassirer JP: Clinical decision analysis by personal computer. Arch Intern Med 1981 (in press).

CHAPTER TWENTY-ONE

Biostatistical Tools: Promises and Accomplishments

E. A. Johnson, PhD

Dramatic promises have been made for the biostatistical tools for classification. Those promises are well-founded. But practically no reports have come out about successful utilization of biostatistical tools for classification in realistic clinical settings, and there probably will not be for some time to come. These two concepts—confident promise and no record of accomplishment—are inconsistent. I will try to explain.

THE TOOLS DO WORK

This is not an appropriate setting for a technical description of classification rules. In most cases, the mathematics involved with describing the rules and proving their behavior is cumbersome. An important review by Solberg[1] summarizes most of the prevalent techniques with a style of writing and a mathematical sophistication aimed at a specialist in clinical chemistry.

All the models for medical decision and interpretation of data mentioned above share one characteristic: the observations consist of multiple symptoms, signs and/or measurements. The elements of an observation are called variables, that is, quantities that vary, and may be discrete or continuous. A variate, or random variable, is a variable that can take any of its possible values with a specified probability as expressed by a frequency function. Observations that consist of multiple variates are called multivariate.

Geometrically, a multivariate observation may be represented by a point in space with as many dimensions as there are variables in the observation. When there are more than three dimensions in the space that we imagine, the term hyperspace is often used. Other terms in common use for the observation are vector or pattern or profile. Related observations (e.g., those obtained on patients with the same disease) are geometrically represented by a swarm or cluster of points, possibly separated from the clusters of observations obtained from other groups of individuals.

The degree to which the symptoms and measurements in the observational vector are useful for diagnosis depends on the degree to which the clusters of the separate disease groups overlap. A diagnosis rule corresponds to the partitioning of the measurement space into regions identified with the various disease clusters. The best possible partitioning of the space corresponds to a classification rule that would have a minimum expected cost of misdiagnosis. This rule is called Bayes' rule. Minimizing the expected cost of misdiagnosis is also the target or the goal of the physician. If he learns the import of these signs and symptoms as best he can, he may attain knowledge equivalent to the boundaries of the space corresponding to the best possible rule, Bayes' rule.

You may ask why one cannot do better. It is because some patients show an atypical pattern. Even though the patient has just suffered a myocardial infarction, she presents signs, symptoms, and enzyme patterns completely consistent with a pulmonary embolism. This would be expected occasionally, if the clusters for myocardial infarction and pulmonary embolism overlap.

The object is to learn Bayes' rule through organized experience. One has to have faith that the same system that generated the cases and their symptom vectors in the past will continue to operate in the future. We hope that our experience is relevant.

If several different classification rules are set before us, there can be only one basis for choice. Which is closest to Bayes' rule? An expert pathophysiologist may impress us with an explanation of why a typical subject responds to a disease in a certain way and provides an observation with a certain profile. Following the line of reasoning he has used to obtain classification rules may be intellectually challenging. The only valid measure of success, however, will be whether this line of reasoning has led him closer to Bayes' rule than others are able to get.

The rules of classification based on biostatistical algorithms have a distinct advantage when it comes to evaluating their performance. The evaluation can be done and has been done. The following quotation of Gordon and Olshen[2] is provided as an example and should not be construed as a specific recommendation of their techniques.

> We study a class of decision rules based upon adaptive partitioning of an Euclidian observation space. The class of partitions has a computationally attractive form, and the related decision rule is invariant under strictly monotone transformation of coordinate axes. We provide sufficient conditions that a sequence of decision rules be asymptotically Bayes risk efficient as sample size increases. The sufficient conditions involve no regularity assumptions on the underlying parent distributions.

In ordinary language, we can count on their technique. Even though we do not know what Bayes' rule is, we can be almost certain that their procedure will converge to it with accumulating experience. The automated algorithms have been studied by theory and simulation. We know what problems are associated with some techniques and not others. We know that rules based on many variables take longer to learn than those based on few variables.

Medicine is a careful and conservative discipline, believing that "The proof of the pudding is in the eating"; we want to see these rules that are based on biostatistical tools perform in a real clinical setting. We must gather some data; establish the rules; test the rules on subsequent cases. This is the only acceptable evaluation in medicine.

When we face up to the fact that few such evaluations have been done, we realize why they have not been done. The necessary record system has not existed except in special, short-term research situations.

THE SYSTEM MUST BE BASED ON RECORDS: RECORDS TO OBTAIN EXPERIENCE; RECORDS TO TEST TENTATIVE RULES

There are three necessary ingredients to the research implied by our discussion. First, a clinical entity must be identified. Second, a protocol must be established to guarantee that the appropriate vector of observations is made on all such subjects. Third, a method must be established for determining the final outcome (diagnosis) for each subject. A record system that provides these ingredients may provide a basis for developing and testing rules of diagnosis. Any record system that does not have the ingredients cannot support both development and testing of rules no matter what the logical basis for the rules. We can safely deduce that the rules based on biostatistical tools have not been adequately tested. Unfortunately, we can also assume that the rules propagated by the expert pathophysiologist have not been adequately tested either.

It has been several years since I had the joy of watching Lawrence Weed, M.D., perform before a group of clinicians. He was pushing for the problem-oriented chart. He would ask for a randomly chosen patient's chart and begin reading aloud from it. He would invite the audience to participate in guessing why certain tests were ordered; what interpretation was put upon their outcome; why certain treatments were initiated. He was careful not to criticize the specific patient management but he pulled no punches in making it clear that there was no basis for learning in the typical chart. I find the order of the words in the title of his book significant: "Medical Records, Medical Education and Patient Care."[3] Medical records come before medical education—that is one of the themes of his book. We will not see a useful evaluation of any system of diagnostic rules until we are willing to support medical education and patient care with adequate record keeping.

The clinical information must go into a condensed computer version of the chart routinely. The pathologist and/or clinical biochemist should be able to process those records to learn the patterns associated with various diagnostic outcomes.

THE OBSERVATION VECTOR IS NECESSARY

Only after experience will it be possible to learn the patterns associated with various diagnoses. To gain the experience, it will be necessary to have test battery results on all subjects. But there would be no justification, using today's standards, for ordering all those tests. You can imagine the objections that would arise. Admission batteries are already under criticism, and there is a general demand for lowering laboratory costs.

We know that the laboratory already does many more tests than are actually ordered. These additional tests are associated with research and development and quality control. It is generally accepted that practice is necessary and that the practice has to be done on real material; the extra cost is considered a justifiable overhead for the sake of excellence. The extra tests and the extra computer processing to learn useful patterns is also justifiable overhead in that excellence will be associated with proper interpretation.

Conn[4] has presented an account of laboratory economics, pointing out that there is very little relationship between laboratory charges and laboratory costs. He refers to the laboratory as a profit center for the hospital. If realistic accounting were done, the concept of more and larger routine batteries would not be so questionable from the financial point of view. Most of the laboratory costs are not directly proportional to the number of tests. The support logistics associated with accommodating spontaneous test requisitions, scheduling specimen acquisition, specimen handling, and reporting results are very expensive. It is our present system that is inequitable. A single test A on one subject may cost five dollars, and a single test B on another subject may cost five dollars, but the usual charge for both tests on the same subject would be ten dollars. The charge actually should be close to five dollars, considering the cost ingredients. Routine batteries will not lead to more requisitions, probably fewer; routine batteries will not lead to more trips for the specimen drawing team, probably fewer; and routine batteries will not lead to more cumbersome records and reporting, probably fewer.

The biostatistical tools automatically develop rules with predictable efficiency. They are unique in this regard. None of the various decision rules, whether based on biostatistical algorithms or medical intuition algorithms, have been proved with extensive trials in realistic clinical settings. Our record systems do not support such research. To quote from Weed:[3]

> The medical record must completely and honestly convey the many variables and complexities that surround every decision, thereby discouraging unreasonable demands upon the physician for supernatural understanding and superhuman competence; but at the same time it must faithfully represent events and decisions so that errors can be detected."

The goals will not be attained until a meaningful accounting system is set up for laboratory charges. According to Conn:[4]

a serious impediment to the most efficient use of laboratory information in the patient-care process.

When we couple reasonably priced test batteries with a record system oriented toward learning, the biostatistical tools for classification will come into their own.

References

1. Solberg HE. Discriminant analysis. CRC Crit Rev Clin Lab Sci 1978;9(3):209-42.
2. Gordon L, Olshen RA. Asymptotically efficient solutions to the classification problem. The Annals of Statistics 1978;6:515-33.
3. Weed LL. Medical records, medical education and patient care. Cleveland: The Press of Case Western Reserve University, 1969.
4. Conn RB. Clinical laboratories: profit center, production industry or patient-care resource? N Engl J Med 1978;298:422-7.

CHAPTER TWENTY-TWO

Test Selection and Early Risk Scale in Acute Myocardial Infarction

Adelin Albert, PhD, Jean-Paul Chapelle, PhD, Camille Heusghem, PhD, Gérard Siest, PhD, and Joseph Henny, PhD

INTRODUCTION

In countries with a high level of medical technology, the costs of clinical laboratory tests have reached a critical point. Faced with such an acute financial situation, health authorities have taken measures to reduce laboratory expenditures. Unfortunately, such decisions are more administrative than medical in nature.

From a medical standpoint the main problem is to know whether this situation can influence the clinical decision-making process. The time has come to take advantage of these difficult economic circumstances to modify the attitude of both biologists and clinicians. Amazingly, they are faced with a paradox: the overproduction and the insufficient use of laboratory data. Well aware of the never-ending developments in the field of biology, clinicians generally ask the laboratory to perform a sufficient number of analyses to protect themselves against any eventuality.[1] Thus both the clinician and the laboratory contribute to the constantly growing amount of irregular requests and irrelevant results that neither one nor the other is able to justify or interpret. Obviously when practiced as such, biology is a waste of competence, time, money, and information.

The dual problems of overproduction and insufficient use of laboratory data have a common source: our inability to extract the real information provided by single and multiple test measurements. In this respect, it is quite clear that various solutions are offered for improving the usefulness and the efficiency of laboratory determinations; for example, selecting the most useful analyses for diagnostic and prognostic purposes, or obtaining a better interpretation of measured values with respect to reference values.[2] Only the first approach is envisaged here.

To extract the maximum amount of semiological information from a given set of laboratory data, one should not only interpret the results on an individual basis, but also account for the correlations existing between the various tests, and evaluate the results from a multivariate viewpoint. This approach also reflects the new philosophy adopted by most leading medical schools in seeking new strategies[3] to upgrade biochemical information with respect to medical diagnosis and prognosis.

In this paper we would like to share some of the exciting horizons open to the biologist that were revealed to us as a result of one of our laboratory experiences and collaborations with clinicians, namely, the establishment of a short-term prognostic index in acute myocardial infarction.

FORMULATION OF THE PROBLEM

A reliable short-term prognostic index available early in the course of an acute myocardial infarction would be most helpful, especially when important decisions, such as early release from the intensive care unit or early treatment by intra-aortic balloon pumping, must be made.[4] Even in the absence of such decisions, separation of patients into high and low risk groups is still valuable in setting up controlled clinical trials. Several prognostic indices for the outcome of patients with acute myocardial infarction (AMI) have been constructed using multivariate analysis techniques.[5,6]

In a prognostic situation, the statistical problem can be formulated as follows: we assume that we have a sample of n patients suffering from a disease D, which has two (or more) possible outcomes: D_1 (for example, remission, survival) and D_2 (for instance, nonremission, death). Outcome D_1 is observed in n_1 patients, outcome D_2 in n_2 patients. For each patient, a vector of p observed variables $X' = (x_1, x_2, \ldots, x_p)$ is available prior to the outcome. The question is: can we predict the outcome of any future patient suffering from disease D on the mere basis of vector X?

Classical discriminant analysis models[7,8] are not always appropriate, for they apply to qualitatively distinct groups, for example, different diseases. In the present situation, the two groups D_1 and D_2 are rather quantitatively distinct, for the difference between them is one of risk.

In this context, we have developed a general prognostic model[9,10] applicable to both discrete and continuous variables, which is able to: (1) assess whether prediction is possible on the basis of vector X; (2) eliminate redundant and irrelevant variables using a stepwise selection procedure based on a log-likelihood ratio criterion; and (3) derive an optimal prognostic index.

SELECTION OF THE MOST USEFUL
BIOCHEMICAL PARAMETERS

Our preliminary investigation was to select the biochemical measurements indicative of the best prediction of risk. In a first study, 100 patients with myocardial infarction were split into two groups according to survival D_1 ($n_1 = 85$) or death D_2 ($n_2 = 15$) at the end of the second week of hospitalization.

We evaluated the predictive value of a large battery of biochemical tests including creatine kinase (CK) and CK-MB, glutamate oxalacetate transaminase (GOT), lactate dehydrogenase (LDH) and its isoenzymes, haptoglobin α_1-acid glycoprotein, glycerol, and nonesterified fatty acids (NEFA). Blood samples were drawn at 4-hourly intervals for 72 hours after admission. The two groups of patients were compared at the peak of CK,[11] occurring early in the course of the disease (mean time: 17 ± 7 hours after admission).

The means and standard deviations calculated in survivors and in nonsurvivors are given in Table 1, together with their statistical significance. From the results, it is clearly apparent that, at CK peak, LDH ($t = 7.2$) is the most significant test for predicting high and low risk patients. LDH_1, expressed in enzyme units, shows about the same power as LDH; however, when expressed either as a percentage of LDH, or as the ratio LDH_1/LDH_2, it appears to be nonsignificant. The peak level of CK possesses a predictive power that is lower than that of LDH measured at the same time. Expressed as a percentage of total CK, the cardiac isoenzyme CK-MB is not statistically discriminating. GOT and α_1-acid glycoprotein also show significant differences between the two groups; NEFA, glycerol, and haptoglobin are without predictive interest, at least at CK peak.

A multivariate analysis was performed on the same sample to determine whether univariate results could be further improved when several parameters were combined. Using the stepwise selection procedure, LDH was selected first, the corresponding error rate being 16%. CK and GOT, selected in that order, added to the predictive power of LDH. By combining them with LDH, the error rate dropped from 16 to 13%. However, the log-likelihood ratio test failed to formally demonstrate the improvement in prediction. Neither the addition of another parameter, nor the replacement of LDH (or CK) by its cardiac isoenzyme LDH_1 (or CK-MB) significantly improved discrimination between survivors and nonsurvivors.

Table 1. Univariate Predictive Power of Biochemical Parameters ($\bar{X}$ ± SD) Recorded at CK Peak in 100 Patients with Acute Myocardial Infarction

Parameter	Survivors ($n = 85$)	Nonsurvivors ($n = 15$)	Predictive Power
LDH (IU/L)	1,213 ± 577	2,434 ± 742	$t = 7.2$ ($p < 0.001$)
LDH_1 (%)	55.3 ± 7.0	54.8 ± 6.1	N.S.
LDH_2 (%)	35.1 ± 5.4	33.8 ± 4.7	N.S.
LDH_1/LDH_2	1.64 ± 0.42	1.67 ± 0.37	N.S.
CK (IU/L)	1,686 ± 982	3,270 ± 1,234	$t = 5.5$ ($p < 0.001$)
CK-MB (%)	10.5 ± 3.2	8.9 ± 2.5	N.S.
GOT (IU/L)	280 ± 149	477 ± 139	$t = 4.8$ ($p < 0.001$)
α_1-acid glycoprotein (mg%)	101 ± 25	116 ± 24	$t = 2.1$ ($p < 0.05$)
NEFA (mE/L)	1.23 ± 0.79	0.91 ± 0.49	N.S.
Haptoglobin (mg%)	318 ± 118	348 ± 147	N.S.
Glycerol (mg%)	3.27 ± 1.75	3.53 ± 1.04	N.S.

A similar statistical study, carried out 4 hours before and 4 hours after the CK peak, confirmed that LDH, CK, and GOT jointly provide optimal predictive information; however, in both instances the error rate (14%) was slightly higher than at CK peak.

It should be mentioned finally that using the same training sample, the predictive power of LDH did not improve later in the course of the disease. The peak of LDH, occurring 16 ± 9 hours after the CK peak, was found to have a mean value of 1,540 IU/L in the survivors and 3,165 IU/L in the nonsurvivors ($t = 6.1$).

CLINICAL FINDINGS AND CONSTRUCTION OF A BIOCLINICAL RISK INDEX

The purpose of the study was to construct a short-term prognostic index usable 24 hours after admission that combines clinical information and laboratory data recorded during the first day of hospitalization.

Having reduced the biochemical information to a simplified form and determined its significance, we proceeded to integrate clinical factors in the study. A new sample of 114 patients with AMI, 95 survivors and 19 nonsurvivors, was considered. Ten parameters were recorded for each patient at the early stage of the disease. The biochemical investigations were (1) CK, (2) GOT, and (3) LDH, all measured at CK peak; the clinical information was (4) sex (0 = male, 1 = female), (5) age, (6) number of previous infarctions (PI = 0, 1, . . .), (7) hypertension (0 = absence, 1 = mild, 2 = severe), (8) smoking habits (0-5 scale), (9) height, and (10) weight.

The stepwise variable selection procedure was applied to all parameters (biochemical and clinical) available at the end of the first day. The results of the selection are shown in Table 2. Again LDH proved to be the best test for predicting the patient's outcome and was selected first; afterward, only age (survivors =

Table 2. Stepwise Variable Selection Applied to the Sample of 114 Patients with Acute Myocardial Infarction (95 Survivors, 19 Nonsurvivors)

Step No.	Variable Selected	Log-Likelihood Ratio $\chi^2_{(1)}$	p-Value	Error Rate (%)
1	LDH	19.0	$p < 0.001$	14.0
2	Age	21.2	$p < 0.001$	12.3
3	Sex	2.6	0.11	11.4
4	PI	4.2	0.04	10.5
5	CK	1.2	0.27	10.5
.	.	.	.	.
.	.	.	.	.
.	.	.	.	.
10	Height	0.0	1.00	10.5

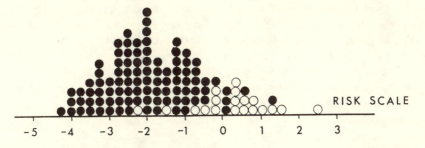

Figure 1. Distribution of the prognostic index R (based on LDH, age, sex, and number of previous infarctions) in the learning sample of 114 patients with acute myocardial infarction. Survivors (n = 95) are indicated by solid circles and nonsurvivors (n = 19) by open circles.

57 ± 12, nonsurvivors = 68 ± 7 years) significantly improved the efficiency of the prediction (χ^2 = 21.2, $p < 0.001$). When adding sex (% female; 10.5 and 26.3) and number of previous infarctions (0.3 ± 0.5 and 0.6 ± 0.7), the error rate dropped from 12.3 to 10.5% and stabilized at that value. These two parameters were included in the prognostic index, although further observations will be required to formally demonstrate their statistical significance.

The prognostic index based on the four selected tests and estimated from the observations of the training sample is given by the equation,

$$R = 0.0012 \text{ LDH} + 0.093 \text{ age} + 0.98 \text{ sex} + 0.57 \text{ PI} - 9.13.$$

This index enables the assessment of the patient's risk from data observable on the first day following admission. Risk, R, was recalculated for all 114 patients of the training sample: the distribution of the values obtained is shown in Figure 1. From that distribution, it is readily apparent that one is confronted with a single population, as initially assumed, with an underlying continuous risk scale. Risk increases as one ranges from negative to positive values. Large positive values of the index are associated with high risk patients, whereas large negative values are associated with low risk patients. Using a threshold value of $R = -1.0$, sensitivity was found to be equal to 90% and specificity to 81%. These results can be considered as very satisfactory, when one recalls that, starting with a large battery of biochemical and clinical parameters, only four variables were finally retained.

This application of discriminant analysis shows how a late and dichotomized assessment of risk can be combined with parameters recorded at the early stage of the disease to evaluate the patient's risk on a single continuous scale of measurement.

CONCLUSION

The use of multivariate statistical methods opens new horizons that were perhaps unexpected for the biologist as well as for the clinician. Undoubtedly this approach reflects one of the logical and inescapable evolutions of clinical chemistry. Confronted with current economic constraints, we have reconsidered our strategies for an improved interpretation of laboratory data. In our opinion, this philosophy should be particularly helpful within the framework of the biologist's collaboration and dialog with the clinician. In the long run, it should prove to be more beneficial for the patient and promote a more rational approach to health care policy.

References

1. Hardison JE. Sounding Boards. To be complete. N Engl J Med 1979;300:193-94.
2. Siest G, Henny J, Heusghem C, Albert A. The use of reference values and the concept of reference state. A contribution to improved laboratory use. Chapter 31 of this volume.
3. Benson ES. Strategies for improved use of the clinical chemistry laboratory in patient care. In: Benson ES, Rubin M, eds. Logic and economics of clinical laboratory use. New York: Elsevier, 1978:245-58.
4. Mulley AG, Thibault GE, Hughes RA, Barnett GO, Reder VA, Sherman EL. The course of patients with suspected myocardial infarction: The identification of low-risk patients for early transfer from intensive care. N Engl J Med 1980;302:943-8.
5. Kitchin AH, Pocock SJ. Prognosis of patients with acute myocardial infarction admitted to a coronary care unit. Br Heart J 1977;39:1163-6.
6. Madsen BE, Rasmussen S, Svendsen L. Short-term prognostic index in acute myocardial infarction. Multivariate analysis by Cox Model. Eur J Cardiol 1979;10:359-68.
7. Anderson TW. An introduction to multivariate statistical analysis. Chapter 6. New York: Wiley, 1958.
8. Anderson JA. Separate sample logistic discrimination. Biometrika 1972;59:19-35.
9. Albert A. Un nouveau modèle général de discrimination. In: Biologie Prospective—4è Colloque de Pont-à Mousson. Paris: Masson, 1978:82-4.
10. Albert A. Quelques apports nouveaux à l'analyse discriminante. PhD thesis: University of Liège, 1978.
11. Chapelle JP, Albert A, Heusghem C, Smeets JP, Kulbertus HE. Predictive value of serum enzyme determinations in acute myocardial infarction. Clin Chim Acta 1980;106:29-38.

CHAPTER TWENTY-THREE

Clinical Algorithms and Patient Care

Harold C. Sox, Jr., MD

INTRODUCTION

The "health manpower crisis" of the mid-1960s led to the deployment of non-physicians in roles that have been traditionally reserved for physicians: the diagnosis and treatment of illness. Teaching these skills to nonphysicians brought about a revolution in clinical teaching methods. Heretofore, medical diagnosis had always been less taught than learned. Physicians-in-training started their clinical work with an extensive knowledge of normal and abnormal human biology. Medical diagnosis was learned, somewhat haphazardly, through caring for a random selection of patients. Nurse practitioners and physician's assistants lack detailed understanding of disease mechanisms. Furthermore, their training is compressed into a much shorter time than physicians' training; yet they are expected to emerge from training as competent clinicians. One solution to this pedagogic problem has been to write down diagnostic strategies for dealing with each of the common problems in medical diagnosis. In this way, the knowledge of experienced physicians could be used to guide the care given by a neophyte clinician. These explicit diagnostic strategies are often called clinical algorithms.

Now, over 10 years later, there is ample evidence that physician's assistants and nurse practitioners can provide safe, effective care for the average office patient.[1] Many trainees learned by using algorithms or protocols, but others did not. Undoubtedly more than one way exists to learn diagnostic strategies for common illness, but the clinical algorithm method is the only one that has been extensively studied. This review summarizes current understanding of the effects of algorithms on learning and patient care, as evidenced by research that has appeared in peer reviewed journals.

DEFINITIONS AND TERMINOLOGY

An algorithm is defined as "a set of step-by-step instructions for solving a problem." This definition, taken from mathematics, has been appropriated by clinicians to describe a set of instructions for solving a medical diagnostic problem. Algorithms specify the information that must be collected, the interpretation of abnormal findings, and consequent diagnostic and therapeutic action. As used in this paper, the term algorithm will refer to written materials used to describe a precise, sequential diagnostic strategy.

The main synonym for clinical algorithm is "diagnostic protocol," a more familiar but less precise term than "algorithm." With the passage of time, though, "clinical algorithm" has come into increasingly common usage by physicians and will be used in this paper.

WHAT DOES AN ALGORITHM DO?

First, an algorithm may serve to guide the management of individual patients:

1. An algorithm defines the types of patients that can be managed by following the algorithm logic. These patients are defined by their age and sex and by whether their complaint fits the subject of the algorithm. In addition, the algorithm logic establishes criteria for early referral of especially sick patients to a physician.

2. An algorithm defines the data to be collected on an individual patient. Certain information must be collected on all patients, usually to screen for the important causes of a symptom. Other data will be collected only on patients who have abnormal findings in the initial, standardized history and physical examination. The algorithm logic specifies the data that are obtained conditional on these abnormal findings. Thus, an algorithm specifies collection of data appropriate to the needs of a specific patient.

3. An algorithm defines the criteria for obtaining consultation from another health provider.

4. An algorithm establishes which clinical findings should lead to diagnostic testing.

5. An algorithm defines the clinical findings that should lead to initiating treatment of a condition.

Second, an algorithm specifies clinical skills that must be acquired and thereby defines curricular goals for training and continuing education of nurse practitioners and physician's assistants. Most algorithms have written documentation for each decision point.

Third, an algorithm can serve as a minimum standard of adequate care for a medical problem. Data collection and clinical decisions on patients may be evaluated by comparison of actual performance to the criteria contained in the algorithm logic.

HISTORICAL BACKGROUND

The term "algorithm" apparently commemorates a ninth century Arabic mathematician, Alkarismi. As used in computer science, it denotes a recursive method for solving a generic mathematical problem. Clinical algorithms were first used in the late 1960s by military corpsmen who were assigned to a military dependents' clinic.[2] Most of the corpsmen had little formal training in the diagnosis and management of disease. Therefore, to maintain tight control over the quality of care provided by the corpsmen, the supervising physicians regularly compared what was recorded in the medical record with the instructions contained in the clinical algorithm. A corpsman who took action not in accord with the algorithms was quickly identified and disciplined.

The first application of clinical algorithms in the training of civilian physician's assistants took place in the training program affiliated with Dartmouth Medical School.[3] The algorithm system used by this program included a checklist medical record form that specified information to be acquired, the algorithm logic (displayed in a branching "yes-no" format), and a series of computer programs that used information recorded on the checklist form to identify discrepancies between the action taken and the action prescribed by the algorithm logic. Similar algorithms were developed by a group associated with Harvard Medical School.[4] The latter group systematically compared the care given by a physician's assistant or nurse practitioner using one of their algorithms with the care given by a physician not using an algorithm. The algorithms developed and validated by this group subsequently appeared in book form.[5] Although the Dartmouth and Harvard groups received many requests for their algorithms, it has not been possible to document the actual extent of their use, either in training programs or in the day-to-day practice of medicine by nurse practitioners or physician's assistants.

Clinical algorithms have influenced several recent developments in health care. First, there has been a resurgence of interest in improving the diagnostic process. Decision points in clinical algorithms have been documented in writing and, wherever possible, by reference to the relevant medical literature. When the literature was searched for clinical evidence to validate diagnostic intuition, little useful information was uncovered, either about the diagnostic value of specific findings in the history and physical examination or about the selection of an optimal diagnostic strategy. That prospective studies of patients with a diagnostic problem could lead to improved strategies was suggested by experience with skull x-rays for head trauma[6] and the management of a sore throat.[7] Many of the clinicians who wrote the original algorithms have continued their interest in diagnostic decision making through the development of empirical decision rules or the use of cost-effectiveness analysis to identify optimal decision strategies.

Second, many practicing clinicians have designed clinical algorithms to fit their own medical practice. Usually, these algorithms have represented a collaboration between a physician and a nurse practitioner or physician's assistant.

Third, when state medical practice or nurse practice acts have been revised to accommodate the expanded role for physician's assistants and nurse practitioners, the language of the law has often mandated the use of protocols or algorithms to guide the selection of diagnostic tests and drugs. Indeed, it is generally agreed that an auditable standard of care should be used by physician's assistants and nurse practitioners. Less agreement exists about how precisely the standard of care should be followed and how often performance should be audited.

For the most part, clinical algorithms have mainly influenced nurse practitioners, physician's assistants, and their physician colleagues. However, federal law has mandated the development of methods for making physicians accountable for their actions. Thus, many physicians have participated in establishing criteria to be used by Professional Standards Review Organizations (PSROs). The criteria have too often been designed to cover every possible clinical contingency; thus these criteria have been unwieldy and insensitive to the nuances of patient care and have often failed to serve their intended purpose. Since algorithms prescribe medical actions that are contingent on specific abnormal findings, the principles used in writing algorithms may be helpful in developing more flexible and more realistic standards of care for physicians. This approach has been brought to its highest development in the use of "criteria mapping" for evaluating care for diabetes mellitus.[8]

WRITING A CLINICAL ALGORITHM

Many practitioners, physicians as well as nurse practitioners and physician's assistants, write their own algorithms or modify published algorithms to fit their own practice. A number of issues must be considered in writing an algorithm for a specific practice setting.[9] The characteristics of the patients is one determinant. The relative frequency of different chief complaints will determine the subject matter of the algorithms. The reliability of the patients will influence the extent of the initial examination and how often the patient should be seen by a physician, since a high frequency of broken follow-up appointments mandates a greater reliance on diagnostic tests and less reliance on "the test of time" to rule out serious disease.

Characteristics of the physician's assistant or nurse practitioner are also important. Their skills may circumscribe the content of the algorithm. Alternatively, the algorithm may define skills that must be taught. Patient care guided by algorithms requires clinical judgment. An experienced provider may require a less detailed algorithm, and would be unlikely to use an algorithm that seriously constrained the exercise of clinical judgment. Algorithms for highly experienced providers should probably focus on the selection of frequently ordered laboratory tests.

Characteristics of the practice setting also will affect the content of the algorithm. If the physician's assistant or nurse practitioner simply serves as a triage agent, the algorithm can be quite brief. Ready availability of a physician to serve as consultant will simplify the algorithm logic. Reliance on simple diagnostic tests will depend on their availability in the practice. Algorithms written for a busy, understaffed practice probably will be simpler and make more extensive use of a brief physician consultation than if the nonphysician provider had the time to function as a substitute for a physician.

Writing a clinical algorithm should occur in several steps. First, the diagnostic problem is chosen. Second, the diseases that cause the problem should be listed and grouped by their medical urgency. Third, for each disease the minimal diagnostic criteria should be listed, together with the indications for physician consultation and laboratory tests. Fourth, the minimal initial examination for all patients should be listed. Fifth, the logic of the diagnostic strategy should be written down. Possible formats include flow sheets with binary decision points,[3] a medical record form that displays the diagnostic logic,[5] or a decision table.[10] Sixth, the reasons for each decision point should be clearly identified in writing, so that the algorithm user will understand and gradually internalize the medical basis of the diagnostic strategy.

HOW ALGORITHMS ARE USED

There are several ways in which algorithms may be used. How particular providers use the algorithm logic will probably change as they gain experience. Some training programs for nurse practitioners or physician's assistants require trainees to use clinical algorithms to learn how to manage common diagnostic problems. The algorithm may simply be used as a visual aid to learning a diagnostic strategy. Alternatively, a training program may require trainees to use the algorithms in patient care, reasoning that the responsibilities of patient care are likely to imprint the lessons contained in the algorithm logic more effectively than passive use.[3,11] The relative effectiveness of these two methods for using algorithms for training has never been tested.

Algorithms often are used to guide and monitor care of patients by graduate nurse practitioners or physician's assistants. How the algorithms are used depends largely on the knowledge and experience of the provider. Providers with little patient care experience and understanding of basic pathophysiology may be required to follow the algorithm logic precisely and be accountable on a daily basis for any actions that contradict the algorithm logic. This use of algorithms will be most effective in practices with minimally trained providers, a predominance of minor illness, and a high rate of personnel turnover. This method is used very effectively in military medicine and is best exemplified by the program at Brooke Army Medical Center.[12] This group uses daily computer-based audit of the function of military corpsmen to assure that care meets the standards set by the algorithms. Alternatively, audit may be performed periodically but less often. The audit may focus on the provider's cumulative performance on recurring or expensive medical decisions. This approach requires less time, reduces any tendency for personnel to feel harassed, and focuses on issues that make a significant difference to the practice. With more sophisticated providers such as nurse practitioners or certified physician's assistants, algorithms are more likely to be used as a standard of care for the practice than as a detailed prescription of what must be done for all patients. However, when clinically significant mistakes are made, the supervising physician and the nurse practitioner or physician's assistant have a standard of care to help resolve disagreements. For a practice with sophisticated nonphysician providers, the collaborative development of an algorithm as a mutually acceptable standard of care may transform cost-ineffective practices into cost-effective and efficient practices.

USE OF ALGORITHMS BY PHYSICIANS

Several studies have shown that physicians will accept guidance from decision-making aids such as decision rules or clinical algorithms. In one report, different types of providers in a university student health service used an algorithm for the management of acute pharyngitis.[13] All providers, including physicians, increased the frequency of recording specific items in the medical record, increased the ordering of specific tests indicated by the algorithm logic, and reduced the inappropriate use of antibiotics. Adherence to the logic of the algorithm improved with time and was unaffected when the frequency of periodic audit was reduced. The physicians used the algorithm system, although their compliance with its logic and their enthusiasm was less than the students'.

Physicians' use of clinical decision-making aids should increase if they recognize their need for assistance. Thus, one use for decision-guidance systems is to help physicians manage problems that they find difficult. One such system helps primary care physicians manage patients receiving cancer chemotherapy.[14] Relatively few primary care physicians have much experience using these toxic drugs, and they are often happy to leave the management of these difficult patients to major medical centers. Frequent visits to a medical center, however, may be very inconvenient for the patient who lives in a rural area. In the chemotherapy management system, the primary care physician had a management protocol form that indicated the data that were to be collected, drug dosages, and appropriate rules for use of the drugs. Compliance with the algorithm was monitored by the investigators, who were located at a major medical center. Seventy-three primary care physicians throughout Alabama delivered appropriate chemotherapy at nearly 97% of 2,612 visits by 195 patients. Disease-free intervals for the patients treated by their primary care physicians were indistinguishable from those of patients treated at the major medical center. This study showed conclusively that primary care physicians will accept guidance from a clinical algorithm when it enables them to give a kind of care that they would have otherwise been unable or unwilling to provide.

Algorithms have been designed to help physicians learn a strategy for diagnostic problems seen commonly in office practice. These algorithms have appeared periodically in *Patient Care* magazine and in a special section of the *Journal of the American Medical Association*.

EFFECTS OF ALGORITHMS ON CARE

1. Educational Effects of Algorithms

Physician's assistants and nurse practitioners will use a clinical algorithm system, at least during their training.[3,11,12] One study has characterized the educational effects of clinical algorithms during the training period.[11] All students had lectures covering the logic and medical content of the algorithms. Physician's assistant students were randomly assigned either to use the clinical algorithm system (checklist medical record form, algorithm, and computer-based audit) in a six-month clinical preceptorship or not to use the system. No significant differences were noted between intervention and control groups in knowledge of general medical facts, management decisions unrelated to algorithm logic, or medical facts related to the algorithms. There were, however, statistically significant differences in knowledge of the algorithm logic and ability to make management decisions related to the algorithm logic. Four months after the students stopped using the algorithm system, they took the National Board of Medical Examiners Physician's Assistants' Certifying Examination. Although there were no differences between intervention and control groups in general medical knowledge, students in the intervention group scored statistically significantly better on patient management decisions than the control students. Thus, algorithm use appeared to have had general effects on clinical decision-making ability that persisted for at least four months. In a second study, periodic written audit of compliance with the algorithm logic had no effect on learning the algorithm logic or algorithm-related facts.

2. Efficiency of Care

Because written standards for patient care are usually conservative and therefore all-inclusive, they may be expected to reduce the efficiency of care. The standard of care for the evaluation of a symptom is usually to "rule out" all the common diseases that may cause the symptom. This standard of care is the classical, safe diagnostic strategy learned by physicians during their clinical training. In practice, this strategy is efficient only because the effort to rule out all diseases becomes increasingly superficial as evidence for one disease becomes increasingly strong. The flexible, branching structure of algorithms can specify a diagnostic strategy that stops when strong evidence is available or continues through the differential diagnosis regardless of the strength of evidence for one disease. In fact, algorithms have usually been written to require the user to seek evidence for all the potentially serious causes of a symptom. Therefore, algorithms may be expected to slow the patient care process, as a penalty for increased diagnostic certainty.

Nonphysician providers using algorithms take about 50% longer than physicians to complete the evaluation of patients with upper respiratory illness[15,16] and abdominal pain, urinary tract infection, and headache.[16] However, they can manage about 50% of patient visits without the need for the physicians to examine the patient. Furthermore, the average time that the physician is required to spend with the patient is reduced to several minutes. Neither of these studies directly measured the effect of algorithms on the process of care. These excellent studies compared a nonphysician provider using an algorithm with a physician who was not using an algorithm. Since the experimental and control groups differed in two ways (type of provider and use of an algorithm), it was not possible to measure the size of the contribution of either of the two variables to the observed differences. These studies prove that the combination of algorithms and a nonphysician provider take somewhat more time than a physician to evaluate a patient, but they do not show that algorithms slow the process of care or affect the amount of information that is obtained.

3. Process of Care

The process of care is what is done to the patient. The process of care may be subdivided into data collection, diagnostic and therapeutic action, and patient counseling. To show that algorithms affect the process of care, care given by nonphysician providers using algorithms must be compared with care given by similar nonphysician providers not using algorithms. As indicated in the preceding section, this research design has not been used in previous studies. However, there is good evidence that algorithms do affect what is done to the patient. Patient records kept by physician's assistant students showed steady improvement in complying with the instructions contained in the logic of an algorithm. Perfect compliance with the algorithm logic for upper respiratory illness occurred in 40% of patients cared for by beginning Dartmouth physician's assistant students; five months later, compliance was perfect in nearly 80% of the patients.[17]

4. Illness Outcome

Several controlled studies have shown that patients cared for by a nonphysician provider using clinical algorithms for respiratory illness,[15,16,18,19] female[16,20,21] and male[22] genitourinary problems, back pain,[23] headache,[16,24] and abdominal pain[16] had clinical outcomes that were indistinguishable from those of patients cared for by a physician who did not use an algorithm.

Illness outcome is an important measure of the effectiveness of patient care, but it is probably insensitive to the quality of care in an ambulatory setting. Most unscheduled visits to an ambulatory drop-in clinic are for illnesses that are essentially self-limited. A relatively small number of patients have illnesses in which serious consequences could result from less than perfect care. Therefore, adverse outcomes will be infrequent, and the probability of detecting a significant difference between intervention group and control group is correspondingly small. Most studies that have shown no difference between intervention and control group have had relatively small numbers of patients, and the investigators have not calculated the probability that a significant difference was present but not detected (type II error).

5. Patient Satisfaction

Patients' satisfaction with their care has been used as a measure of quality of care in most studies of algorithms. For the most part, no difference was noted in patients' satisfaction with care given with or without algorithms.[4,15,18,22] However, satisfaction of patients with care given by nurse practitioners using an algorithm for back pain was statistically significantly greater than satisfaction with physician care for the same problem.[23] These studies do not demonstrate effects of algorithm-directed care on patient satisfaction, because patients' satisfaction could have been due either to the care that was directed by the algorithms or to the characteristics of the provider. Furthermore, patient satisfaction measures patient acceptance of a provider. Although acceptance by patients is important, it does not necessarily reflect delivery of good medical care. Provider-induced changes in patients' health behavior or attitudes should reflect quality of performance more clearly than patient satisfaction. These aspects of care have not been studied.

6. Effects of Clinical Algorithms on the Cost of Care

Since expenditures for diagnostic tests contribute substantially to the cost of medical care, it is logical to propose diagnostic strategies that make sparing yet appropriate use of tests. These strategies can be described in the format of algorithm logic and may be used as the basis for auditing for adherence to more parsimonious practice standards. Several controlled studies indicate that nonphysician providers using clinical algorithms can reduce the cost of care for certain common complaints.

In one study, patients with upper respiratory illness, urinary tract infection, headache, and abdominal pain were randomly assigned to physicians who did not use algorithms or to nurse practitioners or physician's assistants using algorithms.[16] The mean cost per encounter was lower when care was given by a nurse practitioner or physician's assistant than when care was provided by a physician. Nearly all of the difference was accounted for by the salary of the provider; the longer encounter time for nurse practitioners and physician's assistants was more than offset by their lower salary. A small, statistically insignificant reduction in laboratory test costs was seen when care was provided by nurse practitioners or physician's assistants using clinical algorithms. Similar findings were reported for care of upper respiratory illness by physician's assistants.[15]

As with the other studies of algorithms and patient care, these two reports describe the costs of care in two different systems: nonphysician provider with algorithm and physician without algorithm. The effect of the algorithm logic on the costs of care cannot be discerned directly, although random assignment of patients and similar diagnostic test costs certainly suggest that the algorithm logic reflects the standard of practice for physicians. Some investigators have designed algorithms to reduce diagnostic test utilization, but as yet there are no published reports of the potentially very important use of algorithms for improving the cost-effectiveness of the community standard of care.

MEDICOLEGAL ASPECTS

As an explicit statement of a standard of care, an algorithm can serve a purpose in the laws that govern medical practice. Legislators and health professionals are united in their concern for maintaining a high standard of medical practice. Physicians are expected to diagnose and treat disease or to accept responsibility for delegating these tasks to nonphysician clinicians. Substandard care is most likely to occur when providers take more responsibility than their training and experience have prepared them to exercise safely. Explicit rules for task delegation will minimize the chance of irresponsible arrogation of patient care tasks by ill-prepared providers. An algorithm is a written form of task delegation. To assure public safety, state laws governing medical practice by new health practitioners might well require the use of algorithms to express an arrangement between physician and nonphysician clinician about the conditions for ordering a test, prescribing a drug, or sending a patient home without consultation.

A number of state medical practice or nursing practice laws do contain language mandating algorithms to guide certain types of provider behavior. As of 1977, three state nursing practice laws required protocols for test ordering. Eleven states have practice laws that require protocols for prescribing drugs by nurse practitioners.[25] The American Hospital Association's statement on "The Nurse Practitioner in Health Care Institutions" contains among the privileges that may be granted to nurse practitioners the right to "engage in decision making and implementation of therapeutic actions in cooperation with other members of the health care team, as provided in joint protocols."[26] Thus, there is rather widespread agreement that public safety is protected by written guidelines for delegating of certain tasks to new health practitioners. Whether practitioners follow the letter or the intent of the law is not known.

Does a written standard of practice, as expressed in an algorithm, protect a physician from unfavorable malpractice judgments? Does it place the practitioner at extra risk? An algorithm could contain bad clinical judgment. Since no written standard can protect all contingencies, an inexperienced provider could make an error through following an algorithm too closely and ignoring signs of illness not described in the algorithm. To the author's knowledge, an algorithm has not figured in any malpractice action. Since the law is established by precedent in court, it may be a long time before the legal role of algorithms is delineated.

IMPACT OF ALGORITHMS ON PATIENT CARE
IN THE COMMUNITY

As shown by the studies cited earlier, algorithms can have a significant effect on education and care when they are used under the conditions of an experiment in health care delivery. To measure the effect of algorithms on patient care in the community, it is necessary to know how many practices use them and how carefully the algorithm logic is followed. Unfortunately, it can be very difficult to measure clinical algorithm use, since algorithms may influence patient care appropriately without any external evidence of having been used. When algorithms are used to train health care providers, the learning process may require the use of explicit aids such as checklists on which clinical findings may be recorded. The use of algorithms and their effect on the process of care may then be measured by counting checklists and auditing them for compliance with the algorithm logic. Once the student internalizes the algorithm logic, external aids may no longer be used, and the effect of algorithms on patient care becomes exceedingly difficult to measure. As yet, the long-range effects of algorithms on patient care in the community have not been studied. Therefore, there is no accurate information about the pervasiveness of algorithm use or the effect of algorithms on patient care in community practice.

Nonetheless, clear, albeit indirect, evidence exists that algorithms have had a substantial effect. Ten years ago, the word "algorithm" was mispronounced, misused, and derided. Now most primary care providers know what the word means, and professors from distinguished medical schools feel no need to define it when they use it in lectures to students or alumni. Medical magazines, journals, and books use algorithm flow sheets to present a diagnostic strategy in unambiguous terms. The terms "algorithm" or "protocol" appear in state medical practice and nursing practice laws. The original algorithm developers from Dartmouth and, particularly, Harvard have given away or sold tens of thousands of algorithm flow sheets or checklists. When the Harvard group surveyed their clientele several months after an algorithm purchase, they found that nearly all had used the algorithms to help them design their own practice-specific algorithms, and about half of their respondents had made their own medical record checklists. Relatively few practitioners had used the algorithms or checklists without modification (Anthony L. Komaroff M.D., personal communication).

This indirect evidence provides the basis for speculating about how algorithms affect clinical practice in the community. The introduction of a nurse practitioner or physician's assistant into a practice may trigger a decision to define standards by which the new provider is expected to practice. An algorithm format is used to express problem-specific standards for data collection, test ordering, initiation of treatment, and consultation. Algorithms developed in academic centers are used to help define these standards. Thus, along with other factors, algorithms seem to have whetted practitioners' appetite for an organized approach to clinical decision making. Continued research to develop and test diagnostic strategies for more efficient practice seems eminently justified by the demonstrated effects of algorithms on patient care and by community physicians' interest in new methods that will help them to provide accessible, reasonably priced, effective care for their patients.

References

1. Sox HC Jr. Quality of care by nurse practitioners and physician's assistants: A ten-year perspective. Ann Intern Med 1979;91:459-68.
2. Tufo HM, Burger CS. A diagnosis and treatment system for office aides. Patient Care 1970;5:128-37.
3. Sox HC Jr, Sox CH, Tompkins RK. The training of physician's assistants: The use of a clinical algorithm system for patient care, audit of performance, and education. N Engl J Med 1973;288:818-24.
4. Komaroff AL, Black WL, Flatley M, Knopp RH, Reiffen B, Sherman H. Protocols for physician assistants: Management of diabetes and hypertension. N Engl J Med 1974;290: 307-12.
5. Komaroff AL, Winickoff RN, eds. Common acute illness: A problem-oriented textbook with protocols. Boston: Little, Brown and Co, 1977.
6. Bell RS, Loop JW. The utility and futility of radiographic skull examinations for trauma. N Engl J Med 1971;284:236-9.
7. Walsh BT, Bookheim WW, Johnson RC, Tompkins RK. Recognition of streptococcal pharyngitis in adults. Arch Intern Med 1975;135:1493-7.
8. Greenfield S, Lewis CE, Kaplan SH, Davidson MB. Peer review by criteria mapping: Criteria for diabetes mellitus. Ann Intern Med 1975;83:761-70.
9. Sox HC Jr. How to write a clinical algorithm. In: Kallstrom M, and Yarnall S, eds. Design and use of protocols. Seattle:MCSA, 1975.
10. Holland RR. Decision tables: Their use for the presentation of clinical algorithms. JAMA 1975;233:455-7.
11. Wasson JH, Sox HC, Garcia R. A randomized study of the educational effects of an algorithm system. J Med Educ 1979;54:119-21.
12. Wolcott BW. Physician extenders in delivery of non-appointed ambulatory care in the military. Military Medicine 1977;141, No. 5.
13. Grimm RH, Shimoni K, Harlan WR, et al. Evaluation of patient care protocol use by various providers. N Engl J Med 1975;292:507-11.
14. Wirtschafter D, Carpenter JT, Mesel E. A consultant-extender system for breast cancer adjuvant chemotherapy. Ann Intern Med 1979;90:396-401.
15. Tompkins RK, Wood RW, Wolcott BW, Walsh BT. The effectiveness and cost of acute respiratory illness medical care provided by physicians and algorithm-assisted physician's assistants. Med Care 1977;15:991-1003.
16. Greenfield S, Anderson H, Winickoff R, Anderson H, Nessim S. Efficiency and cost of primary care by nurses and physician assistants. N Engl J Med 1978;298:305-9.
17. Tompkins RK, Kniffen WD, Sox HC Jr, Sox CH, Kaplan AD. Use of a clinical algorithm system in a physician's assistants program. In: Walker HK, Hurst JW, Woody MF, eds. Applying the problem-oriented system. New York: Medcom Press, 1973.
18. Winickoff RN, Ronis A, Black WL, Komaroff AL. A protocol for minor respiratory illness. Public Health Rep 1977;92:473-80.
19. Greenfield S, Bragg FE, McCraith DL, Blackburn J. An upper respiratory complaint protocol for physician extenders. Arch Intern Med 1974;133:294-99.
20. Greenfield S, Friedland G, Scifers S, Rhodes A, Black WL, Komaroff AL. Protocol management of dysuria, urinary frequency, and vaginal discharge. Ann Intern Med 1974;87: 452-7.
21. Komaroff AL, Sawayer K, Flatley M, Browne C. Nurse practitioner management of common respiratory and genitourinary infections using protocols. Nurs Res 1976;25:84-89.
22. Rhodes A, McCue J, Komaroff AL, Pass TM. Protocol management of male genitourinary infections. J Am Vener Dis Assoc 1976;2:23-30.
23. Greenfield S, Anderson H, Winickoff R, Morgan A, Komaroff AL. Nurse-protocol management of low back pain: Outcomes, satisfaction and efficiency of primary care. West J Med 1975;123:350-9.

24.Greenfield S, Komaroff AL, Anderson H. A headache protocol for nurses: Effectiveness and efficiency. Arch Intern Med 1976;136:1111-16.
25.Leitch CJ, Mitchell ES. A state-by-state report: The legal accommodation of nurses practicing expanded roles. Nurs Practitioner, Nov/Dec 1977, Vol 2, No. 8, p. 19.
26.American Hospital Association: Guidelines: The nurse practitioner in health care institutions, April, 1979.

CHAPTER TWENTY-FOUR

Improved Clinical Strategies for the Management of Common Problems

Anthony L. Komaroff, MD, Theodore M. Pass, PhD, and Herbert Sherman, DEE

Studies of clinical decision making and laboratory use have concentrated mainly on "expensive" technologies (high unit charges) and/or problems of the hospitalized patient with high-risk illnesses.

Several years ago, we began to investigate these questions with regard to "inexpensive" technologies (low unit charges), primarily in the ambulatory patient with low-risk illness. There were several reasons for doing so:

1. The enormous volume of such technologies means that the total charges are substantial, despite the low unit charge.
2. Ambulatory medical practice may be more susceptible than hospital practice to the inflationary pressures of an expanded health insurance system.
3. There is evidence of a marked variability in the use of these resources, for patients with ostensibly the same clinical problem.

This last reason seems especially compelling. Although physicians usually have a general framework for approaching a particular problem, within that framework, practice is exceedingly variable. Considerable evidence exists that, in the care of patients with the same problem, clinicians differ markedly in their decisions about ordering diagnostic tests, seeking consultation, recommending hospitalization, and prescribing treatment. Such variability strongly suggests that resources are being used inefficiently.

From the Laboratory for the Analysis of Medical Practices, Division of General Medicine and Primary Care, Department of Medicine, Brigham and Women's Hospital, Harvard Medical School, Boston, MA; and the Center for the Analysis of Health Practices, Harvard School of Public Health, Boston, MA.

This research was made possible by Grant HS 02063 from the National Center for Health Services Research, as well as a grant from the Max C. Fleischmann Foundation. Computer support was provided, in part, through a grant from the Esther A. and Joseph Klingenstein Foundation.

But recognizing the possibility that practice patterns are inefficient does not suggest what to do about it. Such variability in practice exists and is accepted for one reason: it is rarely clear that one clinical strategy is superior to any of several others. Therefore, it is rarely clear whether particular practices represent "underutilization" or "overutilization" of resources.

Clinicians will not begin to practice more "cost-effective" medicine until two conditions are satisfied. First, cost-effective clinical strategies have to be identified through careful study, and made known to clinicians. Second, general, nonclinical pressures (economic, social, legal) have to be exerted on clinicians to conserve resources. The second condition without the first is a blunt instrument, possibly discouraging the *necessary* application of resources at the same time that it reduces the *unnecessary* utilization of resources.

The majority of cost-containment efforts are of the latter type: general, nonclinical pressures. Prepayment, group practice, the imposition of "caps" on spending, all create general incentives to conserve resources, or frank constraints on the use of resources.

We are interested in the former issue: the study of cost-effective clinical strategies. We believe it is important to concentrate not only on rationalizing the *system* of medical care, but also medical *practice*. They suggest that we need to introduce efficiencies not only into the structure of our "cottage industry," but also into the clinical management of individual patients.

Our experience with the design and use of explicit cost-effective strategies is preliminary. We will be able to describe only the approach we are taking, and not the results of any of the several studies that are underway.

CURRENT RESEARCH

Decision Analyses in Ambulatory Care

We are currently investigating "cost-effective" clinical strategies for many of the most common conditions in ambulatory care. For each clinical problem—for example, sore throat—we identify what seem to be the "principal management strategies, and their potential consequences, as decision trees. The decision trees require certain *probabilities*, certain dollar *costs*, and certain *health effects* (morbidity or mortality caused or prevented) resulting from an action.

We obtain these probabilities, costs, and health effects values from several places:

1. Intensive search of the published medical literature;
2. The use of information previously collected by our group and others through prospective field studies (described below);
3. The solicitation of opinion from panels of national experts, using the Delphi technique, when empirical data is absent or when published data require expert assessment of their validity.

When the analyses suggest that certain strategies are clearly most cost-effective, we will compare such "superior" strategies to the strategies that appear to be used in current "average" practice, through a special analysis of the National Ambulatory Medical Care Survey data.

More often, though, we expect the analyses to be unable to identify one "superior" strategy with confidence, because there are important gaps in our knowledge about certain probabilities, costs, and/or health effects. In such cases, we will propose a research agenda, with a priority ranking determined from the analyses: the analyses will show which uncertain questions have the greatest effect on the identification of a "superior" cost-effective strategy.

Our work thus far suggests that a common concern about cost-effectiveness studies may not often be valid. Many people view questions of cost-effectiveness as inevitably implying the need to sacrifice some human benefit, in order to save money. This would be true if the only "cost" of taking a medical action were a dollar cost. But we all recognize that attempts to take action, to diagnose and treat the patient, may also *produce* other costs: morbidity, and even mortality. Conversely, attempts to save dollars by *not* taking action may lead to problems down the road: a short-term saving in dollars may wind up costing dollars in the long run.

Thus, both action and inaction can lead to the same kinds of costs: dollars, suffering, and death. There is a trade-off between the costs of trying to diagnose and treat, and the costs of not trying to diagnose and treat. A cost-effectiveness analysis is concerned with discovering which of several alternative approaches to a particular problem is least "costly" in suffering or the chance of death, just as it is concerned with discovering which is least "costly" in dollars. Thus far, none of our analyses has revealed a case in which the patient can only benefit from an approach to diagnosis and treatment, and in which one must ask how much this benefit is worth, in dollars.

We have avoided the "benefit-cost" approach of trying to place a dollar value on suffering and death, thereby reducing all "costs" in the analysis to dollar costs. We are keeping dollar costs, suffering, and the chance of death separate from one another in the analysis. Indeed, we are keeping different kinds of suffering separate from one another.

There are two reasons for this. First, it is conceivable that certain strategies are more cost-effective than other strategies for all types of costs; one strategy may lead to fewer dollar costs, and less suffering, and a lower likelihood of death. If and when that is the case, there is clearly no point in trying to relate these different kinds of "costs" to one another in an inevitably arbitrary manner.

Second, we feel that when it is necessary to make trade-offs between dollar costs and health benefits, these should be made by those responsible for the clinical decision, and by those who will be affected by it, i.e., the clinician and the patient. As analysts, we do not feel it is our role to make these value judgments, but rather to clarify the trade-offs so that those who must make them can do so in a rational manner.

Prospective Field Studies to Obtain Relevant Probabilities

An important aspect of our work is to conduct prospective studies in the field, in order to measure the yield of certain clinical and laboratory information. The features of these studies are as follows:

1. A patient with any of several explicitly designated presenting symptoms is asked to participate in the study, after signing informed consent.
2. The patient is asked to complete a questionnaire seeking past medical history pertinent to the presenting complaint.
3. The patient then is interviewed and examined according to a strict protocol. The protocol explicitly designates the collection of a detailed history and physical examination, which is recorded on a checklist.
4. Certain laboratory tests are ordered whenever a patient has explicitly designated clinical findings, *independent* of the clinician's judgment about the necessity of ordering that test. In this way we intend to control the denominator, in calculating the sensitivity and specificity of a test.
5. Each study patient is followed after the study visit by mail, telephone, and periodic repeat review of his or her medical record.
6. All clinical, laboratory, and follow-up data are entered into our computer.
7. Observer variability, intersite reliability on laboratory tests, and patient consistency in answering questions on the follow-up mail inquiry are all measured.
8. Using both Bayesian and multivariate techniques, we determine the conditional probability of a particular diagnosis given certain explicit combinations of clinical and laboratory findings. As a function of this analysis, the *incremental* gain (or loss) from particular costly procedures such as a laboratory test or time-consuming element of the physical examination (e.g., a speculum vaginal examination) can be calculated.
9. The purpose is to determine the clinical circumstances in which little or no benefit is derived from a particular test, but the cost is high—in terms of practitioner time, patient discomfort and time, or dollars.

We have conducted such a study over a 1-year period in four New England sites: two HMOs and two hospital-based outpatient practices. Approximately 1,300 patients with any of several designated respiratory tract infection symptoms or urinary/vaginal infection symptoms have been evaluated thus far. Ninety-seven percent of all of the data specified on the data collection instruments has been obtained. Reliability checks of the clinical data, selected laboratory tests, and patient follow-up information have been performed.

With the basic clinical data in hand, two further steps remain (as of this writing): first, to determine the final diagnosis as best as is possible in each patient; then to calculate the conditional probabilities of various diagnoses, given certain clinical and laboratory findings.

Determination of the final diagnosis is not straightforward. For instance, in patients with respiratory infections, clinicians generally assume a viral etiology when certain bacterial pathogens (e.g., streptococci) are not isolated by the standard diagnostic techniques. But standard diagnostic techniques do not disclose certain recognized pathogens (e.g., Mycoplasma pneumoniae) or potential pathogens that are treatable with antibiotics. Hence a study of clinical strategies in respiratory infection requires a search for such recognized pathogens, and offers an opportunity to evaluate the role of potential pathogens. We have been collaborating with several laboratories that have special expertise in diagnosing such unusual pathogens.

CONCLUSION

The design of explicit clinical strategies, the use of quantitative techniques, the application of decision analysis, often raise unpleasant spectres of regimentation, "cookbook medicine," mechanization, and dehumanization. In our judgment, such concerns are unjustified—*if* such approaches are properly applied.

Our experience in developing such strategies over the past several years has led us to conclude that, though carefully designed strategies for a given problem can anticipate the relevant information for decision making in *most* patients, such strategies can never anticipate all of the relevant information in *all* patients. Therefore, such strategies should be used to guide, but not to constrain, clinical judgment.

Some critics fear that such explicit strategies may someday be adopted by government bureaucracies, who then will require that such strategies be followed on every patient-clinician encounter. We think that such an unfortunate scenario is quite unlikely, except perhaps for government decisions about the purchase or application of extremely expensive equipment or procedures.

For the vast majority of encounters and procedures, we feel another scenario is much more attractive and much more likely. Increasingly, clinicians will practice in circumstances where general pressures to conserve medical resources are exerted—because they practice in prepaid arrangements, or as part of insurance programs that are forced by government-generated competitive pressures to control costs. An individual clinician, a group of clinicians, or an institution that lives under such a general pressure to conserve needs the clinical information by which choices for resource utilization can be made most efficiently.

Finally, it is important to emphasize that it is not only a desire to contain medical costs that makes such research interesting to us. The explosion of information about pathophysiology, and the proliferation of diagnostic and therapeutic technologies, have made it attractive, perhaps even imperative, to organize this information around the question we face every day: what should we do in caring for a patient with a particular problem? What is a logical approach to the diagnostic workup, and to the plan of therapy?

By helping to organize our knowledge, and thereby to highlight the areas of our ignorance, the investigation of explicit clinical strategies can prove to be important as we face the reality of limited resources.

CHAPTER TWENTY-FIVE

Computer-Based Support for Medical Decision Makers

Homer R. Warner, MD, PhD

Although diagnosis has largely monopolized the attention of people working in the field of computer algorithms for medical decision making, diagnosis is but one of a wide variety of challenging decisions that face the clinician. Listed in the accompanying tabulation are nine kinds of decisions currently being made by HELP, a computer-based system operational at the LDS Hospital in Salt Lake City.[1] In this presentation I would like to discuss examples of each of these nine types of decisions, present a description of the decision tools needed to perform these functions, and discuss the tools we have implemented to initiate the decision process and to direct the decisions to the appropriate destinations.

Kinds of Decisions
1. Screening—normal versus abnormal
2. Limit checking and alarms on raw data
3. Noise recognition
4. Preprocessing and pattern recognition
5. Diagnostic suggestions
6. Patient management decisions
7. Risk evaluation
8. Trigger for diagnostic or therapeutic protocols
9. Evaluation of patient progress

The set of decisions to be made determines the nature of the system design. In screening, the first kind of decision listed here, we have chosen to screen patients being admitted to the hospital for elective surgery. Thus we must gather the data and create the decision logic for recognizing those abnormalities in a patient that might influence his ability to undergo successfully the intended surgery. An electrocardiogram is performed to detect unrecognized coronary artery disease, and this screening becomes even more useful when coupled with a self-administered history designed to recognize angina. Routine spirometry is performed and the data interpreted by algorithms that not only normalize for height, age, and sex, but also categorize the nature and severity of the defect, if detected. Careful follow-up studies have demonstrated the usefulness of this information in patients undergoing abdominal surgery. One hundred percent of patients with abnormal preoperative spirometry develop pulmonary complications demonstrable by x-ray postoperatively, whereas only 40% of patients with normal pulmonary function preoperatively had postoperative pulmonary complications. Screening for evidence of infection, underlying liver or kidney malfunction, anemia, and defects in blood clotting ability are now standard practice in most hospitals and need no justification here. We do not include a chest x-ray as a routine procedure on all patients.

Examples of "limit checking and alarms on raw data" make use of the computer-based decision system as a sophisticated communication device. The computer's role is to assure that a low serum sodium is not only reported immediately on completion of the test, but that the result is acknowledged by someone in a position to do something about it. For instance, we have instituted a nurse-clinician program in which such alarms are systematically logged into a computer file, which may be reviewed on demand by the nurse-clinician. The nurse-clinician then has the responsibility to visit the nursing station of that patient and see that that information is brought to the attention of the nurse, house staff, or attending physician. This kind of follow-up has been appreciated and has, in some instances, significantly altered patient management.

The third category, "noise recognition," is a problem that plagues every clinician. As an example, consider the case of the patient whose initial screening serum creatinine value is flagged as exceeding the upper limits of normal. If this result was unexpected, the physician is faced with the decision as to whether it is an indicator of significant renal dysfunction, or is due to physiologic or laboratory noise. If the test is normal the following day, chances are the flagged deviation represented noise. We have recently completed a study aimed at deriving criteria for making this distinction at the time of the initial measurement by means of other data derived from the same battery of tests. Not only can such efforts aid the physician in solving a frequent and frustrating problem, but also can contribute significantly to the reduction of health care costs.

Another problem in noise recognition that has received a great deal of attention is associated with arrhythmia monitoring in the coronary care unit. Lessons learned from this kind of experience over the past 10 years have been of value in dealing with other kinds of signals as well. For instance, we have learned that it is far more difficult to develop an algorithm to recognize noise due to a loose electrode or contraction of the patient's skeletal muscles than it is to distinguish a normal QRS complex from an abnormal one. In fact, we have learned that if the system alarms the nurse that an arrhythmia has occurred and that alarm is false (due to noise) more than 50% of the time, the nurse will then begin ignoring even the true alarms. This phenomenon, I suspect, has its counterparts in many other areas of decision making where data arrives from a source over which the decision-maker has little control. It is up to the people who know that source to develop models of the noise (defined as the "nonuseful" component of the signal), which can be used as filters to preprocess the information sent to the clinician.

Preprocessing of data by a computer is dependent on either a model of the noise or a model of the signal. One of the most successful preprocessing operations in clinical medicine has been the recognition of electrocardiographic patterns. The models underlying electrocardiography are based on an understanding of the underlying electrophysiology and on empirical correlations with disease evolved over the last 70 years. By turning this tedious preprocessing over to the computer, we have achieved not only standardization and reproducibility in this phase of the decision-making process, but have also made this service directly available to those less skilled in performing it but still in need of the information it can provide.

Other forms of data represent two-dimensional arrays and present a bigger problem for the computer. Computerized axial tomography is an example in which preprocessing makes a major contribution to our ability to deal with a complex signal. Efforts at border detection and parameter extraction from these kinds of signals are also making contributions to medical decision making in areas such as evaluation of left ventricular function.

"Diagnostic suggestions made by the computer," of course, are important. The richest source of medical information is still the patient's history. A sequential Bayesian history program was instituted as an integral part of our patient screening history 8 years ago. This provides diagnostic suggestions to the physician that are based on patient's answers to questions presented on a terminal by the computer. The goal is not to make the primary diagnosis, which is usually already established on these elective surgery patients, but to detect secondary problems that might be relevant to care as the patient undergoes the scheduled surgical procedure. However, the computer will make the correct primary diagnosis in 67% of patients from history alone.

Blood gas reports from our laboratory contain an interpretation of the value as performed by the HELP algorithms. These algorithms reflect the thinking of the pulmonary medicine specialists responsible for that laboratory and, in some cases, include the suggestions for further management of the patient.

In order to facilitate the reporting of the radiologist's interpretation of the results of tests performed in his department, the HELP system provides a list of the most probable interpretations according to information available at the time the film is ordered. The radiologist may then choose from the list of the five most likely interpretations, add modifiers as appropriate, and be assured that results of his decision are immediately available on the terminal at the nursing station. The system accomplishes this with the help of statistics derived from the large patient database. For instance, the a priori probability that any chest film will be normal is 0.35, with the use of a sequential Bayesian algorithm, this probability can then be modified according to other statistics concerning events surrounding the order such as whether the patient is postoperative, the diagnosis on a previous x-ray, the reason for ordering the x-ray, and so forth. Such statistics have been accumulated for the most common x-ray interpretations. Eighty percent of the radiologist's interpretations are chosen from among the five suggested interpretations printed on the requisition by the HELP system.

"Patient management decisions" are some of the most difficult decisions facing the physician and will have perhaps the greatest influence on both the quality and the cost of medical care. For example, consider the decision to admit a patient to the coronary care unit. Opinions vary widely regarding the criteria for this decision, but few would argue that the patient who has been admitted to such a unit, and then has not used any of the special services of the unit, such as antiarrhythmia therapy or treatment for heart failure, really could have done as well at home or in a less intensive or expensive location in the hospital. The problem, then, is to define an algorithm that will permit classification of a patient into one of the two groups, using data available at the time of admission. The HELP system provides the tools for examining the database of a large number of patients. First, each patient is subjected to the criteria retrospectively for the two populations just described. One is called the "test" and one is called the "control." Then criteria are established with the HELP mechanism to define variables that might be used to classify patients, such as initial serum calcium value, or the presence of an old infarct pattern on the electrocardiogram. The distribution of serum calcium values for each of the two populations are then displayed as a histogram for comparison. If differences exist, these histograms are of potential value and are saved for possible use in the decision algorithm. When a number of such variables with different distributions or frequencies in the two populations have been found, tests for independence of the variables within each population are performed. Independent variables are then incorporated into a sequential Bayesian algorithm or a discriminant function for use in the new decision algorithm. The key to this kind of decision making is the data base, which must contain sufficient follow-up information to permit independent definition of the two populations of patients who represent outcomes from the two alternatives to the decision whose criteria are being developed.

"Risk evaluation" is an activity that already has proven particularly amenable to computer implementation. An example is the detection of drug orders or prescriptions that involve undue risk of an adverse reaction for a particular patient. Each time a physician's prescription is entered into a patient's file by a pharmacist via a terminal, any logic contained in the HELP system that involves the drug being prescribed is called in for execution by the computer. If, for instance, digitalis is prescribed and the patient is already getting a potassium-losing diuretic or has a low serum potassium, the system will suggest that a potassium supplement be given. If the pharmacist receives this message, she conveys the information to the physician who wrote the prescription. Eighty percent of the time the computer's suggestions are complied with by the physician. More sophisticated logic involving even models of drug kinetics permits useful consultation regarding dosage as well.

Protocols for management of cancer patients receiving chemotherapy are in widespread use, because it is generally recognized that comparison of patient outcomes under alternate therapeutic regimens will not be meaningful unless rigid definition of group criteria and strict adherence to standardized therapy is accomplished. Already it has been shown that computers are essential aids to this end. Key decisions are being made every day regarding patient management for which we do not have adequate knowledge. Coronary artery disease is a glaring example. Until protocols are in general use in the management of this and many other common problems in medicine, we will not make much headway in improving these decision-making skills. We have implemented, as have others, computer-based protocols for collecting all the data that surround the decision process and as much follow-up data as possible to assess the outcomes of the decision alternatives. Not only does the computer provide a tool for sophisticated data collection as an integral part of medical care, it also provides the means for interaction of the investigator with the data and for implementation of decisions derived from that interaction in the management of subsequent patients.

Many medical decisions involve evaluation of patient progress and its relation to the therapy that a patient is receiving. This kind of decision problem requires a different response from the computer. If the last electrocardiogram showed a myocardial infarction pattern, there is no point in reporting that same interpretation, even though true, for the next ECG. Instead, the physician is interested in changes in the patient's status. The computer system can know this by looking back in the patient record in most cases. The special problems of interpreting serial results require that more than just the last interpretation be saved for future reference. Some derived parameters, and occasionally even raw data, must be preserved for serial interpretation. Otherwise, insignificant changes in one or two parameters may be sufficient to change the classification of the patient based on the current test from that made from the previous test results. If the parameters are saved and used for serial interpretation, that interpretation can be made to reflect the true importance or unimportance of small changes that may have occurred between the two measurements.

Decision Tools

1. To model a sequence of events from a patient's data
2. To express stochastic relationships
3. To express individualized utilities
4. To derive statistics for improving decision criteria
5. To initiate decision process
6. To direct decisions to the appropriate destinations

Listed in the accompanying tabulation are the kinds of decision tools provided by the HELP system to aid in the decision-making tasks just described. First, the system provides a mechanism for modeling an explicit sequence of events using data from a patient's file. At least one time and date is associated with each entry. The choice of which time to log is, of course, based on the kind of decisions that are anticipated from this entry. For instance, most decisions made from a blood gas measurement regarding patient status will relate to the time the sample of blood was drawn, but other times may be needed for quality control decisions.

Since multiple values of a particular variable may be stored in a patient's file during a specified time interval, a variety of modifiers may be used such as first, last, maximum, minimum, average, and nearest to specify the specific information to be used in a decision. For instance, one might specify as an item to be retrieved, as part of a decision to prescribe digitalis, "the maximum heart rate over the period from the onset of atrial fibrillation until now."

The decision tools must allow the user to express not only Boolean and arithmetic relationships, but also stochastic models, in a way that is convenient to specify and easy for another person to understand. We have emphasized Bayesian algorithms that use both binary and continuous variables. The continuous variables may be represented in a HELP decision module in any one of three ways: an equal bin width histogram, an equal bin count histogram, or a set of parameters defining a continuous distribution function for that variable in each of the two populations associated with the decision process.

Just as important as the calculation of probabilities in a decision process is the estimation of utilities that will determine the threshold of probability at which the decision will be made. The HELP system provides for individualizing these utility estimates using patient data such as age, sex, and occupation.

To derive statistics for improving decision criteria, a system called STRATO allows a user to build a HELP decision module to specify criteria for defining each subpopulation of patients from the database to be used in the analysis. This creates a list of patient numbers representing each population. Other HELP modules are then specified for each of the variables to be studied in a population, such as the last serum sodium value before admission to the coronary care unit. The distribution of values for this variable for each of two populations may then be compared by superimposing the histograms and performing a variety of statistical tests. Differences in such distributions, when found, may then form the basis for creation of new decision criteria for an action, such as admitting a patient to the unit.

Decision processes are initiated in the HELP system any time a data item used in a decision is logged into any patient's file. This data-driven feature assures that no item of data will go unheeded, if indeed the system "knows" any way to use it for decision making. Decisions may also be initiated when a specified amount of time has elapsed since a particular event. Thus the absence of expected data can also drive the decision process.

And finally, of course, decisions made by the system must be directed to someone who can use the information. The creator of a HELP module may specify that the decision is to be returned to the program that generated the last data item, stored in one of several temporary files for retrieval on demand by such people as the attending physician, pharmacist, or the nurse-clinician, printed out as part of a laboratory report containing that last piece of data, or printed as an alert at the nursing station printer nearest the patient.

After nine years' experience with the use of a computer-based medical decision support system in a general hospital, we are even more convinced than at the beginning of this effort that the coupling of a medical database to a medical knowledge base is a useful undertaking. It is apparent, however, that many limitations exist to both our ability to gather the needed information from the patient in a standardized way and our fund of knowledge regarding the specific probabilities and utilities. To make the effort successful we need people trained in medicine who are informed about computers and who are motivated to use this powerful tool for the good of patients.

Reference

1. Warner HR. Computer-assisted medical decision-making. New York: Academic Press, 1979.

CHAPTER TWENTY-SIX

INTERNIST: Can Artificial Intelligence Help?

J. D. Myers, MD, Harry E. Pople, Jr., PhD, and Randolph A. Miller, MD

On the basis of the work that we have been engaged in over the past eight years, the question posed in the title can be answered in the affirmative.

Many computer porgrams for diagnosis in medicine have been devised utilizing (a) branching logic techniques, (b) Bayesian analysis, and (c) to a lesser degree, artificial intelligence. These programs have all dealt with circumscribed problems in internal medicine and other clinical fields; none other than INTERNIST has attempted to encompass as broad an area as general internal medicine.

To distinguish clearly the INTERNIST approach from these other approaches to computer-based diagnosis, it is important to clarify what is meant by the terms "problem" and "problem-formation" in this context. Our use of the word "problem" may be considered synonymous with "differential diagnosis," that is, a "problem" is a collection of disease entities, one and only one of which is considered possible in the case being studied; "problem-formation" refers to the process by which appropriate differential diagnoses are evoked for consideration during the course of a diagnostic work-up.

In many computer-based diagnostic systems, the "problem" (so defined) is predetermined, and the program's job is simply to select one of a fixed list of disease entities that best fits the facts of a case. A diagnostic program based on Bayes' rule, for example, requires that problems of differential diagnosis be defined as sets of disease entities that are exhaustive (i.e., all possibilities are included) and mutually exclusive (i.e., one and only one may occur).[1-3]

There are both philosophical and methodological questions associated with the use of Bayes' rules in medical diagnoses; these have been well documented in the literature.[4-6] A major problem is the need to assume that the manifestations of disease are statistically independent so as to reduce the data structuring problem to manageable proportions. A second problem, which bears on the multiple disease issue, is the requirement that for purposes of Bayesian analysis, the set of possible diagnosis must be mutually exclusive and exhaustive.

To deal with complex clinical problems having the potential of multiple diagnoses, some authors have proposed the development of diagnostic programs comprising sets of integrated Bayesian procedures, each dealing with some well-defined subproblem in clinical medicine. Thus the set of all disease entities would be divided into M subsets, not necessarily disjoint, each of which is considered a mutually exclusive and exhaustive "differential diagnosis" list. If M is a relatively small number, it may be feasible to employ a Bayesian decision procedure that attempts to solve all M decision problems simultaneously.[7,8] Alternatively, one may invoke heuristic "activation rules" or rely upon the guidance of persons using the system to select appropriate subproblems for further analysis.[9,10] As this latter approach requires that an initial decision be made concerning the subproblems to be explored, great care must be taken to ensure that the analytical process has the capacity to recover from "false starts." Otherwise, the kinds of difficulties often encountered in branching logic diagnostic systems, discussed in the following paragraph, may limit the usefulness of this approach. We shall return to consideration of this important issue again during the discussion of our plans for INTERNIST-II.

Aside from Bayesian methods, the other approach to computer based diagnosis that has been most extensively studied is the "branching-logic" or "flowchart" method. The essence of this approach is the use of a sequence of discriminating questions that successively narrow the diagnostic possibilities that may be considered for a case under analysis, until ultimately in the limiting case some single diagnosis remains.

Behaviorally, a diagnostic procedure using branching logic would appear to perform in much the same manner as a sequential Bayesian procedure.[11,12] However, major differences exist in the forms of the database and the inferential procedures that are used.

The database for a branching logic procedure is a network, each node of which represents a decision (interrogation) point. Depending on the given initial conditions of a case, the inferential procedure begins at some starting point of the network and then proceeds from node to node, at each point eliciting the discriminating information required by the decision process associated with the node. A decision is then made, on the basis of this result, as to which node is to be considered next.

The major drawback of this method has been its inability to handle new and conflicting information after several previous decisions have been made. As the focus of attention moves through the net, previous nodes or decisions become inaccessible, rendering it impossible to retreat from a given pathway under the influence of new information. In essence the model under certain circumstances may find itself "out on a limb" from which it cannot extricate itself.

Another deficiency of this method is that, unlike the Bayesian procedure described previously and the INTERNIST approach to be discussed subsequently, a diagnostic program based on branching logic is not capable of processing input data presented in random order. The sequence of information input required in the course of a diagnostic study is completely determined by the structure of the decision network, and by the sequence of prior decisions made along the way.

These characteristics of the branching-logic method preclude its use as a general clinical diagnostic tool. However, the method has proved to be extremely useful in certain phases of the diagnostic process; e.g., the staging and analysis of laboratory test data.[13]

Several major investigations have been undertaken during the past few years, seeking to apply the methods of artificial intelligence to problems of medical diagnosis and management. In our own work, the emphasis has been on development of a computer-based diagnostic system for internal medicine. Other studies have focused on the diagnosis and therapeutic management of bacteremia,[14] the differential diagnosis of glaucoma,[15] the management of digitalis therapy,[16] and the taking of the present illness.[17]

Development of the system we now call INTERNIST-I[18] was begun about eight years ago. The system was successfully demonstrated for the first time in 1974 and has been used since that time in the analysis of hundreds of clinical problems. On the basis of extensive testing of this initial INTERNIST system, it has become clear that many aspects of the system's performance could be significantly enhanced if it were possible to handle the various component problems and their interrelationships simultaneously. This has led to the design of INTERNIST-II,[19] a system embodying strategies of concurrent problem-formation that we expect will yield more rapid convergence to the correct diagnosis in many cases, and in at least some cases provide more acceptable diagnostic behavior.

THE INTERNIST KNOWLEDGE BASE

The knowledge base underlying INTERNIST is composed of two basic types of elements: disease entities and manifestations (history items, symptoms, physical signs, laboratory data). In addition, a number of relations are defined on these two classes of elements. To date, some 440 individual disease entities have been profiled incorporating about 3,300 individual manifestations of disease.

A disease is profiled only after extensive study, including a review of published literature, survey of any case series accumulated by faculty members of the University of Pittsburgh School of Medicine, and consultation with clinical experts. Medical students on elective assignment have helped extensively in literature surveys. After study of a disease has been completed, a list of all the manifestations of that disease is drawn up. Manifestations are classified (TYPE) as demographic data, clinical history, symptoms, physical signs, and laboratory data, including radiographic data, isotopic scans, biopsies, etc. Laboratory data are typed into three categories: Lab 0 = routine; Lab 1 = noninvasive, noncostly but not routine studies; and Lab 2 = invasive, dangerous, and/or costly studies.

Each manifestation of a given disease is assigned two numbers, evoking strength (EVOK) and frequency (FREQ). EVOKs ask the question, "How strongly does the manifestation suggest the disease in comparison to all other diseases?" The values for EVOKs range from 0 to 5:

Evoking Strength	Interpretation
0	Nonspecific—manifestation not useful in making a differential diagnosis
1	Diagnosis a rare or unusual cause of listed manifestation
2	Diagnosis causes a significant minority of instances of listed manifestation
3	Diagnosis the most common but not the overwhelming cause of listed manifestation
4	Diagnosis the overwhelming cause of listed manifestation
5	Listed manifestation pathognomonic for the diagnosis

FREQs ask the question, "Given the disease, how frequent is the manifestation?" The values for FREQs range from 1 to 5:

Frequency	Interpretation
1	Listed manifestation occurs rarely in the disease
2	Listed manifestation occurs in a significant minority of cases of the disease
3	Listed manifestation occurs in about half the cases
4	Listed manifestation occurs in a significant majority of cases
5	Listed manifestation is a sine qua non for the diagnosis

An additional third number, IMPORT, is assigned for each manifestation in a global sense, that is, across all diseases, and asks the question, "How important is the manifestation overall in clinical diagnosis?" or "How readily can the manifestation be disregarded vis-à-vis any final diagnosis(es) arrived at?" IMPORTs range from 1 (minimal IMPORT) to 5 (maximal IMPORT).

Other relations are defined on the set of disease entities to record the causal, temporal, and other patterns of association by which the various disease entities are interrelated. These relationships are expressed as LINKs using the same EVOKs and FREQs concepts as described above. These interrelationships can be of various types between disease A and disease B: A predisposes to B (PDIS), A precedes B (PCED), A causes B (CAUS), A and B coincide, exact relationship unknown (COIN), or A and B are part of the same basic disease process (SYST), for example, lupus nephritis or lupus cerebritis as parts of systemic lupus erythematosus. There are also several auxiliary relations defined to express associations among manifestations, such as the derivability of one from another.

When the programming of a disease has been completed and all values have been approved by a principal investigator (JDM), it is checked for accuracy and completeness by analyzing classical ("textbook") instances of the disease. In due time, the disease profile is repeatedly checked by the analysis of additional cases, most of which are difficult diagnostic problems. Diseases as they are programmed are arranged in a hierarchy that is system oriented but based in large part on pathophysiological considerations.

The medical knowledge base in printed form has proven to be a valuable information resource in addition to its serving as the basis for the computer operation of INTERNIST.

PROBLEM FORMATION METHODS AND INTERNIST-I

A major point of departure for the design of the original INTERNIST program was the realization that the task of clinical decision making in internal medicine is ill-structured. In other domains, the task of diagnosis is often viewed as one of pattern recognition or discrimination, that is, a predefined collection of possible classifications (characterizing disease entities or clinical states) is available, one and only one of which is considered possible in the case being studied. A diagnostic problem solver dealing with such a well-structured domain has the fairly straightforward task of selecting that one of this fixed set of alternatives that best fits the facts. Many statistical, pattern recognition, and algorithmic techniques have been used successfully in performing computer-aided diagnosis in these well-structured clinical problem domains.

Primarily because complex cases often involve two or more concurrently active disease processes, no set of exhaustive and mutually exclusive classifications can be developed to structure the diagnostic problem in internal medicine. In principle, it might be argued that this more complex problem domain could be reduced to a simple discrimination task if, in addition to the individual disease entities, one includes appropriate multiple disease complexes in the set of allowable patient descriptors. However, since our experience suggests that as many as 10 or 12 individual descriptors may apply in a complex clinical problem, and considering that a thousand or more individual descriptors of interest exist in internal medicine, the prospect of recording explicitly all possible multiple disease classifications is clearly infeasible.

Our thesis is that, in the absence of explicit structure, the successful clinician engages in heuristic imposition of structure so that effective problem-solving strategies might be selected and used for decision making relative to the postulated problem structure.

In INTERNIST-I, this concept of heuristic imposition of structure is expressed primarily by means of a novel "problem-formation" heuristic. In effect, the program composes dynamically, on the basis of evidence provided, what in context constitutes a presumed exhaustive and mutually exclusive subset of disease entities that can explain, more or less equally well, some significant subset of the observed findings in a clinical case. This heuristic problem structuring procedure is invoked repeatedly during the course of a diagnostic consultation, in order to deal sequentially with the component parts of a complex clinical problem.

The process is as follows. First, the clinical data from a patient are entered into the computer. All positive observations are entered; "significant" negative observations may be entered as desired The evoked disease entities that can explain any or all of the observed findings in a case are weighted individually and assigned scores reflecting their fit with the data. In this scoring process, the evoking strength and importance of manifestations (these are numeric weights recorded in the INTERNIST knowledge base) explained by a disease are counted in its favor; frequency weights count against those disease hypotheses in which the corresponding manifestations are expected but found absent in the case.

Given a ranked list of disease hypotheses, a problem focus is then formulated on the basis of the most highly rated of these items, using the following heuristic criterion: two disease entities are considered to be alternatives to one another (hence part of the same problem definition) if, taken together, they explain no more of the observed findings than are explained by one or the other separately.

The set of alternatives so determined, with scores within a fixed range of the top-ranked disease hypothesis on the list, is then composed into a problem, which becomes the focus of problem solving attention.

When this problem focus contains five or more disease hypotheses, a "RULEOUT" strategy is used. "RULEOUT" asks about manifestations with very high frequency of occurrence in the diseases being processed. Such questions stand a good chance of eliminating one or more of the considered diseases. The level of questions asked is incremented via the TYPE, so that inexpensive items are asked first. Because of the high cost associated with the acquisition of laboratory data, "RULEOUT" mode is not used when the TYPE of questioning has reached the level of laboratory procedures. Instead, the focus is artificially narrowed so that the "DISCRIMINATE" strategy can be used, which normally applies only when two to four disease hypotheses are being considered. In this mode, the top two diagnoses are selected for discrimination; items that count heavily for one hypothesis while counting heavily against the other are the desiderata for questioning. Finally, if the problem focus contains only one predominant model, a "PURSUING" strategy is used. Questions are then selected that are thought to have a good chance of being "clinchers." Manifestations that have a strong evoking strength with respect to the one considered disease are asked. The system continues in "PURSUING" mode until either the initial spread between the two top contenders has reached a conclusive criterion, or until the spread has been reduced to the point that the top node no longer stands alone on the focus list. In the former case, the system "CONCLUDEs" that the considered disease is present; in the latter, processing reverts to the "DISCRIMINATE" mode.

In each mode, a small number of questions are selected and asked. The responses to the set of queries are processed in a manner essentially the same as described above. The program reevaluates all diseases evoked (whether in or out of the current problem focus) on the basis of new information obtained, and then reformulates the problem focus. Depending on which disease entity emerges as most highly rated on successive iterations of the process, the focus of attention may shift from one problem to another, but at any one time, a single problem is under active consideration.

Whenever a problem becomes solved, it is entered into a list of concluded diagnoses; all manifestations explained by that disease are marked "accounted for"; and diseases related to the confirmed diagnosis are given appropriate bonus scores (dependent on evoking strength and frequency of the LINK relationship). If significant patient data remain to be explained after parts of the problem are solved, the process described above is repeated in an effort to discover and confirm additional diagnoses.

CRITIQUE OF THE INTERNIST-I LOGIC

From our observation of clinicians interacting with this model of diagnostic logic, we have come to understand certain important features of this process. The following elements have been found to affect in significant ways both the diagnostic behavior of the system and its potential acceptability to the intended user community.

1. Focus of attention is on the most highly scored disease hypothesis and its competitors.

This feature has both advantages and disadvantages. On the plus side, this focusing scheme tends to single out for consideration that subset of diseases that can account for the most important patient data. Among those selected hypotheses, the more favored are the more common, other things being equal. This results from the use of evoking strength weights of each observed manifestation for each disease hypothesized in the scoring of that disease. Note that the evoking strength weight is in some ways analogous to a posterior probability of disease, given a finding. Hence it necessarily folds in at least subjective estimates of a priori probability, or commonality of disease.

On the negative side, this heuristic mechanism tends to be sensitive to the preponderance of data, as well as to the more relevant measure of specificity and importance. Thus it sometimes happens that important, specific data are temporarily "disregarded" by INTERNIST's problem focusing heuristic whereas less significant facts of the clinical problem are selected for initial investigation on the basis of a large volume of data, much of which might be of limited importance.

A second difficulty, which sometimes arises as a result of the commonality factor, is the selection of a common disease as the diagnosis in situations where actual discriminating points have not been obtained that would set this disease apart from its rarer sister clinical states. Even though such a decision might be rationalized, pragmatically, on the basis that "common things are common," we believe that the clinical user of such a system should be informed of the probabilistic basis of such advice. Because of the compounding of numerous types of influences in the INTERNIST-I scoring algorithm, it would be virtually impossible to reveal in a comprehensible fashion all the factors operative in such a decision.

Another difficulty associated with the emphasis on common disease in INTERNIST-I is the inability of that system to revise its estimate of commonality in cases where the concurrence of multiple interacting disease processes work to alter the odds. By virtue of its single-focus, sequential problem-solving strategy, INTERNIST may not be "conscious" of a concurrent problem in the patient under review, which, if it had been solved first, might have altered (by means of the LINK scoring adjustment referred to earlier) the assessment of likelihood with respect to disease hypotheses in the initial decision set.

2. Sequential problem formation and problem solving.

The major advantage of the single problem focus of INTERNIST-I is the simplicity of control that this permits. By virtue of its frequent reformulation of the problem focus, INTERNIST-I exhibits a responsive "problem hunting" behavior that almost always converges, eventually, on the appropriate conceptualization of a clinical problem. The only difficulty with this approach is that, in complex cases, the program often begins its analysis by considering wholly inappropriate problems on which it may spend an inordinate amount of time. This rarely leads to a false conclusion, but does prolong the sessions of terminal interaction unnecessarily. This phenomenon also dictates the use of a very conservative approach to the patient work-up, as more aggressive strategies might seek costly items of information pertaining to an ill-advised initial conceptualization of a problem.

If, instead of structuring and dealing with decision problems in a sequential fashion, it were possible to structure several problems at the same time, heuristics might be employed to focus attention on the most "solvable" of these, rather than on the one that happens to receive the highest goodness-of-fit rating, as described above. Moreover, the scoring process itself could be made more effective if the findings of a case could be distributed among the several concurrent problem areas in accordance with some notion of relevancy. At present, lacking the perspective of a multiple problem focus, INTERNIST-I assigns credit in the scoring of a disease hypothesis to all manifestations explained by that disease, however rare that association. Hence in a case, say, involving obvious liver and gastrointestinal involvement, the singular focus of INTERNIST-I will invariably favor those hepatic problems that also generate gastrointestinal findings and those gastrointestinal disorders that give rise to hepatic manifestations. The clinician, able to recognize that both problem areas are involved, can attribute findings to the most relevant of these, thereby coming in many cases to a far better ranking of the alternatives in each subproblem. The clinician can also take prior cognizance of the interrelationships among disease entities, to come more quickly to specific hypotheses than would otherwise be the case.

Unfortunately, one of the things that limits INTERNIST-I to the sequential formation and consideration of problems is also one of the features of the system most responsible for its robust behavior, namely —

3. Ad hoc formation of problem structure.

Although the INTERNIST knowledge base includes a hierarchy of disease categories that was originally intended to allow decision making to proceed from general characterization of disease process (via descriptors corresponding to higher level nodes of the hierarchy) to the most specific characterizations corresponding to terminal level disease states, in practice this categorical structure is not actually used to develop problem foci during the course of an INTERNIST-I analysis. Instead, as described previously, the program uses a heuristic partitioning algorithm in order to group together those disease hypotheses "thought" to be competitors to the most highly ranked disease. The reason for using this ad hoc mechanism is that in the real world of clinical practice, individual diseases may present in many different ways. Depending on circumstances, the physician (and the program assisting the physician) must be prepared to structure a decision problem that will serve to discriminate among those hypotheses that seem to be roughly equivalent in explanatory power, in the local context of the available patient data.

Thus, whenever it postulates a problem, INTERNIST-I may group together disease entities from throughout the hierarchy, without regard for the a priori groupings recorded there. If, for example, the only available data concerning a patient pertained to diastolic hypertension, then a problem would be put together cutting across the subareas of endocrinology, nephrology, cardiology, hematology, neurology, and systemic disease. INTERNIST would then seek to narrow this range of alternatives by questioning the user concerning items of information that would subserve one of two "problem-solving" mechanisms. First, data gathered in support of one hypothesis ($H1$) that cannot be explained by another ($H2$) will cause a separation in score between these two hypotheses, which when greater than a specified threshold leads to the conclusion of hypothesis $H1$. A second narrowing mechanism is often brought into play in situations where certain new data are obtained supporting hypothesis $H1$ and other data obtained supporting $H2$. Whenever this happens, these diseases, which formerly were considered to be competitors because they explained the same subset of data, will now no longer be partitioned into the same decision set (the presumption being that since each now can explain some portion of the data not explained by the other, both may be concurrently active). Thus, even with no change in the relative scores, two hypotheses originally thought to be competitors may later be thought complementary, leading the problem formation algorithm to reduce the focus of its decision set accordingly.

Experience has shown that this policy of decision making relative to a postulated problem is one of the great strengths of the INTERNIST system. Diagnostic decisions are rendered whenever sufficient separation is obtained for the leading hypothesis, as compared with its putative competitors. Thus, provided an appropriate differential diagnosis set has been identified, it is possible for the program to come to the correct diagnosis by ruling out all but one of the diagnoses in the set, then recording the remaining contender as its default judgment. In this fashion, the program often manages to solve difficult clinical problems even in the absence of clinching data (obtainable only by biopsy or autopsy, perhaps) that are unavailable at the time of the analysis.

The main difficulty with this decision strategy is that INTERNIST does not, and cannot in its present implementation, question the validity of the postulated problem focus in the context of which its decision-making process is being carried out. As mentioned previously, the program often generates incorrect problem foci at the outset, but the relative ease and frequency with which the problem focus is reformulated generally guarantees that eventually an appropriate decision problem will emerge. Nothing in the logic ensures that this will happen, however, and this sometimes leads to incorrect diagnostic results.

The reason that this difficulty cannot always be overcome within the INTERNIST-I framework is the ephemeral nature of the problems (or decision sets, differential diagnoses) employed there. These ad hoc constructs have no substance outside the context of the particular case in which they emerge. Although clinicians viewing a decision problem formulated by INTERNIST-I may have no difficulty attaching an appropriate label, and may even have very specific ideas about the proper way to work up such a problem, INTERNIST has no access to such problem specific advice.

The only way to make such clinically relevant knowledge available to the program would be to incorporate new knowledge structures containing explicit information about well-structured subproblems, the disease entities they include, criteria useful in ruling these problems either in or out, and specific advice, where useful, concerning the decision process that is to be followed relative to the postulated problem.

To summarize the above critique, in preliminary studies during the past several years, many hundreds of clinical cases have been analyzed using INTERNIST. Although in most cases, satisfactory diagnostic decisions were obtained as a result of these interactions, in some cases the sequence in which various facets of the clinical presentation were handled proved to be inappropriate. At times, the program would fail to attend to significant patient data already known to it, while focusing attention on less important aspects of the problem. More commonly, the program might spend considerable time trying to resolve some component part of a complex problem that could not adequately be dealt with unless other aspects of the problem could somehow be considered simultaneously.

DEVELOPMENT OF INTERNIST-II

Extensive investigation of the phenomena detailed above in the context of INTERNIST-I have convinced us that the basic difficulty is the inadequacy of a hierarchy as a data structure for representing interesting and useful groupings of disease entities. As mentioned previously, it was originally intended that the INTERNIST disease hierarchy would be used to establish "milestones" in a diagnostic work-up, but this has not proved to be the case.

An example might help clarify the nature of the difficulty. Assume that a patient presents with jaundice, pruritis, light colored stools, and on laboratory evaluation is found to have significantly elevated alkaline phosphatase, in short, a fairly typical pattern of cholestatic jaundice. Despite the fact that the INTERNIST hierarchy of disease categories has a node called "cholestasis," it would not do for the program to conclude (or even entertain as a very serious hypothesis) that the patient's real problem is to be found among the diseases cataloged under the "cholestasis" node. The reason for this is that under the heading "cholestasis" are recorded only those disease entities whose predominant mode of presentation is cholestatic. Other diseases that may present variously with some degree of cholestasis are scattered throughout the liver disease subtree and other regions of the hierarchy. For example, alcoholic hepatitis resides under "toxic hepatocellular disease," primary biliary cirrhosis is classified under "hepatic fibrosis," infectious mononucleosis is structured under "infectious lymphadenopathy," and so on.

To overcome the limitations imposed by the strict hierarchical organization of disease categories, two different approaches have been used in adding multifaceted diseases to the INTERNIST knowledge base. In some cases, diseases with protean manifestation lists are subdivided into organ-specific components; for example, hepatic leptospirosis and renal leptospirosis are singled out as separately profiled facets of that systemic infection. In other cases, where a disease might have two or more common modes or presentation that differ in their predominant facets, multiple profiles may be compiled reflecting these differences; these are then recorded in the hierarchy under the appropriate rubrics. Thus hepatocellular viral hepatitis is classified under hepatocellular inflammation, whereas cholestatic viral hepatitis is located under intrahepatic cholestasis; similarly, carcinoma of the head of the pancreas is grouped under extrahepatic cholestasis.

Deciding which approach to use in particular instances is not always an easy choice, and from time to time it has proved necessary to regroup under a single heading what had previously been fragmented components of a disease. Similarly, diseases originally profiled as multifaceted systemic processes have subsequently had to be partitioned into multiple profiles. No one approach seems to be universally acceptable.

It seems clear that what is really needed to deal with the requirement for multiple classification is the introduction of a more general network that can permit direct encoding of any node into as many descriptive categories as necessary. Although such a structure would be fairly easy to implement technically, it is clear that extensive changes in the diagnostic programs will be required to exploit this new facility. In addition, substantial reorganization in the knowledge base may be required in order to achieve the consistency of organization made possible by the new multiple classification network.

To emphasize the significance of this new data structure, higher level nodes of the classification network will no longer be referred to as disease categories but rather as categories of involvement. Thus, in place of the present category called "Disease of Liver and Biliary System," the new classification scheme will have the more encompassing category "Involvement of Liver and/or Biliary System." Under this heading will be references to all diseases presently grouped under the liver subtree, also the leukemias, lymphomas, infectious lympha-denopathies, and other classes of disease not generally thought of as predominantly liver disease but having some potential for expressing hepatic involvement.

Once the enriched classification scheme becomes available, it will be possible to replace the present heuristic problem formation strategy of INTERNIST-I with a "problem evocation" strategy keyed to higher level nodes of the involvements network. Given the typical pattern of cholestatic jaundice cited above, for example, the new INTERNIST will not have to assemble the appropriate differential diagnosis, de novo, by aggregating items scattered throughout the classification structure. Now, the node called "cholestatic involvement" will encompass all and only those diseases comprising this differential.

The process of evocation of appropriate differential diagnoses will be a matter of responding to cues in the patient data by conjecturing the occurrence of one or more nodes of the involvements network, each of which provides a partial description of the clinical problem. For this purpose, it is often unnecessary to go beyond the type of data available on history and physical examination to develop a high level description of the problem being confronted. If the liver is enlarged or distorted, then a hypothesis of liver involvement is clearly warranted; similarly, bronchial breathing can be considered indicative of pulmonary involvement.

By responding to a multiplicity of such cues, the new INTERNIST will be able to evoke and consider simultaneously the many facets of a complex clinical problem. Each such facet can be considered to be an independent differential diagnosis and worked up accordingly. Alternatively, it will be possible to invoke the maxim of Occam's razor and focus attention on that subset of diseases that could explain all (or at least the most significant) of the various types of involvement that have been observed.

To facilitate the synthesis of composite hypotheses that can explain multiple facets of a clinical picture, we intend also to develop a generalized link structure. This can be thought of as a detailed causal network, more extensive than the one now used in INTERNIST, with a planning level of associations used to link high level nodes of the involvements network, where appropriate, on the basis of causal, temporal, or other patterns of interaction. Given a collection of patient data that suggests one or more conclusions with respect to these high level facet descriptors, the generalized causal network can then be used to detect very readily those areas of the disease hierarchy that constitute points of convergence of various chains of reasoning.

For the initial hypothesis formation phase of the process, the detailed substructure of the causal network will be transparent, as only the high level links from one facet descriptor to another will be used. Once some working hypotheses have been structured, however, the detailed substructure of the selected portions of the network can be examined systematically to discover which, if any, of the conjectured top level associations constitute verifiable attribution pathways from specific diseases to the pathological states and manifestations they explain.

Within this framework, it should be possible to develop procedures to handle the difficulties identified so far in connection with our use of INTERNIST-I. Improved focusing methods and attention to the principle of parsimony will be exploited in the postulation of reasonable hypotheses concerning the diagnostic alternatives. Early results, using approximations to the required knowledge structures, suggest that we may indeed expect performance of the new INTERNIST to surpass that of its predecessors. What needs to be done now is a systematic realignment of the knowledge base into the new format, with concomitant development of the expanded capabilities envisioned for the diagnostic planning and evaluative modules.

The above considerations can be emphasized by a recent case run using INTERNIST-I. The case is from the Massachusetts General Hospital (Case 19-1980).[20] (See Appendix, page 265.)

First, all of the positive and negative data provided in the patient's protocol are entered into the computer in the order in which they are presented. In the initial computation many pieces of information are, for the time being, "disregarded." The "considering" list applies only to the leading diagnostic node that has been evoked, namely sinusoidal or postsinusoidal portal hypertension. The system is in the "pursuing" mode, meaning that there is strong evidence for this form of portal hypertension, and clinching evidence will be sought to confirm it. Such evidence was not available (N/A), but nevertheless the diagnosis was concluded.

The computer returns to the "disregarding" list and finds strong evidence for hepatocellular carcinoma at the "pursuing" level. Again, additional positive evidence is lacking, and again the diagnosis is concluded.

The next diagnosis to be concluded is transudative ascites for which ample evidence was present from the beginning, though not mathematically as strong as for either portal hypertension or hepatocellular carcinoma.

Finally, the system turns to the underlying liver disease and attempts to discriminate between Laennec's cirrhosis and postnecrotic cirrhosis. There being no additional information of adequate discriminatory value, the task cannot be accomplished and the system, in a conservative fashion, defers with Laennec's cirrhosis in the first place.

The hepatocellular carcinoma, the portal hypertension, and the transudative ascites are all correct diagnoses. At autopsy the patient did have Laennec's cirrhosis.

The case illustrates several of the deficiencies of INTERNIST-I. The good clinician, knowing that the patient was a chronic alcoholic, and so on, would have postulated a diagnostic complex: Laennec's cirrhosis with hepatocellular carcinoma, complicated by portal hypertension and transudative ascites. Diagnostic effort would have been applied to the complex in toto or in piece.

Second, evidence, which could have been used in the differential diagnosis of the chronic liver disease, was usurped and explained by the hepatocellular carcinoma, for example, the abnormal liver function tests. This occurred because hepatocellular carcinoma happened to precede the chronic liver disease in the serial diagnostic sequence.

Third, sinusoidal or postsinusoidal portal hypertension was diagnosed in preference to presinusoidal portal hypertension on the basis of the greater clinical incidence of the former. In this particular case, the computer analysis was correct, but in the light of the sequence of diseases considered, it could have been wrong.

INTERNIST-II, by forming a diagnostic complex(es) from the beginning and by applying facets of disease, in this case for example hepatocellular injury, to more than one diagnostic entity as appropriate, appears to be able to correct these deficiencies. In addition, undue emphasis is not given to commonality of disease.

References

1. Ledley RS, Lusted LB. Reasoning foundation of medical diagnosis: symbolic logic, probability and value theory and our understanding of how physicians reason. Science 1959; 130:9-21.

2. Nordyke JF, Kulikowski CA, Kulikowski CW. A comparison of methods for the automated diagnosis of thyroid dysfunction. Comput Biomed Res 1971;4:374-89.

3. Patrick EA, Stelmack FP, Shen LY-L. Review of pattern recognition in medical diagnosis and consulting relative to a new system model. IEEE Trans 1974;SMC-4:1-16.

4. Ledley RS. Practical problems in the use of computers in medical diagnosis. Proc IEEE 1969;57:1900-19.

5. Feinstein AR. The haze of Bayes, the aerial palaces of decision analysis, and the computerized Ouija board. Clin Biostat 21:4:482-96.

6. Szolovits P, Pauker SG. Categorical and probabilistic reasoning in medical diagnosis. J Artificial Intell 1978;11.

7. Engle RL, Flehinger BJ, Allen S, Friedman R, Lipkin M, Davis BJ, Leveridge LL. HEME: A computer aid to diagnosis of hematologic disease. Bull N Y Acad Med 1976;52:584-600.

8. Ben-Bassat M, Lipnick E. Diagnosis and treatment in MEDAS. Proc ACM 1977;96-100.

9. Wortman PM. Medical diagnosis: an information processing approach. Comput Biomed Res 1972;5:315-28.

10. Patrick EA, Shen LY-L. A systems approach to applying pattern recognition to medical diagnosis. Purdue Univ Medical Computing Program: TR-EE. 75-12, 1975.

11. Warner HR, Rutherford BD, Houtchens B. A sequential Bayesian approach to history taking and diagnosis. Comput Biomed Res 1972;5:256-62.

12. Gorry GA, Barnett GO. Experience with a model of sequential diagnosis. Comput Biomed Res 1968;1:490-507.

13. Bleich HL. Computer-based consultation: electrolyte and acid-base disorders. Am J Med 1972;53:285-91.

14. Shortliffe E. Computer-based medical consultations: MYCIN. New York: Elsevier, 1976.

15. Weiss SM, Kulikowski CA, Safir A. A model based consultation system for the long-term management of glaucoma. Proc IJCAI-5, Boston 1977:826-32.

16. Silverman H. A digitalis therapy advisor. Project MAC, Mass Inst of Tech, Technical Report TR-143, 1975.

17. Pauker SG, Gorry GA, Kassirer JP, Schwartz WB. Toward the simulation of clinical cognition: taking a present illness by computer. Am J Med 1976;60:981-95.

18. Pople HE, Myers JD, Miller RA. The DIALOG model of diagnostic logic and its use in internal medicine. Proc IJCAI-4, Tbilisi, USSR, Sept. 1975.

19. Pople HE. The formation of composite hypotheses in diagnostic problem solving: an exercise in synthetic reasoning. Proc IJCAI-5, Boston, 1977.

20. Scully RE, ed. Case records of the Massachusetts General Hospital, Case 19, 1980. N Engl J Med 1980;302:1132-40.

Appendix

```
INITIAL POSITIVE MANIFESTATIONS:
SEX MALE
AGE 26 TO 55
MENTAL RETARDATION
THROMBOPHLEBITIS HX
ANTICOAGULANT ADMINISTRATION RECENT HX
EKG Q WAVE [S] ABNORMAL
CHEST PAIN SUBSTERNAL REMOTE HX
DYSPNEA EXERTIONAL
ABDOMEN DISTENTION
FECES GROSS BLOOD
CHEST PAIN SUBSTERNAL AT REST
CIGARETTE SMOKING HX
ALCOHOLISM CHRONIC HX
TACHYCARDIA
TACHYPNEA
WEIGHT GTR THAN 40 PERCENT ABOVE IDEAL
DYSPNEA AT REST
SKIN SPIDER ANGIOMATA
RHONCHI DIFFUSE
RALES LOCALIZED
ABDOMEN FLANK [S] HEAVY BILATERAL
ABDOMEN FLUID WAVE
ABDOMEN FLANK [S] BULGING BILATERAL
PLATELETS 50000 TO 200000
BILIRUBIN BLOOD CONJUGATED INCREASED
AMMONIA BLOOD INCREASED
LDH BLOOD INCREASED
ALKALINE PHOSPHATASE BLOOD INCREASED NOT OVER 2 TIMES NORMAL
EKG SINUS TACHYCARDIA
EKG PREMATURE ATRIAL CONTRACTION [S]
EKG VOLTAGE LOW
EKG ST SEGMENT DEPRESSION WITHOUT RECIPROCAL ELEVATION
EKG T WAVE [S] INVERTED
CHEST XRAY PLATE LIKE DENSITY [IES].
CHEST XRAY LUNG [S] CONGESTED
HEPATITIS B SURFACE ANTIGEN
ASCITIC FLUID PROTEIN 3 GRAM [S] PERCENT OR LESS
FECES GUAIAC TEST POSITIVE
ESOPHAGOSCOPY VARICES
STOMACH ENDOSCOPY GASTRIC VARICES
CELIAC ANGIOGRAPHY LIVER FOCAL HYPERVASCULARITY
CELIAC ANGIOGRAPHY VARICES
ELECTROPHORESIS SERUM ALBUMIN DECREASED
SGOT GTR THAN 400
CPK BLOOD INCREASED
SGOT 40 TO 119
ABDOMEN PAIN COLICKY
ABDOMEN PAIN HYPOGASTRIUM
FECES BLACK TARRY
SYNCOPE OR SYNCOPE HX
ESOPHAGUS BARIUM MEAL VARICES
STOMACH BARIUM MEAL GASTRIC VARICES
```

ABDOMEN XRAY FLUID PERITONEAL CAVITY
STUPOR OR SOMNOLENCE
JAUNDICE
ABDOMEN VENOUS PATTERN CENTRIFUGAL FLOW FROM UMBILICAL AREA
ABDOMEN TENDERNESS RIGHT UPPER QUADRANT
LIVER ENLARGED MODERATE
SPLENOMEGALY MODERATE
FINGER [S] CLUBBED
PROTEINURIA
BILIRUBIN URINE PRESENT
HEMATOCRIT BLOOD LESS THAN 35
FEVER
LIVER RADIOISOTOPE SCAN SINGLE LARGE FILLING DEFECT
LIVER RADIOISOTOPE SCAN IRREGULAR UPTAKE

INITIAL NEGATIVE FINDINGS:
GLYCOSURIA
WBC 4000 TO 13900 PERCENT NEUTROPHIL [S] INCREASED
WBC 14000 TO 30000
RBC RETICULOCYTE [S] GTR THAN 5 PERCENT
PROTHROMBIN TIME INCREASED
ACTIVATED PARTIAL THROMBOPLASTIN TIME INCREASED
UREA NITROGEN BLOOD 30 TO 59
UREA NITROGEN BLOOD LESS THAN 8
GLUCOSE BLOOD 130 TO 300
CALCIUM BLOOD INCREASED
PHOSPHATE BLOOD INCREASED
ELECTROPHORESIS SERUM GAMMA GLOBULIN INCREASED
AMYLASE BLOOD INCREASED
ANTIBODY HEPATITIS B SURFACE ANTIGEN
ALPHA FETOGLOBULIN INCREASED
ALPHA 1 ANTITRYPSIN DECREASED
ASCITIC FLUID CYTOLOGY POSITIVE
STOMACH ENDOSCOPY DIFFUSE INFLAMMATION
STOMACH ENDOSCOPY ULCER CRATER
DUODENUM ENDOSCOPY ULCER CRATER
STOMACH BARIUM MEAL ULCER CRATER
DUODENAL BULB BARIUM MEAL ULCER CRATER
LEG [S] EDEMA BILATERAL SLIGHT OR MODERATE
ABDOMEN XRAY FREE AIR PERITONEAL CAVITY
ABDOMEN TENDERNESS REBOUND LOCALIZED

DISREGARDING: ABDOMEN PAIN COLICKY, ABDOMEN PAIN HYPOGASTRIUM, CHEST PAIN
SUBSTERNAL AT REST, DYSPNEA AT REST, DYSPNEA EXERTIONAL, ABDOMEN FLANK [S]
HEAVY BILATERAL, ABDOMEN FLUID WAVE, ABDOMEN TENDERNESS RIGHT UPPER QUADRANT,
FEVER, FINGER [S] CLUBBED, JAUNDICE, LIVER ENLARGED MODERATE, RALES LOCALIZED,
RHONCHI DIFFUSE, SKIN SPIDER ANGIOMATA, STUPOR OR SOMNOLENCE, WEIGHT GTR THAN
40 PERCENT ABOVE IDEAL, ALKALINE PHOSPHATASE BLOOD INCREASED NOT OVER 2 TIMES
NORMAL, BILIRUBIN BLOOD CONJUGATED INCREASED, BILIRUBIN URINE PRESENT, CHEST
XRAY LUNG [S] CONGESTED, CHEST XRAY PLATE LIKE DENSITY [IES], EKG Q WAVES
ABNORMAL, PROTEINURIA, SGOT 40 TO 119, SGOT GTR THAN 400, ABDOMEN XRAY FLUID
PERITONEAL CAVITY, AMMONIA BLOOD INCREASED, ASCITIC FLUID PROTEIN 3 GRAM [S]
PERCENT OR LESS, CPK BLOOD INCREASED, ELECTROPHORESIS SERUM ALBUMIN DECREASED,
HEPATITIS B SURFACE ANTIGEN, LIVER RADIOISOTOPE SCAN IRREGULAR UPTAKE, LIVER
RADIOISOTOPE SCAN SINGLE LARGE FILLING DEFECT, CELIAC ANGIOGRAPHY LIVER FOCAL
HYPERVASCULARITY

CONSIDERING: AGE 26 TO 55, SEX MALE, ABDOMEN VENOUS PATTERN CENTRIFUGAL
FLOW FROM UMBILICAL AREA, FECES BLACK TARRY, FECES GROSS BLOOD, SPLENOMEGALY
MODERATE, FECES GUAIAC TEST POSITIVE, HEMATOCRIT BLOOD LESS THAN 35,
ESOPHAGUS BARIUM MEAL VARICES, PLATELETS 50,000 TO 200,000, STOMACH BARIUM
MEAL GASTRIC VARICES, CELIAC ANGIOGRAPHY VARICES, ESOPHAGOSCOPY VARICES,
STOMACH ENDOSCOPY GASTRIC VARICES

PURSUING: SINUSOIDAL OR POSTSINUSOIDAL PORTAL HYPERTENSION

PLEASE ENTER FINDINGS OF AUSCULTATION ABDOMEN
*GO

ABDOMEN BRUIT CONTINUOUS PERIUMBILICAL?
N/A

PRESSURE HEPATIC VEIN WEDGE INCREASED?
N/A

PLEASE ENTER FINDINGS OF ARTERIOGRAPHY ABDOMEN
*GO

MESENTERIC ARTERY SUPERIOR ARTERIOGRAPHY VARICES SMALL INTESTINE?
N/A

CONCLUDE: SINUSOIDAL OR POSTSINUSOIDAL PORTAL HYPERTENSION

DISREGARDING: ABDOMEN PAIN HYPOGASTRIUM, CHEST PAIN SUBSTERNAL AT REST,
DYSPNEA AT REST, DYSPNEA EXERTIONAL, ABDOMEN FLANK [S] HEAVY BILATERAL,
ABDOMEN FLUID WAVE, RHONCHI DIFFUSE, SKIN SPIDER ANGIOMATA, STUPOR OR
SOMNOLENCE, WEIGHT GTR THAN 40 PERCENT ABOVE IDEAL, CHEST XRAY LUNG [S]
CONGESTED, EKG Q WAVE [S] ABNORMAL, ABDOMEN XRAY FLUID PERITONEAL CAVITY,
AMMONIA BLOOD INCREASED, ASCITIC FLUID PROTEIN 3 GRAM [S] PERCENT OR LESS,
CPK BLOOD INCREASED, LIVER RADIOISOTOPE SCAN IRREGULAR UPTAKE

CONSIDERING: ABDOMEN PAIN COLICKY, ABDOMEN DISTENTION, ABDOMEN TENDERNESS
RIGHT UPPER QUADRANT, FEVER, FINGER [S] CLUBBED, JAUNDICE, LIVER ENLARGED
MODERATE, RALES LOCALIZED, TACHYCARDIA, TACHYPNEA, ALKALINE PHOSPHATASE
BLOOD INCREASED NOT OVER 2 TIMES NORMAL, BILIRUBIN BLOOD CONJUGATED
INCREASED, BILIRUBIN URINE PRESENT, CHEST XRAY PLATE LIKE DENSITY [IES],
EKG SINUS TACHYCARDIA, PROTEINURIA, SGOT 40 TO 119, SGOT GTR THAN 400,
ASCITIC FLUID OBTAINED BY PARACENTESIS, ELECTROPHORESIS SERUM ALBUMIN
DECREASED, HEPATITIS B SURFACE ANTIGEN, LDH BLOOD INCREASED, LIVER
RADIOISOTOPE SCAN SINGLE LARGE FILLING DEFECT, CELIAC ANGIOGRAPHY LIVER
FOCAL HYPERVASCULARITY

PURSUING: HEPATOCELLULAR CARCINOMA

ABDOMEN BRUIT CONTINUOUS RIGHT UPPER QUADRANT?
N/A

ABDOMEN BRUIT SYSTOLIC RIGHT UPPER QUADRANT?
N/A

CELIAC ANGIOGRAPHY LIVER FOCAL HYPERVASCULARITY SURROUNDED BY RADIOLUCET ZONE?
NO

DISREGARDING: ABDOMEN PAIN HYPOGASTRIUM, CHEST PAIN SUBSTERNAL AT REST,
DYSPNEA AT REST, DYSPNEA EXERTIONAL, ABDOMEN FLANK [S] HEAVY BILATERAL, ABDOMEN
FLUID WAVE, RHONCHI DIFFUSE, SKIN SPIDER ANGIOMATA, STUPOR OR SOMNOLENCE,
WEIGHT GTR THAN 40 PERCENT ABOVE IDEAL, CHEST XRAY LUNG [S] CONGESTED, EKG Q
WAVE [S] ABNORMAL, ABDOMEN XRAY FLUID PERITONEAL CAVITY, AMMONIA BLOOD INCREASED,
ASCITIC FLUID PROTEIN 3 GRAM [S] PERCENT OR LESS, CPK BLOOD INCREASED, LIVER
RADIOISOTOPE SCAN IRREGULAR UPTAKE

CONSIDERING: ABDOMEN PAIN COLICKY, ABDOMEN DISTENTION, ABDOMEN TENDERNESS RIGHT
UPPER QUADRANT, FEVER, FINGER [S] CLUBBED, JAUNDICE, LIVER-ENLARGED MODERATE,
RALES LOCALIZED, TACHYCARDIA, TACHYPNEA, ALKALINE PHOSPHATASE BLOOD INCREASED
NOT OVER 2 TIMES NORMAL, BILIRUBIN BLOOD CONJUGATED INCREASED, BILIRUBIN URINE
PRESENT, CHEST XRAY PLATE LIKE DENSITY [IES], EKG SINUS TACHYCARDIA, PROTEINURIA,
SGOT 40 TO 119, SGOT GTR THAN 400, ASCITIC FLUID OBTAINED BY PARACENTESIS,
ELECTROPHORESIS SERUM ALBUMIN DECREASED, HEPATITIS B SURFACE ANTIGEN, LDH BLOOD

INCREASED, LIVER RADIOISOTOPE SCAN SINGLE LARGE FILLING DEFECT, CELIAC ANGIOGRAPHY
LIVER FOCAL HYPERVASCULARITY

PURSUING: HEPATOCELLULAR CARCINOMA
CONCLUDE: HEPATOCELLULAR CARCINOMA

DISREGARDING: ABDOMEN PAIN HYPOGASTRIUM, CHEST PAIN SUBSTERNAL AT REST,
RHONCHI DIFFUSE, SKIN SPIDER ANGIOMATA, STUPOR OR SOMNOLENCE, WEIGHT GTR
THAN 40 PERCENT ABOVE IDEAL, CHEST XRAY LUNG [S] CONGESTED, EKG Q WAVE [S]
ABNORMAL, AMMONIA BLOOD INCREASED, CPK BLOOD INCREASED, LIVER RADIOISOTOPE
SCAN IRREGULAR UPTAKE

CONSIDERING: DYSPNEA AT REST, DYSPNEA EXERTIONAL, ABDOMEN FLANK [S] BULGING
BILATERAL, ABDOMEN FLANK [S] HEAVY BILATERAL, ABDOMEN FLUID WAVE, ABDOMEN
XRAY FLUID PERITONEAL CAVITY, ASCITIC FLUID PROTEIN 3 GRAM [S] PERCENT OR
LESS

CONCLUDE: TRANSUDATIVE ASCITES

DISREGARDING: ABDOMEN PAIN HYPOGASTRIUM, CHEST PAIN SUBSTERNAL AT REST,
RHONCHI DIFFUSE, STUPOR OR SOMNOLENCE, WEIGHT GTR THAN 40 PERCENT ABOVE
IDEAL, CHEST XRAY LUNG [S] CONGESTED, EKG Q WAVE [S] ABNORMAL, AMMONIA
BLOOD INCREASED, CPK BLOOD INCREASED

CONSIDERING: ALCOHOLISM CHRONIC HX, SKIN SPIDER ANGIOMATA, LIVER RADIOISOTOPE
SCAN IRREGULAR UPTAKE

DISCRIMINATE: MICRONODAL CIRRHOSIS [LAENNECS], MACRONODAL CIRRHOSIS
[POSTNECROTIC]

PLEASE ENTER FINDINGS OF INSPECTION GENITALIA MALE
*GO

TESTIS [ES] ATROPHY?
N/A

PLEASE ENTER FINDINGS OF PALPATION ABDOMEN
*GO

LIVER FINE NODULE [S]?
N/A

PLEASE ENTER FINDINGS OF PALPATION SALIVARY GLAND [S]
*GO

PAROTID GLAND [S] ENLARGED?
N/A

LIVER DISTORTED OR ASYMMETRICAL?
NO

LIVER BOSSELATED?
NO

PLEASE ENTER FINDINGS OF JAUNDICE HX
*GO

JAUNDICE CHRONIC PERSISTENT HX?
NO

DISREGARDING: ABDOMEN PAIN HYPOGASTRIUM, CHEST PAIN SUBSTERNAL AT REST,
RHONCHI DIFFUSE, STUPOR OR SOMNOLENCE, WEIGHT GTR THAN 40 PERCENT ABOVE
IDEAL, CHEST XRAY LUNG [S] CONGESTED, EKG Q WAVE [S] ABNORMAL, AMMONIA
BLOOD INCREASED, CPK BLOOD INCREASED

CONSIDERING: ALCOHOLISM CHRONIC HX, SKIN SPIDER ANGIOMATA, LIVER
RADIOISOTOPE SCAN IRREGULAR UPTAKE

DISCRIMINATE: MICRONODAL CIRRHOSIS [LAENNECS], MACRONODAL CIRRHOSIS
[POSTNECROTIC]

PLEASE ENTER FINDINGS OF BLOOD COUNT AND SMEAR
*GO

RBC TARGET [S]?
N/A

LIVER EDGE HARD?
N/A

PLEASE ENTER FINDINGS OF LIVER BIOPSY/ASPIRATE
*OMIT

DEFERRING

Section VI. Research Initiatives Toward Effective Decision Making and Laboratory Use

CHAPTER TWENTY-SEVEN

Research and Operational Strategies: An Overview

Ellis S. Benson, MD

One of the most important developments in recent years with respect to the clinical laboratory has been the dawning realization that more is required of a laboratory test than the assurance of technical validity. We in laboratory medicine now know that we have responsibilities that go beyond the assurance of the reliability of test results. The concepts "diagnostic sensitivity" and "diagnostic specificity" have been with us for many years but it was not until Galen and Gambino[1] rediscovered and popularized these concepts in 1975 that we paid much attention to them. Use of these concepts, and that of "predictive values," has helped to focus attention on the *diagnostic* effectiveness of tests in specific diagnostic and management situations. Since issues of cost have risen sharply and the clinical laboratory is viewed as a limited resource, concerns have multiplied about the usefulness of laboratory tests and other diagnostic technologies.

Escalating health care costs is a public policy issue of major importance in the United States today, and the cost of clinical laboratory services is a leading element in this rise. Yet careful analysis shows that unit costs of laboratory tests have not increased over the past few years and may even have decreased to some extent, indicating increased efficiency in a "labor-intensive" field, probably owing largely to automation. Increased costs can be ascribed to increased input volume (expanded utilization of services) and increased input variety (introduction of new services).[2,3]

Our own analysis indicates a constantly increasing use of laboratory tests per hospital bed, patient, patient day, and other similar denominators.[4] I believe this to be another indication of a general trend toward increase in "intensity of care" at all levels of care. The President's Council on Wage and Price Stability in a staff report on rising health care costs in 1976 concluded that the escalating rise in health care costs was due largely to a *change in product*,[2] in other words, a change in the style and character of services provided by hospitals and doctor's offices. Finkelstein[5] and Griner,[6] in studying utilization of laboratory services in hospital care, have concluded that there has been a *change in style* in the use of the laboratory, on the part of physicians, toward more intensive use.

These changes may not be bad, economically or medically, but the repeated observation that these changes have occurred and are continuing calls for intensive study of their significance, especially in the face of escalating costs and limited resources. Since the laboratory is indeed a limited resource, its use must be measured to meet real needs.

J. M. G. Wilson[7] recently has placed the problem in the following perspective:

> Automation in clinical chemistry is a powerful tool. Like many innovations, it is posing some problems as well as resolving some. Its use in population screening is leading to a search for better methods of indicating the significance of laboratory tests and to a vigorous examination of the clinical value of the ever increasing number of tests.

Two general reactions to the changes I have just described have developed. Some critics decry the destructive effect of technology on the art of medicine. Others have suggested that if we returned, in effect, to an earlier day when laboratory services were more restricted and requisitioning of laboratory tests more difficult, we would see better use.[8-10] We know from experience that poor service chills demand quite rapidly. Rationing, quotas, tariffs, and negative incentives are varieties of this approach and have their advocates.[10,11] Such methods, however, have rarely worked well and have sometimes "backfired" when consumers have discovered that, because of them, they were denied access to valuable services. A Canadian experience, in which a check was placed on diagnostic service requisitioning by each physician based on an average for that specialty, failed when ceilings quickly became floors.[10]

A second approach is typified by Dr. Stead's suggestions at this conference (see Chapter 4) that technology may be made to enhance the art as well as the science of medicine. This position is supported by Drs. Myers, Weed, Warner, and others who have taken part in this conference. This conference has emphasized routes toward more rational and prudent use of diagnostic technologies as the approach of choice to problems of utilization and cost. First, education has been stressed, at all levels of the physician's career, by Griner, Burke, Goldfinger, and Eisenberg. Second, laboratorians-pathologists and others are called to become more involved with the clinical tasks of medicine to be better prepared to guide rational use.

Finally, the need is urgent to develop and put into operation a strong research agenda directed toward improved use of laboratory tests and laboratory information. Attractive research initiatives may lie along the following avenues.

SCREENING AND PROFILING

Admission screening and profiling are test selection strategies whose effectiveness must be further studied. Since these approaches add much to the laboratory's workload through the follow-up investigations they generate, often because of false positive test results, it is important to analyze their worth critically.

Not so long ago, the initial examination of a patient admitted to medical care included a thorough medical history, a complete physical examination, and a few basic fairly simple laboratory examinations. Depending on what was uncovered by this preliminary examination, the physician went on in a logical stepwise fashion to conduct or request a number of additional examinations to confirm or reject diagnostic possibilities. The advent of automation in the clinical laboratory, especially multichannel analysis, introduced many additional tests at the beginning of the diagnostic process (admission) and along its route. It was reasoned that if these analyses could be provided rapidly, accurately, and economically they might accelerate the diagnostic process and thus shorten hospital stay. Unfortunately many of the batteries were constructed on the basis of laboratory (or manufacturer's) convenience rather than clinical usefulness or logic.

What has been the product of this strategy? Has the diagnostic process been accelerated and has length of stay been shortened? Studies thus far indicate that the answer is "no." Carmalt and Whitehead,[12] Whitehead and Wooten,[13] and Leonard et al.[14] all reporting from England, found that use of an admission screening battery had no effect on length of stay in hospital. Leonard and associates[14] furthermore found a much increased volume of laboratory tests on screened patients when compared with controls.

Recently, Durbridge et al.[15] reporting from Australia, in an extensive study found a low yield of significant information from routine admission biochemical screening in a general hospital population. They concluded that this approach is cost ineffective as a case finding technique. A number of studies have cast serious doubts on the effectiveness of biochemical screening as a case finding instrument in unselected hospital patients.[16-18]

Werner and Altshuler,[19] on the other hand, have argued persuasively that the screening approach provides a database for subsequent clinical investigation. It may detect unsuspected disease in a small number of patients; it reassures others and thus may be cost effective, depending on how these various factors are judged. Their argument comes down to the following dictum: "Good medical care is enhanced by acquisition of a comprehensive database."

Obviously the screening approach, especially routine admission biochemical screening, demands more study. Unfortunately, it has been put into widespread use before satisfactory studies have justified such use. Studies thus far would indicate that the yield does not justify the expense when biochemical screening is applied as a routine measure to unselected patients on admission to hospital or clinic. Screening of selected categories of patients such as newborns, the aged, and other high risk categories is probably an entirely different matter. At any rate, the burden of proof is now on those who would advocate routine admission screening and other screening or profiling protocols; such advocates must justify the worth and cost effectiveness of these procedures before they are put into widespread use.

2. EVALUATING THE EFFECTIVENESS
OF LABORATORY TESTS

As evidenced by the experience with admission screening and profiling, new technology is often introduced into widespread use without adequate evaluation of its diagnostic effectiveness and cost effectiveness. Similarly, old technology replaced by new is retained and the technological pool is consistently expanded. The repertoire of laboratory tests, especially in clinical chemistry, has grown very long over the past three decades; furthermore, overlap between tests in diagnostic significance and use is appreciable.

Before new tests are placed into widespread use, their diagnostic and cost effectiveness should be clearly established and their advantages over existing technologies delineated. Furthermore, old, replaced technologies should be dropped from the laboratory's repertoire.

Methods for evaluating laboratory tests on the basis of their reliability and diagnostic and cost effectiveness are now available[20,21] but need more study and application to actual clinical circumstances. As noted previously, Galen and Gambino[1] made a notable contribution to this subject by their reintroduction of the concepts of diagnostic sensitivity, diagnostic specificity, and predictive values of laboratory tests. Using these formulations, the value of a given laboratory test can be assessed in a specific diagnostic problem, and tests of low discriminant value can be dropped from use in relation to that problem. Galen[22] has recently applied this approach to the assessment of the value of serum haptoglobin assay in the differential diagnosis of anemia (Chapter 28).

3. DECISION ANALYSIS

This conference has been based on the assumption that improved laboratory use will come through an improved understanding of the clinical decision-making process. Decision analysis offers a framework for assessing the value of individual laboratory tests in the solution of specific problems.[23]

Decision analysis can also be useful in in the development of *algorithms* and *diagnostic protocols*. Diagnostic protocols (see Sox, Chapter 23) are step-by-step instructions ("recipes") for handling specific diagnostic problems. Algorithms are sequential branching strategies for solving specific problems. Diagnostic search and exclusion algorithms have been developed by a number of investigators and have been used, for example, in analyzing cases of hypercalcemia[24] and in the evaluation of acid-base disorders.[25] They are especially useful where a quite methodological approach to a diagnostic problem has been established. They tend to lend themselves well to computer-assisted reasoning but are too rigid and arbitrary for many physician users.[26]

4. ARTIFICIAL INTELLIGENCE

A number of investigators have proceeded from decision analysis to the task of attempting to apply artificial intelligence techniques to the clinical decision-making process, in the hope of developing acceptable and effective interfaces between physicians and diagnostic programs.[27-31] This effort has been represented in this conference by several presentations, including those of Paul Johnson (Chapter 6) and J. D. Myers, H. E. Pople, and R. A. Miller (Chapter 26).

The efforts to apply artificial intelligence techniques are of great interest beyond the practical goal of successful computer-assisted diagnosis. The light they may shed on how successful clinicians arrive at diagnostic and management decisions will be of help to those in the clinical laboratory, who are attempting to fit their work in the provision of tests and test results most effectively into the clinical decision process.

5. SURVEILLANCE OF LABORATORY USE

Professional Standards Review Organizations (PSROs) and medical audits are attempting to review the quality of care to establish standards of care. A New Mexico study has emphasized peer review through the PSRO process as a mechanism of surveillance of laboratory use.[32] Disappointingly, over a 4-year period, the study showed no net savings through peer review. In general, retrospective manual chart review, the method used, seems to be too "labor intensive" to be applied to laboratory medicine to any significant extent.

Wheeler et al.[33] used an algorithm for the diagnosis of anemia as a means of monitoring laboratory use. These authors by retrospective chart analysis, using their algorithm in which a low hemoglobin value was the entry portal, judged appropriate and inappropriate behavior of physicians in the use of the laboratory.

Computer-based surveillance and monitoring thus might provide individual physician profiles of laboratory use. Physicians showing weak planning logic could be identified and appropriate educational programs applied.

Assuredly, further attention to the development and testing of surveillance systems seems worthwhile. Initiatives along these lines and others may lead to more logical, economical, and prudent use of clinical laboratory resources in patient care.

References

1. Galen RS, Gambino SI. Beyond normality. New York: John Wiley & Sons, 1975.
2. Council on Wage and Price Stability: The problem of rising health care costs. Washington, DC: Executive Office of the President, 1976;116.
3. Benson ES. Strategies for improving the use of the clinical chemistry laboratory in patient care. In: Benson ES, Rubin M, eds. Logic and economics of clinical laboratory use. New York: Elsevier North-Holland, 1978;245-58.
4. Benson ES. Initiatives toward effective decision making and laboratory use. Hum Pathol 1980;11:440-8.
5. Finkelstein SN. Technological change and laboratory test volume. In: Benson ES, Rubin M, eds. Logic and economics of clinical laboratory use. New York: Elsevier North-Holland, 1978;225-34.
6. Griner PF. Use of laboratory tests in a teaching hospital: long term trends, reduction and use and relative cost. Ann Intern Med 1976;90:243-8.

7. Wilson JMG. Current challenges and problems in health screening. J Clin Pathol 1976; 26:555-60.
8. Burke MD. Clinical problem-solving and laboratory investigation: contributions to laboratory medicine. In: Benson ES, Stefanini M, eds. Progress in clinical pathology Vol. VIII. New York: Grune and Stratten, Inc., 1981;1-24.
9. Engel GL. Are medical schools neglecting clinical skills? JAMA 1976;236:861-3.
10. Ashley JSA, Parker P, Beresford JC. How much clinical investigation? Lancet 1972;1: 890-3.
11. Mechanic D. Future issues in health care: social policy and the rationing of health services. New York: The Free Press, 1979.
12. Carmalt MHB, Whitehead TP. Patient investigation by biochemical profiles. Proc R Soc Med 1971;64:1257-63.
13. Whitehead TP, Wooten IDP. Biochemical profiles for hospital patients. Lancet 1974;1: 1439-43.
14. Leonard JV, Clayton BE, Colley JRT. Effect of admission screening on work load. Br Med J 1975;2:662.
15. Durbridge TC, Edwards F, Edwards RG, Atkinson M. Evaluation of benefits of screening tests done immediately on admission to hospital. Clin Chem 1976;22:968-71.
16. Alvin RC. Biochemical screening—a critique. N Engl J Med 1970;283:1084-7.
17. Korvin CC, Pearce RH, Stanley J. Admissions screening: clinical benefits. Ann Intern Med 1975;83:197-203.
18. Williams BT, Dixon RA. Biochemical testing for acute medical emergencies in four district general hospitals. Br Med J 1979;1:1313-15.
19. Werner M, Altshuler CH. Utility of multiphasic biochemical sceening and systematic laboratory investigation. Clin Chem 1979;25:509-12.
20. Buttner H. Optimization of laboratory testing. In: Benson ES, Rubin M, eds. Logic and economics of clinical laboratory use. New York: Elsevier North-Holland, 1978:91-102.
21. Statland BE, Winkel P, Burke MD, Galen RS. Quantitative approaches used in evaluating laboratory measurements and other clinical data. In: Henry JB, ed. Clinical diagnosis and management by laboratory methods. 16th ed. Philadelphia: W. B. Saunders, 1979:525-55.
22. Marchand A, Galen RS, Van Lente F. The predictive value of serum haptoglobin in hemolytic disease. JAMA 1980;243:1909-11.
23. McNeil BJ, Adelstein SJ. Determining the value of diagnostic and screening tests. J Nucl Med 1976;17:439-46.
24. Bricetti AB, Bleich HL. A computer program that evaluates patients with hypercalcemia. J Clin Endocrinol Metab 1975;41:365-73.
25. Bleich HL. Computer evaluation of acid-base disorders. J Clin Invest 1969;48:1689-96.
26. Crosby WH. Algorithms: medicine, chess and war. JAMA 1977;238:1847.
27. Gorry GA. On the mechanization of clinical judgment. In: Weller SJ, ed. Computer application in health care delivery. New York: Grune and Stratton, 1976.
28. Shortliffe EH. Artificial intelligence and medical decisions. New York: Elsevier North-Holland, 1976.
29. Kulikowski CA. Problems in the design of knowledge bases for medical consultation. Proceedings First Annual Symposium on Computer Application in Medical Care. Washington, DC: October 3-5, 1977.
30. Pauker SG, Gorry GA, Kassiser JP, Schwartz WB. Towards the simulation of clinical cognition. Am J Med 1976;60:981-90.
31. Elstein AS, Shulman LS, Sprafka SA. Medical problem solving: an analysis of clinical reasoning. Cambridge: Harvard University Press, 1978.
32. Brook RH, Williams KN, Ralph JC. Use, costs and quality of medical services: impact of New Mexico peer review system. Ann Intern Med 1978;89:256-65.
33. Wheeler LA, Brecher G, Sheiner LB. Clinical laboratory use in evaluation of anemia. JAMA 1977;238:1847-56.

CHAPTER TWENTY-EIGHT

The Predictive Value Model and Patient Care Decisions

Robert S. Galen, MD, MPH

The predictive value model has been applied by a number of investigators to the evaluation of a single test to optimize its screening or diagnostic function. In fact, however, it is rare to use the result of a single test as the final arbiter of a medical decision. The predictive value model can be expanded to deal with multiple tests. We have applied the predictive value model in evaluating multiple tests used either in series or parallel fashion. These two approaches to laboratory testing, series and parallel, will be explored relative to the sensitivity, specificity, and predictive value of each strategy, with the use of data from ongoing studies in our laboratories. We have developed a simple APL procedure that is a convenient and general method for specifying arbitrary combinations of variables, and for evaluating the success with which any such combination rule can classify subjects or cases into two classes defined by a criterion variable: member or nonmember. The rule entered by the user is an APL Boolean expression whose arguments are the names of variables and appropriate constants. The output consists of the basic fourfold decision matrix and predictive value calculations. This interactive program has proved quite simple to use, facilitating the manipulation of variables and providing an empirical approach to gaining optimal results from laboratory tests both in terms of test sequence and interpretation.

THE PREDICTIVE VALUE OF LABORATORY DIAGNOSIS

Sensitivity, specificity, predictive value, and efficiency define a laboratory test's accuracy.[1] Sensitivity indicates the frequency of positive test results in patients with a particular disease, whereas specificity indicates the frequency of negative test results in patients without that disease. The predictive value of a positive test result indicates the frequency of diseased patients in all patients with positive test results. The predictive value of a negative test result indicates the frequency

Table 1. Determination of Predictive Value of Laboratory Tests

	No. with Positive Test Result	No. with Negative Test Result	Totals
No. with disease	TP	FN	TP + FN
No. without disease	FP	TN	FP + TN
Totals	TP + FP	FN + TN	TP + FP + TN + FN

Definitions

TP = True positives: number of diseased patients correctly classified by the test.

FP = False positives: number of nondiseased patients misclassified by the test.

FN = False negatives: number of diseased patients misclassified by the test.

TN = True negatives: number of nondiseased patients correctly classified by the test.

Sensitivity = positivity in disease = expressed as percent $\dfrac{TP}{TP + FN}$ x 100.

Specificity = negativity in health, or absence of a particular disease, expressed as percent = $\dfrac{TN}{FP + TN}$ x 100.

Predictive value of positive test = percent of patients with positive test results that are diseased = $\dfrac{TP}{TP + FP}$ x 100.

Predictive value of negative test = percent of patients with negative results that are nondiseased = $\dfrac{TN}{TN + FN}$ x 100.

Efficiency of test = percent of patients correctly classified as diseased and nondiseased = $\dfrac{TP + TN}{TP + FP + FN + TN}$ x 100.

of nondiseased patients in all patients with negative test results. The efficiency of a test indicates the percent of patients correctly classified (diseased and nondiseased) by the test. (See Table 1.)

In screening for disease, we are most interested in the predictive value of the positive result. These results represent patients who will be presumptive positives for a particular disease and undergo diagnostic work-ups. Of this group, those patients who turn out not to have the disease will be defined as false positives. In the discussion that follows, predictive value will be used to refer to the predictive value of the positive test result. A marked change in predictive value occurs when a change occurs in the prevalence of the disease in the population

Table 2. Predictive Value as a Function of Disease Prevalence*

Prevalence of Disease	Predictive Value
1%	16.1%
2	27.9
5	50.0
10	67.9
15	77.0
20	82.6
25	86.4
50	95.0

*For laboratory test with 95% sensitivity and 95% specificity

under study. For example, we could know from a test's sensitivity and specificity that it was positive in 95 percent of diseased patients and negative in 95 percent of nondiseased patients. Table 2 demonstrates the change in predictive value that occurs for this test with changing prevalence of disease. It can readily be seen that a particular test has a higher predictive value when the disease occurs with a higher prevalence. This explains why a good diagnostic test often fails as a screening test when the drop in prevalence is quite marked. When clinical judgment is used in ordering laboratory tests, the patient suspected of having a particular disease is placed in a new population with a high prevalence or probability of disease. Therefore, the test performs much better.

Figure 1 illustrates how sensitivity and specificity are altered by the selection of an upper limit of normal for a particular test. If we studied patients admitted to the hospital with the diagnosis of "rule out sepsis," divided the population into septic and nonseptic according to blood culture findings, and then expressed with the white blood cell count for each group as a frequency distribution, we would find the classical overlapping distribution seen in Figure 1. It is impossible to select a cutoff point for white blood cell count that would afford complete discrimination between the two groups. At any cutoff point, one must sacrifice sensitivity for specificity and vice versa. Herein lies the major flaw of laboratory diagnosis, in that the tests are not sensitive and specific at the same time. Looking at multiple laboratory tests improves the predictive value somewhat, but the trade-off between sensitivity and specificity always remains. If we wanted to select a cutoff point for the test illustrated in Figure 1, We could choose any point in the overlapping region. Table 3 lists several cutoff points with the sensitivity, specificity, and predictive value associated with each.

COMBINATION TESTING

In reality, it is rare to use the result of a single test as the final arbiter of a medical decision. If we are going to use more than one test, a number of questions

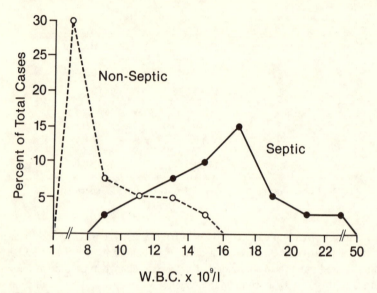

Figure 1. Selection of an upper limit of normal based on the sensitivity and specificity of a laboratory test:

Prevalence of sepsis   = 50%

Upper limit of normal = 8 x 10^9/L
Sensitivity   = 100%   Specificity = 60%

Upper limit of normal = 16 x 10^9/L
Sensitivity   = 50%   Specificity = 100%

need to be answered. Which tests should we use? In what sequence should they be performed? How many tests are enough in a profile or battery of tests? How should the results be interpreted? To begin with, let's consider situations where we use two tests. Two independent tests in a screening or diagnostic situation can be used in three different ways: (1) Test A is applied first and all those with

Table 3. Referent Values and Associated Predictive Values
for Test (WBC Count) Illustrated in Figure 1

Referent Value (Cutoff Point)	Sensitivity	Specificity	Predictive Value
8 x 10^9/L	100%	60%	71.4%
10	95%	75%	79.2%
12	85%	85%	85.0%
14	70%	95%	93.3%
16	50%	100%	100.0%

Disease prevalence = 50%

Table 4. Hypothetical Data for Two Tests, A and B

| | Test Results | | | | |
	A+B−	A−B+	A+B+	A−B−	TOTALS
Disease	190	40	760	10	1,000
Nondisease	9,800	4,850	100	84,250	99,000
Totals	9,990	4,890	860	84,260	100,000

a positive result are retested with test B (series approach: [++] = +). (2) Test B is applied first and all those with a positive result are retested with test A (series approach: [++] = +). (3) Tests A and B can be used together and all those with positive results for either or both tests are considered to be positives (parallel approach: [+−] = +, [++] = +, [− +] = +).

Which approach or sequence is best? This depends on the testing situation and the sensitivity and specificity of the individual tests and their combinations. For the sake of this discussion, we will examine the hypothetical data presented in Table 4.

The sensitivity of test A is (190 + 760)/1,000 = 95%. The sensitivity of test B is (40 + 760)/1,000 = 80%. The sensitivity of the series combination (A and B positive) = 760/1,000 = 76%, but the sensitivity of the parallel combination (A or B positive) is (190 + 40 + 760)/1,000 = 99%. With parallel testing, the combined sensitivity is greater than the individual sensitivities of the contributing tests.

Similarly, the specificity of test A is (4,850 + 84,250)/99,000 = 90%. The specificity of test B is (9,800 + 84,250)/99,000 = 95%. The specificity of the series combination is (9,800 + 4,850 + 84,250)/99,000 = 99.9%, since A+B−, A−B+, and A−B− are all interpreted as negative results in series testing. The specificity of the parallel combination is 84,250/99,000 = 85.1%, since only A−B− is considered a negative response.

Parallel testing results in the highest sensitivity but the lowest specificity, whereas series testing results in the lowest sensitivity but highest specificity. Table 5 summarizes these findings.

Table 5. Combination Testing for Hypothetical Data

	Test(s)	Sensitivity (%)	Specificity (%)
Single	A	95.0	90.0
Single	B	80.0	95.0
Series	A and B	76.0	99.9
Parallel	A or B	99.0	85.1

Table 6. Hemolytic Disease Study

Test	Sensitivity	Specificity	Predictive Value	Efficiency
Haptoglobin	83%	96%	87%	93%
LDH	83%	61%	40%	66%
LDH isoenzymes	58%	93%	74%	85%
Haptoglobin *and* LDH isoenzymes*	50%	100%	100%	88%
Haptoglobin *or* LDH isoenzymes†	92%	89%	73%	90%

*Series interpretation
†Parallel interpretation

Both sequences, using the series approach, produced the 1,255 positives with 760 true positives in the group. However, the latter sequence (B then A) is considered more effective, since fewer patients required retesting to achieve the same end result. This analysis assumes that both tests cost about the same to perform in the laboratory. If two tests are going to be used in series, the optimal sequence can be determined using the predictive value model as described here.

For tests run in parallel (A and B determined simultaneously), but considered positive if *either* component is positive, and negative only if *both* are negative, the sensitivity is higher and the specificity is lower than in comparable series testing. The sensitivity is increased because some diseased patients are positive on one test, but not on the other. Similarly, there are more false-positive results in nondiseased patients. The parallel approach outlined above has the highest sensitivity. It detects the greatest number of diseased patients in the population. However, it also produces the greatest number of false positives. In this case the predictive value is so low (6.3%) that this test might be unacceptable for any disease. Of all the approaches, the parallel approach requires the most laboratory work, since both tests are performed on all patients in the population.

The above relationship can be demonstrated with actual data from a study of haptoglobin, lactic dehydrogenase (LDH), and LDH isoenzymes in the diagnosis of hemolytic disorders.[2] One hundred hospitalized patients were evaluated to fulfill the physician's request for a serum haptoglobin. The laboratory then performed LDH and LDH isoenzyme determinations. A hematologist classified these 100 cases, without knowledge of the haptoglobin, LDH, or LDH isoenzyme data, into two major groups: hemolytic disease and other (nonhemolytic disease). Twenty-four patients were classified as having hemolytic disease: patients with autoimmune hemolytic anemia (Coombs' test positive), autoimmune hemolytic anemia (Coombs' test negative), pernicious anemia, mechanical hemolytic anemia, and hypersplenism. The remainder, or 76 patients, were classified as having other diseases including "nonhemolytic" hematologic disorders such as iron deficiency anemia and bleeding. The remainder represented a broad spectrum of disease states. Table 6 summarizes the sensitivity, specificity, predictive value, and

Table 7. Hemolytic Disease Study

	Haptoglobin Results		
	⩽ 25 mg/dl	> 25 mg/dl	TOTAL
Hemolytic disease	20	4	24
Other	3	73	76
Total	23	77	100

Sensitivity = 83%; specificity = 96%; predictive value = 87%; efficiency = 93%.

efficiency of these procedures used as single tests and in combination with each other. Haptoglobin was determined nephelometrically and considered positive at a concentration less than or equal to 25 mg/dl. LDH activity was considered positive at 250 IU/L. LDH isoenzymes were separated in cellulose acetate and scanned fluorometrically. LDH isoenzymes were considered positive when LDH_1 activity exceeded LDH_2 activity (a "flipped" LDH pattern).

The highest efficiency (overall correct classification) is achieved by simply using haptoglobin alone. The predictive value table for haptoglobin is presented in Table 7. It is interesting to explore the four cases of hemolytic disease that were "false negatives," that is, patients who did not have depressed haptoglobin levels. These turned out to be two patients with hypersplenism and two with pernicious anemia. On the other hand, three "false positives" occurred, that is, in nonhemolytic cases in which patients showed depressed haptoglobin levels. These turned out to be patients with ovarian carcinoma, cirrhosis, and sarcoid.

The contrast between series and parallel testing is demonstrated quite nicely by the combined use of haptoglobin and LDH isoenzymes. Although the efficiency is essentially the same, a series approach requiring both tests to be positive has a predictive value of 100%. The sensitivity, however, is only 50% and half of the cases would go undetected. A parallel approach requiring either test to be positive actually has the highest sensitivity of the tests listed (Table 6).

If we consider hematological profiles interpreted in a parallel fashion, we see that they have extremely high sensitivity, but low specificity. Because of the high sensitivity, these profiles, when negative, have a very high negative predictive value. For that reason they are used by clinicians to exclude or rule out with a high degree of probability a variety of diagnoses. Later on in the diagnostic work-up, series testing is performed, which is highly predictive of the presence of a particular disease because of its high specificity. As clinicians follow their own algorithms for working up a patient, the probability continues to increase as they receive more information.

In making patient care decisions relative to laboratory testing, it is essential that the laboratory have at its disposal simple ways of analyzing data sets. With this in mind, we have been working with Dr. Carl Helm, Professor of Biomathematics and Community Medicine of the College of Medicine and Dentistry of New Jersey, to develop a general purpose data analysis system. Techniques for ad hoc data analysis are not new, but using APL offers particular advantages relative to the ease with which variables can be manipulated and new variables created. It may not be obvious to the non-APL user, but the capability of executing an APL expression, which is entered as a text string, provides great generality in defining trial classification rules. The ease of use and formating of the output are designed to facilitate the use of the predictive value model in designing test strategies and evaluating the usefulness of laboratory tests. The widespread use of computers in laboratory medicine should permit this type of approach to data analysis to become routine in the next few years.

References

1. Galen RS, Gambino SR. Beyond normality: The predictive value and efficiency of medical diagnoses. New York: John Wiley & Sons, Inc., 1975.
2. Marchand A, Galen RS, Van Lente F. The predictive value of serum haptoglobin in hemolytic disease. JAMA 1980;243:1909-11.

CHAPTER TWENTY-NINE

Use of a Laboratory Database to Monitor Medical Care

Charles H. Altshuler, MD

A database composed primarily of comprehensive laboratory information may be used as a clinical decision support system. In this presentation, I hope to show how the system may be used to identify and correct some deficiencies in practice, and how it can be used to study some of the more important factors affecting hospital care costs.

METHODS

Since 1968 the laboratory at St. Joseph's Hospital—a 580-bed general acute care general hospital—has offered a programmed accelerated laboratory investigation (the PALI). This system was designed to exploit developments in laboratory automation and information handling; during the time in which it has been in use, we have accumulated a relatively comprehensive database on a small digital computer. An interpretative information retrieval system was also employed to help the physician use these data. Both systems have been the subject of previous reports.[1,2]

In an effort to determine the diagnostic content of this laboratory data, we merged the laboratory information with diagnostic and administrative data obtained from PAS (Professional Activities Service, Ann Arbor, Michigan) and the merged information was stored on the hospital mainframe, a Burroughs 6700. In this manner, separate annual databases were developed. Since there were approximately 20,000 discharges from the hospital each year and the study began with all patients discharged in 1975, the data available for study in 1979 were derived from around 80,000 hospital admissions over a 4-year period. (Each admission in the system is treated as a separate transaction so that the same patient admitted three times is handled as three separate admissions.)

In late 1979 and early 1980, as part of a general restructuring of the database, we merged all of the data over the period of 1975-1978 and then added the information from 1973, 1974, 1979, and 1980. Thus, the database available at the present time contains information relating to 170,000 inpatient encounters over a 7½-year period.

Certain additional cost information was entered at the end of 1976 and drug profile data for one year were added in 1977. Microbiologic data became available on a routine basis beginning in January, 1978; these data also were added to the database. (The hospital charges include the pathologists' component but not other physicians' fees.)

At the outset, software was developed to enable searches on:

1. Diagnosis(es);
2. Laboratory test(s);
3. Results of ranges of test results;
4. Age;
5. Sex, color;
6. Date of discharge;
7. Drugs;
8. Costs or any combination of the above.

Subsequently, the search parameters were expanded to include admission frequency, outcome, procedures, physician, type of service, source of payment, and patient identification.

RESULTS

When we searched the database using parameters designed to identify patients with IgA myeloma, the diagnoses were not always made (Figure 1). This impression was confirmed by examination of the medical records. This difficulty with diagnosis was not limited to proteins but applied equally well to any disease that may be characterized by laboratory information. It is of interest that for the most part, the diagnoses are overlooked by specialists dealing with a problem outside their area of expertise.

Not only is the program helpful in the evaluation of the diagnosis, but certain determinations, including those of drug levels, permit an estimation of how well some therapeutic practices are carried out. These studies pertain particularly to the use of theophylline, anticonvulsants, antibiotics, digoxin, other cardiac drugs, and so on. A "lab test frequency" report for patients on both quinidine and digoxin is shown in Figure 2. This study was designed to identify those patients who might show the effects of the interaction between the two drugs.

The major conclusion from these studies is that there is plenty of room for improvement, with regard to both diagnostic and therapeutic practices. When one studies the patient's medical records and consults with the physicians in an effort to learn the reasons for the shortcomings observed, several factors become apparent; the findings should be no surprise to any physician actively engaged in medical practice. The major problems seem to be:

Selective Test Report

Selection and Conditions

```
          Lab Test IgG  052/01   Range:      .00     799.00
          Lab Test IgA  052/02   Range:   451.00    9999.00
          Lab Test IgM  052/03   Range:      .00      59.00
```

Patient No.	Visit	Age	Sex		Admission date	Discharge date	Total Charge	Lab Charge
082871	01	85Y	F	White	12/10/77	12/23/77	2740.00	466.00

```
Fin DX: 782.0 GI bleeding NEC           052/01 IgG  12/10    600.00
Oth DX: 562.1 Diverticulosis colon      052/02 IgA  12/10   1360.00
Oth DX: 412.9 Chr ischemic hrt dis NEC  052/03 IgM  12/10     25.00
Oth DX: 599.5 Urin tract infection NOS  Bacti Urine 12/16 No organisms found
Oth DX: 401.0 Benign hypertension
Maj OP: T92.4 Proctosigmoidoscopy
Oth OP: T99.6 Radioisotopic scan
Oth OP: T98.4 Intravenous pyelography
Oth OP: T97.6 Physical therapy
```

398811	01	71Y	M	White	11/21/77	12/05/77	2872.00	724.00

```
Fin DX: 185.0 Malignant neo prostate    052/01 IgG  11/20    470.00
Oth DX: 203.0 Multiple myeloma          052/02 IgA  11/29   1700.00
Oth DX: 519.6 Lung Disease NEC          052/03 IgM  11/29     25.00
Oth DX: 775.7 Lymphadenopathy NOS       Bacti Bronch 12/02 Normal flora
Maj OP: T32.1 Excision lesion bronchus  Bacti sputum 12/02 Beta strep Group B
Oth OP: T99.8 Ultrasonic diagnostic
Oth OP: T99.6 Radioisotopic scan
Oth OP: T96.7 Bone marrow aspiration
```

Figure 1. Selective test report for patients with IgA myeloma.

Lab Test Frequency Report - Search on Lidocaine, Procainamide, Quinidine and Prim
Same When Present Along with Digoxin

Medical # 214765		Length of Stay 16 Days		Visit 3	Discharge 01/31/79		Admission 01/15/79	

	Age	Sex	Race	Service	Total	Lab	Payment	Discharge status
	80Y	M	White	Cardiology	4824.00	937.00	Medicare	Home Self Care

Diagnosis

```
Final   427.31  Atrial fibrillation       ICD9CM
Other   789.0   Abdominal pain            ICD9CM
Other   E942.0  Adv eff card rhyth regul  ICD9CM
Other   414.0   Coronary atherosclerosis  ICD9CM
Other   496.    Chr airway Obstruct NEC   ICD9CM
Other   428.0   Congestive heart failure  ICD9CM
Other   389.9   Hearing loss NOS          ICD9CM
```

Surgical procedures

```
Major   0087.73  Intravenous pyelogram     ICD9CM  Day 014
Other   0088.76  Dx ultrasound-abdomen     ICD9CM  Day 014
Other   0092.02  Liver scan/isotope funct  ICD9CM  Day 015
Other   0092.05  C-Vasc scan/isotope funct ICD9CM  Day 015
```

Lab tests

Hist test Number	Test Name	Units	Low Value	High VAlue	---First --- Date Value	---Last--- Date Value	Total
04010110	Quinidine	Mg/l	3.00	3.00	01/24 3.00	01/24 3.00	1
07150110	Digoxin	Ng/ml	.50	4.00	01/15 .50	01/28 3.40	7

Figure 2. Laboratory test frequency report.

1. Data are inadequate.
2. Some of the diagnoses were missed because the laboratory data became available after the patient was discharged from the hospital.
3. Previous diagnoses were sometimes overlooked on new admissions.

4. The diagnostic significance of previous laboratory work on previous admission had sometimes been overlooked.
5. The trend of some laboratory changes may not have been appreciated.
6. There is a sensory overload of the physician.
7. The physician has a lack of knowledge.
8. Appropriate ongoing therapy has not been ensured.
9. Too many physicians are caring for the patient, without anyone effectively correlating these efforts.

The availability of the data and the identification of our practice deficiencies make it possible to correct some of the operational weaknesses. Some of the things we can do to accomplish this goal might be the following:

1. With regard to "inadequate data," we can help in the systematic investigation of the patient by involving the laboratorians more actively.
2. With regard to late arriving data: (a) we can send a summary report of all laboratory data to the doctor's office when all data are available, and (b) we can provide a computerized discharge audit evaluation.
3. With regard to overlooking previous diagnoses: a summary report of all previous diagnoses at the time of admission can be provided.
4. With regard to missing the significance of previous laboratory work: a computerized evaluation (historical audit) of the significance of laboratory work done in each of the previous admissions might be provided.
5. With regard to missing the significance of certain laboratory trends: (a) we can provide a serial report of selected laboratory results in all previous admissions, and (b) messages composed by using data derived from more than one hospital episode might be generated.
6. With regard to sensory overload of the physicians, we can (a) provide for a systematic investigation of the patient, (b) create a current file, so as to be able to supply messages in time to affect critical clinical decisions, (c) encourage direct communication between physicians and responsible laboratorians, (d) provide a summary message at the time of discharge, and (e) create an "alert" file.
7. With regard to lack of knowledge on the part of the physicians, we can (a) create a convenient information retrieval system, (b) merge the information retrieval system with CME efforts, (c) promote effective CME efforts based on identified practice weaknesses, (d) determine the efficacy of educatory efforts, and (e) use the database for practice quality control purposes.
8. With regard to continuity of care problems: (a) periodic computerized reminders to physicians and, perhaps, to patients if desired, can be provided, and (b) we can create and use alert files.
9. With regard to the lack of a "coordinating physician," we must (a) support the concept of a designated "coordinating" physician, (b) supply summary reports and messages for each of the physicians, and (c) when

desired, create messages addressed to the coordinating physician that differ from those of the other attending physicians.

Rapidly rising health care cost has been a stimulus for the widespread re-examination of our modes of practice and, as a result, many health planners have offered corrective proposals, often involving some action by the government. It is necessary, therefore, to ask whether we can afford to use the laboratory to help in the care of the patient.

The availability of computerized information of the type described allows us to study the problem of costs in a systematic and objective way. The data-base makes it possible to determine the cost impact of (a) the diagnosis; (b) any complications of secondary diagnoses; (c) repeated hospitalizations caused by missing or delaying a diagnosis; and (d) chronic illnesses or self-inflicted or self-aggravating illnesses for which no effective therapeutic modalities are available, and so on.

For example, Figures 3, 4, and 5 illustrate the single episode costs of missing or delaying a diagnosis. Similarly, the repeated hospitalization costs for some diseases in which no effective therapeutic modalities exist; the cost implications for readmissions; the cost implications of self-inflicted of self-aggravating diseases; and the effect of the outcome of disease may be determined. The net result of these studies suggest that good medicine is cost effective except in those instances of fatal disease and self-limiting disease. We must use the data to help in the care of the patient: we cannot afford to do otherwise.

How might this be done? First, it is imperative that pathologists and other laboratorians be encouraged to help clinicians with the utilization of the laboratory information; second, it is essential, imperative, to stop throwing this valuable information away. Then, we must put the data into a retrievable form. Next, we must obtain the diagnoses and other patient administrative information and merge them with the objective clinical information. Lastly, we must see to it that regional computer facilities are provided so that use studies can be carried out. It is apparent that we have a unique opportunity now to improve medical care in a cost effective way.

```
                         Selected Historic Information MB

Medical #     Discharge  Admission  Age  Sex  Race  Service   Total    Lab    Payment   Visit   Dischg Stat

033992 Inpat  01/14/79   01/10/79   48   F    W     ENT       858.00   61.00  Bl Cross  7       Home Self
                                                                                                Care

        Diagnosis
              Final   473.0   Chr maxillary sinusitis        ICD9CM
              Other   471.9   Nasal polyp NOS                ICD9CM
              Other   473.2   Chronic ethmoidal sinusitis    ICD9CM

        Surgical Procedures
              Major 0021.31   Intranas les destruction       ICD9CM    Day 001
              Other 0022.39   Ext maxillary antrot NEC       ICD9CM    Day 001
              Other 0022.63   Ethmoidectomy                  ICD9CM    Day 001

        Lab tests
    Test Nbr      Test Name          Units   Date    Value
    05180225   CBC:HGB               GM/     1/10    12.10
      05210225  CBC:Hematocrit       %       1/10    37.00
      05240225  CBC:RBC              M       1/10     3.30
      05250125  CBC:MCV                      1/10    112.00
```

Figure 3. Selected historic information on patient with elevated mean cell volume (MCV).

```
                            St. Joseph's Hospital

Pathology Laboratory

03 39 92 X
M. B.                      Age:  48   Sex:  F
Dr. L. D.                  LOC:  OP

F Individual RPT printed 21 Mar 1980:  12 Feb 79/12 Feb 79      Page 02

---------------------------------------------------------------------------

LDHISO:              Total LDH    F1      F2      F3      F4      F5
                         IU       %       %       %       %       %
     Lo Norm            100     17.0    28.0    19.0     5.0     5.0
     Hi Norm            225     27.0    38.0    27.0    16.0    16.0

13 Feb 08 Hr            205     32.7H   32.9    16.0L    8.8     9.6

---------------------------------------------------------------------------

B12 Binding Protein: Vita B12    UBBC    TBBC    % Sat   UA-Bin  UB-Bin  %U-A
                     Pf/Ml    PG/ML   PG/ML                 PG/ML   PG/ML
     Lo Norm            400      900    1300    25.0                      17.0
     Hi Norm            800     1600   2400H    35.0                      24.0

13 Feb 08 Hr           240L     1363    1603    15.0L     514     849    38.0H

---------------------------------------------------------------------------

Std Quant:           Title       Result    Lo Norm    Hi Norm    Units

12 Feb 11 Hr         ESR         16           0          20      MM
12 Feb 11 Hr         Creat       0.9L        1.0         2.0     MG/100ML
12 Feb 11 Hr         ETR         0.87L       0.90        1.10    Ratio
12 Feb 11 Hr         T4Totl      2.4L        4.5        12.5     UG/100ML
12 Feb 11 Hr         T4Feee      0.3L        0.8         2.3     NG/100ML
13 Feb 08 Hr         Folacd      13.8        1.9        14.0     NG/ML
```

Figure 4. Laboratory values at subsequent admission of same patient as in Figure 3.

```
                       Selected Historic Information MB

Medical #    Discharge  Admission  Age  Sex  Race  Service    Total    Lab   Payment  Visit  Dischg Stat
033992 Inpat  03/31/79   02/16/79   48   F    W    Medicine  8480.00  1024.00  Bl Cross    8   Home Health
                                                                                                Srv
      Diagnosis
            Final   281.0  Pernicious anemia          ICD9CM
            Other   535.0  Gastritis/duodenitis NOS   ICD9CM
            Other   244.9  Hypothyroidism NOS         ICD9CM
            Other   336.8  Myelopathy NEC             ICD9CM
            Other   266.2  B complex defic  NEC       ICD9CM


      Surgical Procedures
            Major   0045.13  Sm bowel endoscopy NEC      ICD9CM   Day 012
            Other   0093.09  Other Dx patient procedure  ICD9CM

      Lab tests
Test NBR   Test Name    Units   Date   Value
05180225   CBC:HGB      GM/     2/16   12.70   2/23  12.30   2/27   12.10   2/28   12.10
05180225                        3/09   11.80   3/19  12.40   3/25   12.40
05210225   CBC:Hematocrit  %    2/16   38.00   2/23  37.00   2/27   35.00   2/28   36.00
05210225                        3/09   36.00   3/19  37.00   3/25   38.00
05240225   CBC:RBC             2/16    3.10   2/27   3.00   2/28    3.50   3/09    3.20
05240225                        3/19    3.40   3/25   3.60   2/23    3.00   2/27    3.00
05240225                        2/28    3.50   3/09   3.20   3/19    3.40   3/25    3.60
05250125   CBC:MCV            2/16   122.00   2/23 123.00   2/27  117.00   2/28  103.00
05250125                        3/09   112.00   3/19 109.00
```

Figure 5. Final diagnosis and laboratory value trends for same patient as in Figures 3 and 4.

In summary, certain considerations must be stressed: (a) Comprehensive medical information is a valuable medical resource. (b) Good medicine is cost effective. (c) Improvement in data utilization is essential if we are to save meaningful sums of money in health care. (d) Unless the effectiveness of a proposed change in practice can be demonstrated objectively, it is wise to proceed with caution, since many current proposals for change in the health care system appear to be naive, and could be counterproductive.

References

1. Altshuler CH, Bareta J, Cafaro AF, Cafaro JR, Gibbon SL. The PALI and the SLIC system. CRC Crit Rev Clin Lab Sci 1972;3:379-402.
2. Altshuler CH, Bareta J, Cafaro AF, Cafaro JR, Hollister WN. AIDE (Accessible Information for Diagnosis and Evaluation): An Information Retrieval System. Grune and Stratton, Inc., 1975.

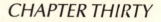
Doctor Billing in a Federal Institution

Joyce A. Campbell, MD, and
Michael T. Makler, MD

INTRODUCTION

This study was designed to determine whether a weekly bill delivered to interns containing the total number and cost of tests would affect laboratory use at a federal institution. Previous studies have suggested that lack of awareness of laboratory costs[1-3] and overuse of laboratory tests[4-6] account for a substantial amount of the costs generated by house staff at private and teaching hospitals. Various educational programs have been described to reduce overutilization of the laboratory.[7-10] This study was also designed to examine the questions of the level of cost awareness and the priorities interns use in ordering laboratory tests.

METHODS

The subjects were 22 interns from the Department of Medicine at the University of Oregon Health Science Center who were randomly assigned to two groups composed of ten experimental (eight male, two female) and twelve control (ten male, two female) interns.

Five hundred twenty-five patients were cared for during the total period. The study was divided into three periods. The first period, designated the pretrial period, allowed baseline data to be gathered as well as to establish the level of cost awareness and the importance placed on reasons for ordering tests. The second period, the actual billing period, lasted 10 weeks for each intern. During this period only the experimental interns received the weekly bills with attached questionnaires relating to their laboratory use. The controls were billed but the bills were not delivered or seen by this group. In the third period, the posttrial

Supported by the Veterans Administration Health Services Research and Development Service and the Medical Research Foundation of Oregon.

period, both the experimental and the control interns were reexamined about cost awareness and their reasons for ordering tests. In this third period, a resident and a staff physician were asked to examine a random sample of the charts from the patients cared for by the experimental interns, and to answer the same questions that the experimental interns had been asked to answer weekly on the experimental intern questionnaire.

The bill delivered to the experimental interns consisted of a computer printout with the intern's name, the patient's name, a list of 25 procedures, the first 7 days of the patient's hospitalization, the cost per test, the total number of tests, and the total cost of the tests. These costs were based on units derived for laboratory procedures by the College of American Pathologists.

Before and after the billing period, all 22 interns were requested to take a quiz asking them to estimate the cost of 20 common laboratory tests and to grade (from 1+ to 5+) the reasons for ordering these tests.

RESULTS

The case mix of the study is presented in Table 1. The experimental and control interns cared for predominately male white patients over the age of 60 who had been previously admitted to this institution for chronic medical conditions such as heart, liver, and lung disease. Thirty-two percent of these patients had a history of alcoholism.

Table 2 reports data obtained from interns during the pretrial period of the study. During this period, the average mean test per patient of the experimental group was 16.7 tests per week, compared with 31.6 tests per week for the control group. This difference was found to be not significant by the unpaired t-test. The skewing of the baseline data was caused by two intern controls' having had single patients with very high laboratory utilization.

Data collected from the experimental and control group during the 10-week billing period are presented in Table 3. The average number of tests and cost per

Table 1. Case Mix of Patients*

	Experimental Interns (10)	Control Interns (12)
Age	61 years	63 years
Percent		
Male	97%	100%
Married	46	48
White	96	98
Previous admissions	71	64
Chronic diseases	62	53
History alcohol abuse	31	33

*Based on 112 of 172 patients of experimental interns and 113 of 181 patients of control interns.

Table 2. Baseline Period Number and Cost of Tests

	Mean of Experimental Group (10) (n = 81 patients)	Mean of Control Group (12) (n = 91 patients)
Intern mean number of tests per week	16.7*	31.6‡
Intern mean cost per week	$122†	$247§
Intern median number of tests per week	15.4	26.6
Intern median cost per week	$107	$217

*SD =   6.00
†SD = $24.69
‡SD =   48.50
§SD = $217.42

Table 3. Billing Period (10 Weeks) Number and Cost of Tests

	Mean of Experimental Group (10) (n = 172 patients)	Mean of Control Group (12) (n = 181 patients)
Intern mean number of tests per week	15.1*	15.6‡
Intern mean cost per week	$108†	$113§
Intern median number of tests per week	11.1	13.2
Intern median cost per week	$77	$91

*SD =   2.05
†SD = $19.69
‡SD =   3.49
§SD = $26.90

week were 15.1 tests and $108 for the experimental group and 15.6 and $113.00 for the control group. There is no statistically significant difference between these.

To evaluate whether the experimental and control groups ordered different types of tests, utilization of four commonly ordered laboratory procedures was compared. Table 4 demonstrates the results. There is no difference between the average number of tests per patient week ordered for the 12 chemistry panel, 6 electrolyte panel, complete blood cell count (CBC), or white blood cell (WBC) differential.

To attempt to determine whether the patterns of utilization of tests were different between the experimental and control groups, chemistry and hematology ratios were derived from the number of 12 chemistry panels/the number of 6 electrolyte panels, and the number of white cell differentials/the number of CBC profiles, respectively. These ratios were identical, as is shown in Table 5.

Table 4. Rate of Ordering (average number of tests per patient week)

	Experimental (10) (n = 172 patients)	Control (12) (n = 181 patients)
SMA 12 Chemistry Panel	1.48	1.30
SMA 6 Electrolyte Panel	2.62	2.12
WBC Differential	1.44	1.65
Coulter CBC Profile	2.06	2.33

Table 5. Laboratory Utilization Ratio

	Experimental (10)	Control (12)
Chemistry ratio (12/6)*	0.56	0.61
Hematology ratio (Diff/CBC)†	0.70	0.71

*Average number SMA 12 Chemistry Panels / Average number SMA 6 Electrolyte Panels

†Average number WBC Differentials / Average number Coulter CBC Profiles

During the billing period, experimental interns answered questionnaires, attached to each bill, designed to elicit the reasons for ordering the tests. They also were asked to identify unnecessary tests as well as tests that they felt they had failed to order. Of 209 completed questionnaires, the experimental interns assigned 3,103 tests to 11 categories. Close to 40% were ordered for therapeutic monitoring, 26% for routine reasons, and 14% and 7% to establish either a primary or secondary diagnosis. (Routine in this study was defined as tests ordered regardless of admitting complaint.)

In addition, the experimental interns identified 405 of the 3,103 tests (13%) as unnecessary. The questionnaires also suggested that an additional 17 tests were required that were not ordered. A resident and a staff internist reviewed 20 charts of patients cared for by the experimental interns. They independently noted that 17.9% and 19.8% of the tests ordered were unnecessary. The resident noted two omitted tests, and the internist noted seven. They both assigned reasons for ordering similarly to interns.

In both the pretrial and posttrial period, the experimental and control interns were asked to estimate the costs of 20 laboratory tests. The results are presented in Table 6. During the pretrial and posttrial period no significant difference was seen in the accuracy of estimates. Both groups were 25% accurate before and after the billing period. However, in terms of relative importance of factors used in ordering tests, experimental interns graded cost significantly lower after the study (from 8 to 11) (Table 7).

Table 6. Cost Awareness (comparison estimates with costs)

| | Percent Accurate* | |
	Pretrial	Posttrial
"Billed" tests		
Experimental interns (10)	26	29
Control interns (12)	23	22
Tests not "billed"		
Experimental interns (10)	15	26
Control interns (12)	18	24

*Within ± 25% costs

Table 7. Relative Importance of Factors
in Ordering Laboratory Tests

Group	Factor
Pretrial	
Experimental interns (10)	1 Establishing primary diagnosis
	2 Establishing secondary diagnosis
	3 Therapeutic monitoring
	.
	.
	.
	8 Cost
Control interns (12)	1 Establishing primary diagnosis
	2 Therapeutic monitoring
	3 Establishing secondary diagnosis
	.
	.
	.
	9 Cost
Posttrial	
Experimental interns (10)	1 Establishing primary diagnosis
	2 Establishing secondary diagnosis
	3 Therapeutic monitoring
	.
	.
	.
	11* Cost
Control interns (12)	1 Establishing primary diagnosis
	2 Therapeutic monitoring
	3 Establishing secondary diagnosis
	.
	.
	.
	9 Cost

*Significant by *t*-test

DISCUSSION

This study demonstrated that medicine interns at a federal hospital who were receiving weekly laboratory bills on their patients did not reduce laboratory use. The results also show that when these interns were compared with the control group rotating at the same time but not receiving bills, no significant difference was seen in the ordering patterns. The experimental interns found approximately 13% of their tests were unnecessary, retrospectively. This figure was confirmed in a random sample study by a faculty internist and a senior resident.

Our initial hypothesis had been that billing would affect laboratory utilization. The results clearly demonstrate that this is not the case. In fact, awareness of the cost of laboratory tests at this hospital has resulted in an even lower grading of cost by the experimental interns. The reasons why billing does not affect utilization are complex. The interns, attending a seminar after completion of the study noted that this was a federal institution, in which there was no obvious motivation to cut costs. Others suggested their primary concern was the care of the patient and that cost in itself had a low priority.

The study clearly demonstrates that awareness of costs of tests did not improve, despite weekly billing. It also shows that the most frequent reason for ordering tests is therapeutic monitoring. Finally, as far as we are aware, this billing system is the first ever established in a federal institution. It has allowed our staff to monitor laboratory use and to derive a total cost figure for the amount of laboratory tests performed. We have also derived two laboratory utilization ratios to compare qualitative ordering patterns between physicians individually, or in groups, by specialty.

References

1. Skipper JK, Smith G, Mulligan JL, Garg ML. Physicians' knowledge of cost: The case of diagnostic tests. Inquiry 1976;XIII: 194-8.
2. Kelly SP. Physicians' knowledge of hospital costs. J Fam Pract 1978;6:171-2.
3. Dresnick SJ, Roth WI, Linn BS, Pratt TC, Blum A. The physician's role in the cost containment problem. JAMA 1979;241:1606-9.
4. Griner PF, Liptzin B. Use of the laboratory in a teaching hospital. Implications for patient care, education and hospital cost. Ann Intern Med 1971;75:157-63.
5. Dixon PH, Laszlo J. Utilization of clinical chemistry services by medical housestaff; an analysis. Arch Intern Med 1974;134:1064-7.
6. Eisenberg JM, Goldfarb S. Clinical usefulness of measuring prothrombin time as a routine admission test. Clin Chem 1976;22:1644-7.
7. Eisenberg JM, Williams SV, Garner L, Viale R, Smits,H. Computer-based audit to detect and correct overutilization of laboratory tests. Med Care 1977;XV:915-21.
8. Schroeder SA, Kenders K, Cooper JK, Piemme TE. Use of laboratory tests and pharmaceuticals: variation among physicians and effect of cost audit on subsequent use. JAMA 1973;225:969-73.
9. Eisenberg JM. An educational program to modify laboratory use by housestaff. J Med Educ 1977;52:578-81.
10. Griner PF. Use of laboratory tests in a teaching hospital: long-term trends. Reduction in use and relative cost. Ann Intern Med 1979;90:243-8.

CHAPTER THIRTY-ONE

The Use of Reference Values and the Concept of Reference State: A Contribution to Improved Laboratory Use

Gérard Siest, PhD, Joseph Henny, PhD, Camille Heusghem, PhD, and Adelin Albert, PhD

The concept of "normal values" is beset by many ambiguities, mostly related to definition and selection of "normals." To avoid these ambiguities and their attendant confusion, Dybkaer and Gräsbeck[1] in 1969 introduced the concept of "reference values." These authors recommended that the term "normal value," with all its ambiguities and misconceptions, be discarded. They defined reference values as a set of values of a certain kind of quantity attainable from a single individual or a group of individuals corresponding to a stated description. This description must be spelled out in detail and available if others are to use the reference values.

Reference limits (which usually include 95 percent of the subjects) serve essentially to describe reference populations. Decision limits are based on clinical experience and take into account reference values and also other information, for example, the prevalence of the specific disease considered.

The concept of reference values may lead to better interpretation of laboratory results and thus improved use of the clinical laboratory in patient care.[2,3] One of the clear advantages of the "reference value" concept is that it avoids consideration of the "normal" and the "normal state" as the standard of comparison and substitutes a reference base that can be more or less strictly defined, depending on the situation under study. The concept of "reference values" requires a firm understanding of biochemistry and physiology of human beings in various states of health.[4] Although it introduces a larger degree of complexity than the early "normal values" concept, it also allows us to more clearly demarcate descriptive limits and relate reference limits and decision limits (Figure 1). The laboratory should provide the clinician reference distributions specific for

We wish to thank the Caisse National d'Assurance Maladie for its financial support.

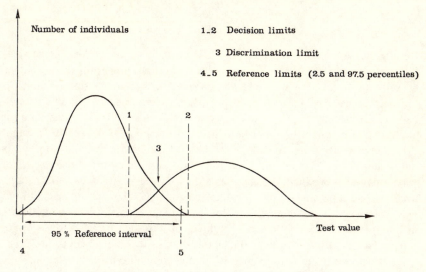

Figure 1. Reference, decision, and discrimination limits.

each case, allowing the physician to set decision limits and to evaluate risk in proceeding to diagnosis and treatment.

When one measures a specific serum constituent in a supposedly healthy individual, a value is obtained that must be placed in relationship to other values. This decision is made easier if values from three population types are available: (1) values obtained from individuals in the general population, unselected, and not having modified their usual living conditions; (2) values obtained from healthy individuals under carefully described conditions (these are the reference values for this particular situation); (3) values obtained from heterogeneous populations, that is, populations where several factors were not sufficiently controlled. The term usual values applies to heterogeneous populations, grouped through reasons of convenience (for example, medical students, blood donors) and to ill populations (for instance, hospitalized patients). In spite of the great variation of values, knowledge of unhealthy population distributions is very useful.

Use of the term reference values, with no other precision, implies that the values are obtained from healthy subjects, controlled for the principal known sources of biological variation. But the term "reference values" also can be used for healthy subjects in relation to particular states in which a biological variation may be expected, such as a woman using oral contraceptives, an astronaut immobilized in a space capsule, and 20- to 30-year-old men on high-protein diets. In each of these instances, the subject is presumed healthy but has specific characteristics that will have an effect on many serum constituents.

THE REFERENCE STATE

Results obtained at the Center for Preventive Medicine of Vandoeuvre-Les-Nancy, added to those already provided in the literature from other centers, have led us to propose the following concept of a reference state.[5] Since it is known that certain factors (notably sex, age, weight, medication, and alcohol) have a bearing on variation in many serum constituents, the reference state for adults of a population should be described with these factors taken into account. For example, the reference state might be described as follows: 20 to 30 years old, male, not obese, not on medication, not consuming more than a liter of wine a day or more than 10 cigarettes a day, fasting for 10 hours. Under standardized conditions the samples are obtained and measurements are made. In this way, reference values are obtained for a population class. Then, theoretically, differences noted in a given subject subsequently tested should be due only to genetic factors, if the environmental factors described above are controlled.

Reference values so obtained will allow comparisons of populations on a regional, national, or international basis. Measured values for individuals in the reference state could be included on the health record of each individual used as a means of assessing health at a future time.

USE OF POPULATION REFERENCE VALUES

Population reference values are obtained either "a posteriori" by selection from a large population or "a priori" by direct measurement of biologic constituents of a small sample population carefully selected.[6]

The protocol for developing population reference values has to be very well defined. The following steps are necessary: (1) List all biological variations. (2) Choose criteria for the defined group. (3) Exclude from the reference sample individuals who may produce bias that cannot be controlled. (4) Prepare individuals in a standardized way for sampling. (5) Treat the biological specimen in a standardized manner. (6) Carry out the analysis under appropriate well-defined and carefully standardized conditions.

There are two ways of using reference values once they are produced: an isolated value may be compared with them (for example, to determine whether a given patient is healthy or not); or reference values may be compared among themselves.

The use of reference values as a standard of comparison is part of traditional clinical decision making and medical diagnosis. The comparison of groups can be used in epidemiology in a study of the effects of certain medications, for example, or in comparison of materials and methods between two laboratories.

Use in Epidemiology and Anthropology

Examples of this type of use include the following: (1) measurement of important physiological variation; (2) measurement of the importance of envi-

Table 1. Alkaline Phosphatases: Classification of the Different Variables
Calculated with the Median Values

Variable	Sex	Percentage
Age		
Between children (4 to 5 years) and adults		
(30 to 60 years)	Males	74 %
	Females	79
20-30 to 60-100 years	Males	13
	Females	44
Menopause		
(45 to 55 years)		21.1
Socioprofessional categories		
(heavy workers)	Males	20
Sex		
Between males and females (20 to 30 years)		19
Overweight		
(20 to 40 years)	Males	2.5
	Females	10
Oral contraceptives	Females	7.5
Height		
(20 to 40 years)		
Between small and middle subjects	Males	2
	Females	2.5
Between tall and middle subjects	Males	0
Exercise		
Before/after	Males	1.3
Meals		
Before/after	Males	0.4
Analytical variations		
Day to day, CV	Males	4.9

ronmental factors in serum constituents; (3) classification of biological variation (see Table 1); (4) study of genetic differences; (5) comparison of populations; (6) transferability of reference values; (7) comparison of procedures for obtaining reference values; (8) definition and representativeness of a reference sample; (9) prevalence of the reference state; (10) study of risk factors; and (11) study of prevalence of known illnesses.

Use of Reference Values in Laboratory Testing

1. Validation of existing tests:[7] A comparative study of reference values between a healthy population and a population of sick people allows us to class tests according to their discriminatory power. In Lamberg's study,[8] measurement

of T_3 was found to be the most specific test for hyperthyroidism, whereas the measurement of cholesterol showed only a very minor distinction between healthy and sick populations.

2. Strategy for the choice of tests: Knowledge of biological variation is important in the selection of new tests and new examinations. A satisfactory test will increase the discrimination between a healthy individual and a sick individual.[9] A test designed to survey the health state in the population must be sensitive to environmental factors to detect their effects early.[7]

3. Use in the study of drug effects: Since intra- and inter-individual variations in the effects of drugs on biological parameters are very great, it is impossible at this time to standardize this factor of variation. Therefore, drugs must be excluded in establishing reference states. On the other hand, for certain types of drugs and for certain limited aims (for example, for the use of oral contraceptives), it is worthwhile to know the effect of the agent on a defined population. A careful questioning at the time of sampling is necessary to determine whether drugs are being used.[10]

Use for Comparison of Methods and Instruments

Population reference values are useful in the evaluation of laboratory techniques and methods in the following ways: (1) for comparison of reference values on a regional or national basis; (2) for the evaluation of new methods or instruments; and (3) for definition of analytical variability and analytical goals in testing as a function of biological variability.

DISCUSSION

The general concept of reference values can be applied to individuals[7] or groups and can be utilized in multivariate analysis.[11] In health, as in illness, the results of one test are not independent of the results of other tests and a multivariate approach is desirable as an aid to interpretation. Clinicians should become familiar with the concept and use of reference values. In this way, the medical decision process will be improved.

To facilitate the use of reference values, in early 1975 we proposed creation of a reference data bank.[12] This bank would store information on biological variability of healthy subjects and could be used to provide better and more specific reference values. To improve the use of reference values, we have proposed two charts, one showing biological variations (Table 2) and the other, pathological variations (Table 3).[13] We believe that knowledge of healthy and ill subjects will advance if reference values are used to reduce errors of classification; and reference values will provide better measures of health without increasing costs.[14]

References

1. Dybkaer R, Gräsbeck R. Theory of reference values. Scand J Lab Invest 1973;32:1-7.

Table 2. Gammaglutamyltransferase: Biological Variations

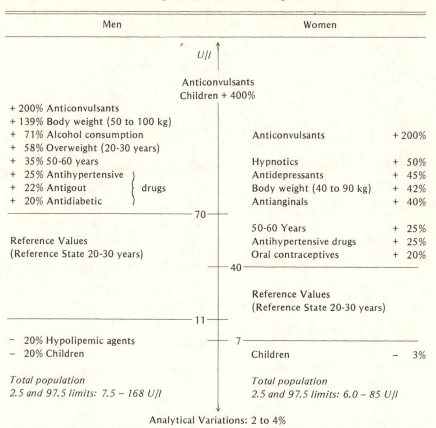

Men	Women

U/l ↑

Anticonvulsants
Children + 400%

+ 200% Anticonvulsants
+ 139% Body weight (50 to 100 kg)
+ 71% Alcohol consumption   Anticonvulsants   + 200%
+ 58% Overweight (20-30 years)
+ 35% 50-60 years   Hypnotics   + 50%
+ 25% Antihypertensive)   Antidepressants   + 45%
+ 22% Antigout   } drugs   Body weight (40 to 90 kg)   + 42%
+ 20% Antidiabetic   )   Antianginals   + 40%
                        — 70 —
                                   50-60 Years   + 25%
Reference Values   Antihypertensive drugs   + 25%
(Reference State 20-30 years)   Oral contraceptives   + 20%
                        — 40 —

                                   Reference Values
                                   (Reference State 20-30 years)
                        — 11 —
− 20% Hypolipemic agents   — 7 —
− 20% Children
                                   Children   −   3%

Total population   *Total population*
2.5 and 97.5 limits: 7.5 – 168 U/l   *2.5 and 97.5 limits: 6.0 – 85 U/l*
                        ↓
Analytical Variations: 2 to 4%

The values correspond to the percentage calculated with the median values.

2. Gräsbeck R, Siest G, Wilding P, Williams GZ, Whitehead TP. The concept of reference values. Clin Chim Acta 1978;87:459F-65F.
3. Siest G, Bretaudière JP, Buret J, et al. Le concept de valeurs de référence en biologie clinique. Commission Valeurs de Référence de la Société Française de Biologie Clinique. Ann Biol clin 1977;35:269-70.
4. Métais P, Agneray J, Ferard G, et al. Biochimie clinique. II. Biochimie métabolique; Ville-urbanne: Simep, 1980.
5. Siest G. Reference values in human chemistry. Symposium 4: New concepts in the interpretation of laboratory data II. In: Abstracts of the ninth international Congress of Clinical Chemistry. Toronto, 1975:8.
6. Siest G. Strategy for the establishment of healthy population reference values. Proceedings of the workshop on Reference Values in Helsinki, May 1980. In: Reference values, current state of art. Sussex: J. Wiley & Sons (In Press).
7. Siest G. Les valeurs de référence en biologie. Utilisation et intérêt particulier en médecine préventive. Path Biol 1975;1:63-70.
8. Lamberg BA, Heinonen OP, Viherkoski M, et al. Diagnosis of hyperthyroidism. Statistical

Table 3. Gammaglutamyltransferase: Pathological Variations

Men	Women

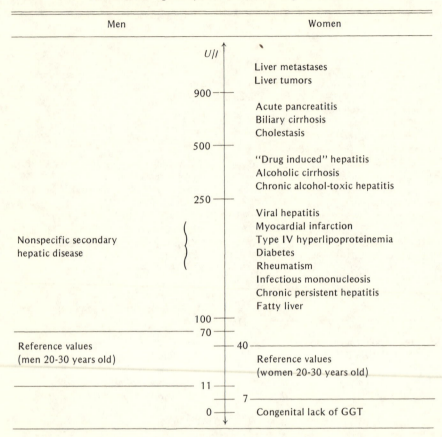

evaluation of laboratory and clinical criteria. Acta Endocrinol [Suppl] (Kbh) 1970;146: 7-42.

9. Harris EK. Criteria for judging whether combinations of measurements can reduce variability. In: Abstracts of the 8th international congress on Clinical Chemistry. Copenhagen, 1972: Scand J Clin Lab Invest 1972;29:Suppl 126.

10. Siest G, Galteau MM, Notter D. Notions générales concernant l'effet des médicaments sur les examens de laboratoire. Commission Effet des Médicaments sur les Examens de Laboratoire de la Société Française de Biologie Clinique. Ann Biol Clin 1981;39:91-98.

11. Albert A. Une approche nouvelle de l'utilisation des valeurs de référence. In: Siest G, Galteau MM, eds. Compte rendus du 4éme colloque de Pont-áMousson "Biologie Prospective." Paris: Masson, 1980:157-60.

12. Siest G, Floc'h A, Poulizac H, Senault R. Du concept de valeurs de référence. In: comptes rendus du symposium "Information systems in the field of health." Council of Europe, 1976:42-100.

13.Siest G, Henny J, Schiele F. Variations biologiques et valeurs de référence des constituants plasmatiques. Aide à l'interprétation. In: Interprétation des examens de laboratoire. Valeurs de référence et variations biologiques. Basel: Karger, 1981.

14.Albert A, Chapelle JP, Heusghem C, Siest G, Henny J. Test selection and early risk scale in acute myocardial infarction (Chapter 22 of this volume).

CHAPTER THIRTY-TWO

The Nominal Group Process Reports

To promote a synthesis of ideas and experience related to medical decision-making and laboratory use, the contributors of each major section joined in two nominal group process (NGP) sessions.

BACKGROUND AND FORMAT

NGP is a structured group process strategy, developed in 1968 by André Delbecq and his associated at the University of Wisconsin.[1] It has been widely used for program planning in health, social service, education, industry, and government organizations. The term "nominal" denotes a key feature of the strategy. During the *first phase*, participants are in each other's presence, but do not interact verbally. Instead, they generate *ideas in writing* in response to a question. Thus, the participants are a group in name only, or "nominally." The *subsequent three phases* include: (1) *round-robin listing* of ideas in brief phrases on a flip chart; (2) *serial discussion* of each recorded idea for clarification; and (3) individual *voting* to reach a group consensus on priorities for program planning.

Research and experience have shown NGP to be more effective than interactive groups for needs assessment, problem identification, and exploration of the components of problem solution. There are several particularly important *benefits* associated with NGP.

- As compared with interacting groups, research has demonstrated that NGP results in a greater number of *high quality ideas*. Several explanations have been suggested. The silent writing period maximizes participant involvement in idea generation and avoids distractions while ideas are being generated. NGP avoids the tendency of interacting groups to focus early on a particular train of thought. People seem comfortable in sharing only fairly well-developed ideas in a newly formed group. The round-robin procedure increases participants' willingness to share risky ideas.

- There is *balanced participation* among members of the group.
- There is a *focus on ideas* rather than individuals.
- NGP results in *group decisions* and *quantitative data* (the voted priorities) and *qualitative data* (clarifications of ideas in the discussion phase).
- NGP results in *high participant satisfaction*, due to balanced participation, group accomplishment of the task, and a sense of closure.

In spite of these theoretical benefits of NGP, in this instance the results of the process were obtained with some controversy and concern about the scientific validity and effectiveness of the approach, the significance of consensus, and the minimal time allotted for the activity. Each group was asked to develop a prioritized key issue list and to provide a list of strategies in pursuit of the top one or two issues. The final result was a product of a mere two to three hours of interchange and did not allow for more deliberate and considered judgment. Clearly, a well-reasoned statement of strategy, resources, and impediments would require considerably more time and might result in a book itself, a task well beyond the scope and intent of the brief encounters. In spite of the deficiencies in the approach, the prudent reader may gain insights from the four synopses presented in this chapter as indicators of directions that seem worthy of more thoughtful attention.

Each group summarized the results of their deliberation in a somewhat different style. To preserve as much of the value of the groups' efforts as possible, the synopses are presented with only minor modifications.

MEDICAL DECISIONS, TECHNOLOGY, AND SOCIAL NEED

Participants: D. Fenderson (Chair), A. Albert, H. S. Frazier, S. J. Reiser, G. Siest, E. A. Stead

Summary by: D. Fenderson, PhD

The question posed to the group was "What are the most important problems and issues to address in using medical technology to improve the quality and efficacy of health care?" In the second session, as for each of the three other groups, the participants were asked to identify strategies for implementing the priority issue identified in the first session, and to list resources available for and possible impediments to strategies selected.

The original list consisted of 14 specific items that through discussion, were reduced to 12. This list represented several dimensions and levels of specificity. It was reorganized into an outline to provide a measure of consistency and integration as a basis for other discussion.

I. Strategic Objective: Develop *Usable* Information
   A. *Clinical "library"* — a cumulative record of medical experience especially with chronic disease, permitting more accurate estimation of disease course and prognosis, and leading to an increasingly clearer understanding of the —
   B. *Relationship of "inputs" to "outcomes"*
   C. *Test data* to help guide their use. Perhaps "package insert" type of information on tests could be given, including appropriate and questionable uses, and *sensitivity/specificity* for various purposes
   D. *Policy information*
   E. *"Perverse" and other incentives*
   F. *Generalizable rules* and algorithms as diagnostic and prognostic aids

II. Means
   A. *A clinical decision support structure* and interface system (initial cost will be high)
   B. *New clinical team*, linking clinicians with laboratory experts
   C. *A system to capture data* "as it goes by" on a continuing basis

III. Downstream Issues
   A. *Analysis and display of data* in time, place, and manner to be useful in deciding which diagnostic and therapeutic procedures to use in a given circumstance
   B. *Ethical issues*
   C. *Educational strategies*

DISCUSSION

The medical schools and affiliated teaching institutions would seem to be the appropriate setting for the development of such an informational and analysis system. But clearly these facilities are not equipped to do so. They do not include epidemiologists and biostatisticians as part of the health care team, and a general support system for this level of clinical decision analysis does not exist. The present infrastructure is inadequate. Such a system would need to be pervasive within the clinical departments. No financial support has been provided for epidemiologists and biostatisticians as clinical team members, and in many environments, such a team configuration would be greeted with restrained enthusiasm.

The controlled clinical trial, although very important to such a system, also faces a number of constraints that preclude massive and universal use. Substantial preliminary work could be done, however, with the use of a continuing collection and analysis of data plus repeat trials to screen, focus, and select the most crucial problems for controlled clinical trials. The proposed system would involve a continuing evaluation system at the interface between clinical care and data.

This concept might be explored through demonstration projects in academic centers, which have the interest, personnel, and resources to make such projects possible. Such a plan must be close to clinical practice and to the faculty in clinical departments if it is to succeed. A system cannot be externally imposed on physicians who are resistant to it. The dangers of central, large-scale financing have been mentioned. Perhaps a more auspicious starting point is to do studies that clearly demonstrate discontinuities in the present arrangements, and let the system respond. Again, the danger exists that the status quo is so well rewarded that change may not be possible without some major disturbance of the equilibrium. Incentives in the current system are of several types, including "perverse incentives" that are resistant to change. How does one get this change of thinking into the system? Where do we get the people with the tools (skills) required for this new team arrangement? And what forces will help to bring about this change?

Change is inevitable. Cost-benefit or cost-effectiveness studies will demonstrate discrepancies between rational models of clinical decision making and current procedures. Another driving force is the expense of the present system. A third driving force is the logic of tracing incremental change over time, demonstrating a "compounding effect" of the serial display of accumulated experience.

It is generally believed that from a national and public frame of reference, such a system of usable information would "pay" in the long run. Perhaps the post-World War II strategy for scientific research might be instructive with regard to large-scale demonstrations in this area. Congress, the National Center for Health Services Research, and other national groups have for some years recognized the importance of this kind of investigation, but a balance of impeding forces exists, forces that are not clearly understood.

The Health Care Financing Administration (HCFA) has fiscal resources for studies of the type envisioned but, under current policies, does not support this kind of activity. It tends to support policy studies based on available data rather than new enterprises.

THE PROCESS OF CLINICAL DECISION MAKING

Participants: G. A. Gorry (Chair), A. S. Elstein, P. E. Johnson, J. P. Kassirer
Summarized by: G. A. Gorry

In recent years, important advances have been made in studying and understanding the decision-making process. These studies, for the most part, have not dealt specifically with decisions related to the choice and use of clinical laboratory tests. What approaches can be used to study the role of clinical decision-making models in ensuring effective use of laboratory tests?

The discussion of this panel placed particular emphasis on the organization of investigative and educational studies of the interface between clinical decision making and the laboratory. In general the discussion focused on the two broad types of studies, descriptive and normative.

The rapid growth of the scientific knowledge that underlies the practice of medicine has produced a marked degree of specialization among practitioners, so the proper integration of diverse information in medical decision making is an increasing challenge to clinicians and laboratory physicians alike. Despite the paramount importance of decision-making strategies in medical practice, little is known about them. Hence, while it is axiomatic that the ways in which physicians make decisions is related to their use of laboratory services, it is difficult at present to link directly the choice of particular laboratory studies to the expectations of their worth and the analysis of their results, which are such integral parts of the decisions made in clinical medicine.

In recent years, a number of efforts have been made to formulate explicit principles of sound clinical judgment and to introduce normative decision-making procedures into the clinical arena.[2-4] Such methods, of which decision analysis is perhaps the most prominent, are derived from assumptions about how clinical decisions ought to be made. Other studies, mostly in cognitive psychology and the field of computer science known as artificial intelligence, have been aimed at discovering how experienced clinicians actually do solve problems.[5-8]

The confluence of these two general areas of research has produced a new, more scientific view of medical decision making. The value of such efforts for people interested in laboratory utilization is perhaps more potential than actual at present, because neither normative nor descriptive studies of clinical decision making have had much of a demonstrable effect upon the use of laboratory services. To date, even more extensive studies of decision making in radiology have not had any significant influence on the use of radiologic procedures.

Descriptive Studies

As the name connotes, descriptive studies are aimed at providing good descriptions of the ways in which clinicians deal with the uncertainty that characterizes the clinical environment. The reflections of experienced clinicians on their own problem-solving processes have suggested some principles that may help the younger physician in analyzing clinical problems. The difficulty with these introspective statements is that they are often very general and do not provide proper guidance for the kinds of explicit decisions that need to be made.

The inadequacy of unaided introspection in explicating clinical judgment means that we must seek other investigative tools if we are to add much to our store of knowledge. As a result, researchers in the field of problem solving have turned to the use of computer programs to test psychological theories because computer science provides a substantial number of well-defined and experimentally implemented concepts for "thinking about thinking," only a few of which have identifiable analogs in traditional psychology.

In the descriptive approach, a favored procedure is to have the clinical problem solver think aloud as he proceeds through a task. The recorded introspection, together with the sequence of moves actually taken, provides the data to be analyzed by the researcher to develop an account of clinical reasoning. Through the use of protocol analysis, that is, the study of the transcripts of verbalized problem-solving behavior, detailed descriptions of the diverse problem-solving strategies of physicians can be obtained. One possible hazard of this approach is that the verbalizations may be treated as a true account of the reasons for a particular sequence of action. This assumption may well be questioned, for it is surely clear that people do not always know the reasons for their actions or if they do, they do not always choose to articulate them. We need not assume, however, that statements made by physicians concerning their problem-solving activities are either complete or wholly accurate, but only that the transcript of their verbalized problem-solving behavior is a rich source of clues regarding thought processes underlying the performance.

Hypotheses concerning thought processes may be derived from this analysis and stated precisely in the form of computer programs that can be tested through the use of simulation. The advantages of this use of the computer as a "psychological laboratory" are great. In contrast to an English language description of a psychological theory, the computer program embodiment of the theory is an unambiguous representation. The program and hence the theory can be tested by tracing the sequence of the actions the program takes in response to various test cases. These actions are the "predictions" of the theory as it applies to the specific situation represented by the test case. Inadequacies in the theory often are uncovered rapidly in this way, and so, on the whole, this approach is quite appealing.

The use of such "process-tracing" studies was thought by the group to offer considerable promise in explaining those aspects of clinical decision making that bear on the use of laboratory tests. Although the collection and analysis of protocols is a tedious undertaking, it is a way to identify the knowledge and decision-making procedures used by clinicians when they are required to assess the information embodied in a particular test result. It is thought by the group that many of the differences in observed behavior among clinicians in regard to laboratory use may be attributable to differences in knowledge concerning the important aspects of the tests involved—for example, the accuracy of the tests or the way in which the interpretation of the test needs to be modified in the presence of certain clinical features of the case. Without a clear understanding of the knowledge employed by clinicians in choosing and interpreting the diagnostic tests, it will be difficult to infer how choices of diagnostic tests are made.

Consider the following basic scheme for each project. A subject physician is presented a certain amount of factual information about a particular case. The clinician is asked to discuss interpretations of those facts and to indicate those diagnostic hypotheses he or she is actively considering. The physician then is given the opportunity to seek further information in order to confirm or to eliminate diagnostic hypotheses. To gain such additional information, he or she must choose particular diagnostic tests and discuss the reasons for the selections made. Then, the results of the test are provided and the physician is asked to discuss the ways in which those results affected the opinions previously held. The entire session with the physician is tape-recorded and a transcript of the session is prepared.

By appropriate variation of this simple experimental procedure, a great deal of data could be gathered concerning how physicians use laboratory information. By using a series of cases with a given group of physicians, the role of factual knowledge could be elucidated. By altering aspects of a particular case, the influence of certain social and cultural factors upon the physicians' use of laboratory services could be investigated. Again, by manipulating the facts in a single case, it should be possible to identify the role that certain psychological factors play in clinical decision making. Finally, the development of skilled reasoning about laboratory information could be studied through the presentation of a given case to physicians at different points in their training.

We also need research on the effectiveness of decision analysis in clinical problem solving. By confronting physicians with simulated problem-solving tasks that contain uncertainty and then collecting verbalized data, we may gain insight into the most effective role for decision analysis. Process tracing and decision analysis can be complementary: process tracing reveals the decision tree (the alternatives) whereas decision analysis makes explicit the consequence of choice.

It is obvious that many variations on these themes could be pursued, and in the light of recent work on clinical decision making, it is reasonable to expect some interesting results. However, it seemed to the group that both clinicians and laboratory physicians would be key participants in such research. The laboratory physician can help immensely with the definition of experimental setting. The clinicians can aid in the analysis of the protocols gathered. Additionally, it is important to have associated with any such project at least one individual who has some previous exposure to this kind of research. Therefore, a major impediment to the pursuit of process-tracing studies as they pertain to laboratory use seems to be the relative scarcity of research teams with the proper mix of experience and skills. On the other hand, the analytic skills required are not particularly difficult to master, and it is reasonable to assume that prospective research teams who have access to problems and subjects could be trained in research techniques by individuals with more experience in process-tracing studies.

Prescriptive Studies

Explicit principles of sound clinical judgment and normative decision-making procedures can be derived from assumptions about how clinical decisions *ought* to be made. The discussion group felt that efforts to introduce formal methods for evaluating the information content of laboratory tests into the spectrum of undergraduate, graduate, and continuing medical education should be encouraged. For example, one of the potentially powerful aids to clinical decision making is decision analysis, a formal theory for making decisions in the face of uncertainty. The methods of decision analysis are technical, having solid groundings in mathematics, but the appreciation of them does not require an extensive mathematical background. Indeed most of the value of decision analysis can be gained through the study of its rudiments, which are easily understood by any physician with an interest in clinical decision making‚and a little patience. This makes the introduction of decision analytic methods into clinical practice a reasonable goal. Because decision analysis fits certain clinical decision-making problems so well, experienced physicians may see its principles are more precise versions of those they apply but that in general cannot explain in detail. For the student, the framework that decision analysis provides is useful in organizing a growing clinical experience and in hastening the development of clinical judgment.

It has been said that decision making comprises three principal phases: finding occasions for making a decision; finding possible courses of action; and choosing among courses of action. For the most part, decision analysis deals with the last of these phases, the choice among alternative course of action. Therefore, decision analysis is most useful in situations in which the options available to decision makers can be clearly described. Although this requirement restricts substantially the range of problems for which decision analysis is appropriate, a large number of important clinical problems, many involving laboratory tests, can be formulated in such a way that decision analysis can be used in solving them. In fact, a number of clinical problems that share certain "structural" features have been analyzed formally. An example of such a problem is one in which a physician must respond to a test result that is highly suggestive of a diagnosis he previously thought very unlikely. Once a physician has been taught a general approach to the revision of diagnostic probabilities, he is better able to address a specific instance of such a problem.

In the majority of medical schools and programs of graduate medical education, few teachers are prepared to provide explicit aid in problem solving beyond offering guidance about what to do or not to do in a particular case. Except in a few sharply circumscribed situations, teachers are seldom able to explain the principles they themselves apply to problems. Whether in simulated situations or in dealing with actual patients, the young physician learns about making decisions by making decisions. In these circumstances, it is difficult to integrate decision analysis into clinical practice without the acceptance and continued support of the teachers involved. Therefore, it may be necessary to teach the teachers in order to have a lasting effect on more than a few students, and the teachers may be relatively resistant to change.

There is, however, some evidence that a gradually increasing number of educational programs are being planned and implemented that should extend the appreciation and use of decision analysis and heuristic problem-solving strategies in the medical community. At present, these innovations are in the nature of educational experiments. They await adequate evaluation, in itself a difficult problem.

Clear demonstrations of the practical value of decision analysis in medicine are lacking. Whether doctors who understand decision analysis practice better medicine is an unresolved question. Therefore, the challenge is to bring together clinicians who teach students or other physicians, laboratory physicians who see the laboratory use that follows from clinical decisions, and decision analysts who can help create a limited and controlled setting in which to assess the success of an educational intervention. With the proper combination of people, such settings can be established, but the discussion group recognized the patience and care that would be required. It was felt that the value of clear demonstrations of the effective use of decision analysis would be sufficiently great to warrant the effort required.

In the same general vein, the discussion group favored the study of computer-based aids to clinical decision making. Programs embodying principles and procedures of decision analysis could be made available to students and physicians in clinical settings to help them select and interpret laboratory procedures. Such programs would be particularly helpful, if they had access to the latest, most detailed data on test results in various groups of patients. Physicians also might learn general approaches to decision problems in medicine from the use of such programs.

In summary, although we recognize the difficulties in mounting experimental programs such as those suggested above, we feel that the studies of clinical decision making done to date strongly suggest that similar studies focused on laboratory use will yield important results. We expect that as laboratory physicians become more familiar with the approaches used to study and improve clinical problem solving, they will find ready use for them in addressing their own concerns.

CLINICAL DECISION AND THE CLINICAL LABORATORY —THE INTERFACE

Participants: D. S. Young (Chair), C. Altshuler, E. S. Benson, J. A. Campbell, D. P. Connelly, S. N. Finkelstein, R. S. Galen, W. A. Gliebe

Summary by D. S. Young

The question posed to the group related to the general increase in use of laboratory tests in the recent past: "What approaches can be used to foster the appropriate use of laboratory tests in clinical decision making, so as to enhance appropriate use of clinical and economic resources?" Members of the group were clinical laboratorians and others involved in health care studies. Although all except one of the group were physicians, none were clinicians.

In the brief time available to identify the most important approaches to be used, the five top-ranked were these:

- Teach medical students better in the field of laboratory medicine.
- Educate laboratory directors to play an active role in interpreting results.
- Teach clinical residents proper laboratory use.

- Define the usefulness of each test.
- Computerize laboratory data.

Thus, the emphasis is on improved education, and the top three responses were initially ranked as of equal importance. When voted upon again, the top two choices were again ranked of equal importance.

About 50 different responses were provided by the group and although some of these were similar, many different concepts were voiced and could provide a means for addressing the increased use, with questionable effectiveness, of clinical laboratory services.

These included (in order of number of votes received) the following:

1. Provide a programmed accelerated laboratory investigation (PALI) scheme as devised by Altshuler.[9]
2. a. Heighten awareness in educators and students that overuse of, or dependence on, clinical laboratory information is an important concern.
   b. Document the level of laboratory use at present, because some of the current concerns are based only on impressions.
   c. Develop algorithms for clinicians to order appropriate laboratory tests in given situations.

3. a. Develop mechanisms to inform physicians privately of their ordering patterns in comparison with their peers.
   b. Reemphasize the "art" of medicine at all levels of training.
   c. Find and implement new methods of teaching that really affect laboratory use.
   d. Teach pathology residents proper laboratory use so that they, during training and subsequently, can effectively teach this to others.

4. a. Include justifications with orders for some or all laboratory tests.
   b. Develop appropriate education materials for medical students.
   c. Merge laboratory data, when reported, with diagnoses and charges to patients.
   d. Experiment with different reimbursement procedures.

5. a. Identify reasons for inappropriate ordering of laboratory tests.
   b. Improve methods of surveillance of laboratory use.
   c. Publicize charges of tests to patients.
   d. Inhibit the ordering of a repeat test until the results of the same test ordered previously have been received by the requesting physician.
   e. Develop protocols, which must be adhered to, for the introduction of new tests into routine practice.

6. a. Identify areas requiring continuing medical education for utilization of laboratory tests.
   b. Improve medical record keeping.
   c. Provide incentives (financial and other) to physicians for not ordering laboratory tests.

The underlying theme affecting most of the suggestions is the need for improved education of users of the clinical laboratory. Only a small number of administrative remedies were deemed to be appropriate for addressing the presumed overordering. However, one problem identified is our lack of quantitative information on the magnitude of overuse of the laboratory. Much of the information that we have is derived from impressions of individuals concerned with the proper use of laboratory services, but even these impressions have not been quantified or ranked in order of importance.[10]

Only the first two approaches to presumed inappropriate use of the clinical laboratory were addressed by the group.

Teaching Laboratory Medicine to Medical Students

The most important strategies to teach laboratory medicine in a better way to medical students were identified as:

1. Having pathologists teach improved utilization of the laboratory;
2. Recruiting better individuals into the field of laboratory medicine to serve as role models;
3. Having laboratory rounds on wards as a clinical elective;
4. Teaching laboratory use in the senior year at medical school;
5. a. Teaching decision analysis; and
   b. During teaching of laboratory medicine, providing case studies including both clinical and laboratory applications.

The first two strategies appeared to the group to be much more important than the others, judging by the voting of the group. Several other strategies that ranked only slightly lower than some of those in the priority list included:

1. Simulation of case studies;
2. Stimulation of a laboratory medicine focus in the National Board of Medical Examiners examinations;
3. Inclusion of electives in laboratory medicine in laboratories of different sophistication;
4. Problem oriented discussion of cases in curriculum;
5. Adoption by more teachers of the content and style of the courses put on by Drs. Burke and Ward;
6. Fellowship periods in laboratory medicine made available to students;
7. Development of algorithms for logical testing as a base from which students could be encouraged to develop their own;
8. Adoption elsewhere of methods of teaching of laboratory medicine in centers where they have been demonstrated to be successful; and
9. Teaching of computer applications in medicine.

The recommendations focused mainly on improved teaching by laboratorians and in effect excluded further involvement in the teaching of laboratory medicine. The recommendations did not hinge on administrative changes to any extent and the only major change that would be required in existing medical school curricula would require the shifting of some of the teaching of laboratory medicine into the senior year, an already very crowded period for the medical student. The other recommended administrative change would require some consideration of the discipline of laboratory medicine in the National Board examinations. The other recommendations are, in theory at least, within the capabilities of existing departments of pathology or laboratory medicine, if enough adequately trained and motivated staff are available.

Resources

To teach laboratory medicine effectively, departments of laboratory medicine (or their equivalent) must have a commitment to do this teaching. The commitment must be made by the chairman of the department and be supported by the faculty. The medical school must also recognize that laboratory medicine is an important facet of the medical student's training and must juggle existing time to allow some to be set aside for rounds to be presented by residents and the faculty. Student laboratories should also be used for computer instruction. The laboratories should generate with computers patterns to correlate laboratory data with diseases. A model for this is the recent publication by Friedman et al.,[11] which lists those diseases that alter specific tests and those tests that are affected by specific diseases.

Impediments

The major impediments to the introduction of a new teaching program are the attitudes of the staff. Even when it is admitted that teaching is currently inadequate, there may be a reluctance to foster and accept change. Many of the staff in departments of laboratory medicine or pathology, although physicians, have become too laboratory, as opposed to clinically, oriented and probably could not respond to the clinical challenges required in conducting rounds and being "real" physicians again.

The curriculum committee in any medical school must feel convinced that laboratory medicine is a part of medicine important enough to have time created for its teaching. In most instances this will mean that time would be taken away from other disciplines, which will probably be regarded as unacceptable. Many clinical departments regard interpretation of laboratory data as within their purview and will oppose any suggestion that they do not teach laboratory use and data interpretation adequately.

The major problems will arise from the need of departments of laboratory medicine to make the commitment to teach when they probably lack the right individuals to do this, and may not even be staffed to do this well and continue to provide a high level of service. The staff of most departments recognize that a major new teaching effort will require much preparation, without there necessarily being many good programs that could be emulated.

Educating Laboratory Directors to Play an Active Role in Interpreting Results

The group believed that laboratory directors must become more active as physicians. Four strategies appeared to be most important and received considerably more votes than the others:

1. The laboratory director should attend clinical rounds.
2. Competitive financial incentives should be provided to the laboratory directors to encourage them to become actively involved in the interpretation of data.
3. The committee of chairmen of pathology departments should endorse and actively encourage this role for laboratory directors.
4. Surveillance systems should be set up to identify abnormal test results that would then stimulate the laboratory director to study these and communicate them to clinicians.

Other strategies to educate laboratory directors that were considered included:

1. Merging of laboratory data with clinical data so that the laboratory director becomes more involved with the latter;
2. Development of databases uniquely for laboratory directors so that they must be consulted for certain decisions;
3. Direct involvement of laboratory director in patient-care decisions;
4. Development of diagnostic algorithms with the aid of laboratory directors;
5. Arrangement of laboratory data in a retrievable form by laboratory directors;
6. Identification of successful models for education of laboratory directors, synthesis of techniques, and encouragement of implementation;
7. Study of techniques, and encouragement of implementation;
8. Limitation of the number of tests that clinicians can order without approval of the laboratory director, ensuring consultation between the clinicians and laboratory directors;
9. Social contacts of laboratory directors and clinicians, so that their expertise in test-ordering and interpretation might become apparent;
10. A system of further elaboration of results that could involve the laboratory director when abnormal results were produced; and
11. Introduction of a column, or feature, written by laboratory directors, into a leading medical journal to demonstrate their expertise.

Resources

The resources for the recommended strategies already exist, except for numbers 2 and 3. All the other strategies could be implemented with the good-will and cooperation of laboratory directors and clinicians. There is no docu-mented evidence that patients are diagnosed earlier or treated better when labo-ratorians interpret laboratory data for clinicians than when the latter do it them-selves. Without such evidence it is unlikely that financial support will be made available as an incentive to laboratory directors to do this. It might well be ar-gued that some of the reimbursement of pathologists is now based on the as-sumption that they are actively involved in the interpretation of data.

The committee of chairmen of pathology departments does not have the influence over individual medical schools or departments of laboratory medicine or pathology that would ensure that a pronouncement by the committee had much influence on individual laboratory directors, or on their becoming involved in data interpretation and assistance to physicians in using laboratory services better.

Impediments

In almost all hospitals, the potential for laboratory directors to become in-volved in data interpretation already exists. A small number may be involved in doing this, probably because of their own background training and interests. Most laboratory directors entered the field of pathology because of a lesser inter-est in clinical medicine than in laboratory medicine or pathology. It is thus likely that their own attitudes to change their ways would be the biggest impediment to improving their assistance to physicians in the interpretation of laboratory data.

If it is necessary for laboratory directors to become an interface between the laboratory and clinicians for reporting of abnormal data, there may be a de-lay in the reporting of such results, which would ultimately lead to a deterior-ation of the medical service.

Summary

Both to improve teaching of medical students and to foster a greater in-volvement of medical directors in ensuring proper laboratory use, we need to at-tract appropriately qualified and motivated individuals into the field of labora-tory medicine. Without this personal motivation, we are unlikely to accomplish either of the two most important approaches to enhance the appropriate use of laboratory tests in clinical decision making. Even if the goals were accomplished, change is likely to occur only slowly.

MEDICAL EDUCATION AND LABORATORY USE

Participants: P. F. Griner (Chair), M. D. Burke, J. M. Eisenberg,
S. E. Goldfinger, L. L. Weed
Summary by: M. D. Burke

Introduction

The question posed was: What approaches to medical education can be used to ensure effective use of laboratory tests in patient care?

Following the nominal (silent writing) phase of the process, 19 responses were elicited in round-robin fashion. These are shown verbatim in Table 1. Further discussion and clarification of these responses led to the group consensus that no more than six ideas were contained within the original 19 responses. These revised ideas were then voted on and a priority approaches list was generated.

Attention was then directed to the strategies, resources, and impediments attending each priority. Because time was limited, the round-robin and balloting phases of the nominal group process were confined to ranking strategies for that approach given top priority.

Priority Approaches

1. Develop methods for disseminating the data required for clinical decision making.
2. Formalize systematic teaching of the principles and practice of laboratory usage and interpretation.
3. Educate and recruit needed faculty.
4. Reinforce desired physician behavior, i.e., operant conditioning techniques.
5. Improve the clinical and laboratory database.
6. Conduct a public education campaign.

Strategies, Resources, and Impediments

Priority Approach 1—Data Dissemination

Strategies are ranked as follows: (1) data displays (when available); (2) laboratory resource persons; (3) publication of laboratory costs; and (4) newsletters, etc.

Resources mentioned by the group include written materials (tests, manuals, publications), clinical-laboratory interaction (lectures, rounds, conferences, courses), computer systems, the existing database (patient records, laboratory records), and laboratory personnel.

Impediments are resistance on the part of clinical faculty, lack of time and money, lack of an adequate database, poorly developed methods of data acquisition and/or retrieval, and the traditional "clinician-chemist" communication gap.

Priority Approach 2—Formal Teaching

Strategies are acquisition of curriculum time, indoctrination of medical

Table 1

1. Use of guidance tools—no more memory (tools in real care)
2. Patient management problems
3. Faculty development
4. Improvement of database necessary to promote quantitative clinical reasoning
5. Systematic instruction of medical students
6. Teach formal decision analysis
7. Implement behavioral modification techniques
8. Make data available in practical and usable form
9. Participation by laboratory people in clinical discussions (teaching and research)
10. Teach epidemiological principles
11. Public education campaign
12. Feedback of utilization patterns to clinicians
13. Teach principles of clinical health economics
14. Formal lectures
15. Patient conferences
16. Newsletters
17. Continuing education
18. Publicize cost of diagnostic tests
19. Provide MDs with their patients' bills

students with resident reinforcement, continued education of practicing physicians, and the training of clinically oriented laboratory teachers.

Resources are the faculty (clinical and laboratory), and the necessary knowledge embodied in epidemiology and in economic and decision theory.

Impediments are lack of curriculum time, lack of money, apathy, disinterest and lack of knowledge on the part of the faculty, and the difficulties inherent in convincing students and practicing physicians of the importance attached to epidemiological principles and decision theory.

Priority Approach 3—Faculty Education and Recruitment

Faculty goodwill is mentioned as a resource. Lack of money and entrenched traditional views prevalent among existing faculty are identified as impediments.

Priority Approach 4—Behavior Modification

Strategies mentioned include incentives, penalties, and feedback approaches. The internal drive of trainees is identified as a resource, with lack of time and ethical considerations as impediments.

Priority Approaches 5-6—Improved Database and Public Education Campaign

Computer-based systems and networks of physicians collecting data constitute resource suggestions for an improved database. The difficulty inherent in acquiring large numbers of data is regarded as an impediment. One participant pointed out that the cooperation of insurers should be regarded as a resource for a public education campaign. However, the time-consuming and expensive nature of such a campaign is regarded as an impediment.

Conclusions

Data must be made available to users in usable form. Curriculum time must be allocated for teaching effective use of laboratory tests. Faculty sensitive to the needs of clinical decision making must be recruited and trained.

More intelligent and intensive use of men and machines will be required to gather, retrieve, and disseminate usable data. Little is likely to be achieved without alteration of the entrenched view that equates science with technology-intensive medical practice and—by inference—considers clinical decision making to be the reverse.

References

1. Delbecq AL, VandeVen AH, Gustafson DH. Group technique for program planning: a guide to nominal group and delphi processes. Glenview, IL: Scott Foresman and Company, 1975.
2. Lusted LB. Introduction to medical decision making. Springfield, IL: Charles C Thomas, 1968.
3. Pauker SG, Kassirer JP. Therapeutic decision making: A cost-benefit analysis. N Engl J Med 1975;293:229-34.
4. McNeil, BJ, Keeler E, Adelstein SJ. Primer on certain elements of medical decision making. N Engl J Med 1975;293:211-15.
5. Kassirer JP, Gorry GA. Clinical problem solving: A behavioral analysis. Ann Intern Med 1978;89:245-55.
6. Elstein AS, Shulman LS, Sprafka SA. Medical problem solving: An analysis of clinical reasoning. Cambridge, MA: Harvard University Press, 1978.
7. Shortliffe EH. Computer-based medical consultations: MYCIN. New York: Elsevier/North Holland, 1976.
8. Pauker SG, Gorry GA, Kassirer JP, Schwartz WB. Toward the simulation of clinical cognition: Taking a present illness by computer. Am J Med 1976;60:981-96.
9. Altshuler CH. The usefulness of laboratory information in medical monitoring. In: Young DS, Uddin DE, Nipper H, Hicks JM, eds. Clinician and chemist: The relationship of the laboratory to the physician. American Association for Clinical Chemistry, Washington, DC, 1979:284-96.
10. Griner PF. Current practices in laboratory utilization in the teaching hospital: possible impact of education programs. In: Young DS, Uddin DE, Nipper H, Hicks JM, eds. Clinician and chemist: The relationship of the laboratory to the physician. American Association for Clinical Chemistry, Washington, DC, 1979:307.
11. Friedman RB, Anderson RE, Entine SM, Hirshberg SB. Effects of disease on clinical laboratory tests. Clin Chem 1980;26:1D-476D.

Appendix
Discussion

Discussion

PANEL ONE

Participants: J. P. Kassirer (Chair), B. J. Andrew, A. S. Elstein, G. A. Gorry,
P. E. Johnson, A. L. Komaroff, J. M. Murray, and E. A. Stead

E. Stead: I don't think doctors think as we've been told they think. I don't
think doctors do anything but count on their memories. They lay down patterns.
They check data against those patterns. Inasmuch as they can remember the patterns, they do well. Inasmuch as they get them mixed up, they do poorly. You
take simple data and it gets you so far. You can have a list of everything that
might be extended from that pattern, but that's all doctors do. They don't do
very complex things.

Question: To what degree do national board questions using new evaluation
techniques take into account the problems noted by Elstein that experts in referral centers get a biased view of medical care and thus of procedures needed to
explore a given clinical decision?

B. Andrew: Actually I think there are a couple of pieces to the question. One relates to who is setting the standard—who is scoring the test questions and determining what constitutes the right answers or the best answers. This problem is
one that we encounter not only for new evaluation techniques, but for the techniques that we have been using for some time. It's extremely important to try to
call upon a group of experts that represents a variety of what are the well-known
differences and perspectives within the health care setting. We find that many
times different physicians coming from different kinds of academic medical centers have different opinions about what constitutes appropriate courses of action.

327

Those who are primarily based in community health care settings have different perspectives. One of the interesting things about watching a committee talk through a process such as this is that you find that there is a great deal of commonality of overlapping perspective that makes the scoring of simulations or test questions easier for those particular items. There are, in fact, some test items that are thrown out because one can't get consensus from a group of reasonably qualified individuals. Those questions don't represent appropriate challenges for students. One of the interesting things about these more complex simulations is that you don't have to do anything with them—that is, you don't have to score them. You let people proceed as they would and you allow for a great many differences in style. You score performance only on those things on which you can get substantial consensus representing key and crucial decisions in patient care. So the development of complex simulations, I think, will actually refine our scoring procedures and force us to focus on those things that are the key elements of decision making.

Question: I am interested and surprised that so far we have ignored the effect of legal processes on physician behavior. This needs to be discussed in terms of undergraduate, graduate, and continuing educational processes. Please do so.

J. Murray: I have a very simple answer to that—I don't think we should have anything to do with that sort of thing, personally. I don't think we should let the medico-legal world determine how we should do our tests and how we should use them at all. I don't think it has any place in the management of patients. Whether or not we should be scared of malpractice, we should do the best we can with what we've got and ignore that.

A. Elstein: Perhaps it's easy for me to speak because I'm not going to be sued. It is my impression, and I guess the impression of my physician colleagues with whom I've spoken about these matters, that the issue of medical malpractice, being sued for errors of omission or commission, is something of a red herring. They think that many physicians in training seem to be using that issue as a justification for why laboratory tests ought to be done: we ought to do these laboratory tests not because we really think there is any valuable information that we're going to get from them, but because we might be sued if we didn't. It seems to me that that is a relatively easily answered objection and I think that the fact that it is offered as a defense for testing indicates that we've gotten into the kind of climate that Dr. Reiser alluded to this morning. We have gotten into the climate in which the evidence of one's senses and the evidence of verbal testimonies are no longer trusted and that evidence derived from laboratory tests is regarded somehow as perfect information, obtained at no cost and given to us free of error. The paradoxical thing is that every pathologist and every radiologist knows that both of those assertions are not true. The difficulty that we've had in getting physicians in training to realize that these tests do cost money and that they do have their own error rates, indicates how pervasive the test technology has become. I really regard the legal defense as an easily surmounted subterfuge for a much more pervasive cultural attitude toward this kind of information.

A. Komaroff: I would echo that. You cannot dismiss the real fear that many practicing physicians have of malpractice, but I do think that it's more often the excuse than the reason. I also would like to think that the kind of investigations that are being described here in these next several days where the actual risks and benefits of doing a diagnostic test are measured to a more precise degree than we have done in the past will serve as reasonable evidence in a court of law. It's not just how many dollars you are willing to spend for a benefit. But you can show in a court of law, given the low probability of a disease in an individual patient, that the patient had more to lose in risks from the diagnostic test than the gain from the possible discovery of a very unlikely disease. So I would like to think that that kind of argument with numbers attached to it would carry some weight in a court of law.

E. Stead: You're much better off if the record shows that you thought of the test and you said these are the reasons that we're not going to do it.

Question: Have you tested your model, your simulator, and your subjects with an item of deliberate misinformation, such as an erroneous lab result?

P. Johnson: We've constructed what are called "garden path" cases. These are cases in which we provide an initial piece of information that leads to the elicitation of a "foil" disease. And then later, we've provided information that's intended to get the physician thinking back on the track. What's required in order for one to avoid the garden path is to have enough knowledge so that one can override the seductiveness of the early cue. When we've done that kind of thing, what we've discovered typically is that medical students tend to be very often quite confused by that kind of case and don't end up doing anything. Individuals at the middle level, trainees so to speak, tend to be very seduced by that kind of case—they go for the foil information; they will commit themselves to a diagnosis of valvular stenosis and not even think of subvalvular stenosis because the initial cue has been so dominant. Experts tend to see both the foil and the later information. They are careful, get the information sorted out, and end up with the correct diagnosis. The simulation under those conditions tends to perform like a trainee, that is to say the simulation can be seduced just like trainees can be. Under those conditions we've gone back and tried to discover what it was about the piece of laboratory data or clinical information that led to the erroneous conclusion.

Question: If you alter the sequence of the data that you give to the people, and the simulator—what happens?

P. Johnson: That tends to destroy the simulation's thinking. It also tends to give medical students and some trainees a lot of difficulty. Experts, it turns out, are much more robust than we thought they would be under such conditions. We did a couple of studies where we asked individuals at the end of the session to give us back the data of the case. We didn't think physicians would be able to do that. But the more expert the subject the more completely they could give us back everything we told them. We asked one of the experts how he could do that. The physician said, "Well, you have to understand that I'm not really remembering very much. The way I do this is I know what the disease is because I just diagnosed it. And then, of course, I know all those things that should be true of that disease, and I just gave you back normal values for the rest. So I'm not really remembering very much at all." If you don't know as much, you have a lot more trouble with that kind of problem.

Question: All studies presented today analyze clinical behavior in the usual environment, where hypotheses evolve initially from patient interviews. Are there studies that presented laboratory data first? Does this approach aid or hinder correct hypothesis formation?

J. Kassirer: I don't know of any specific studies, but I can tell you of my own experience. I'm a nephrologist and do a lot of work in electrolytes and in acid-base disorders. The house staff are often trying to get information about electrolyte and acid-base problems and will frequently simply put up a bunch of numbers on the board. I'll end up talking about them for a half an hour. I can tell you that you can make very adequate diagnostic hypotheses on the basis of just some numbers. How widely representative that is, I can't tell you.

Question: What is the expected cost effectiveness of developing artificial intelligence for clinical decision making?

A. Gorry: I really don't know. I'm inclined to say that there are some decided benefits for having computer programs that make clinical decisions. But one would have to look at these programs from a number of different vantage points. I should think that some of the programs that are currently available, such as the program INTERNIST developed by Drs. Myers and Pople at Pittsburgh, are the harbingers of computer programs that may well have a substantial impact on various aspects of clinical medicine. Whether their use would be cost-effective or not, I think, depends in large part on the development of methods for assessing cost and benefits we do not yet have. The development of computer programs that reputedly embody methods for making clinical decisions has done at least one thing. It has focused much additional attention on clinical decision making as it is done by clinicians. Once one takes statements about how things are thought to be done by clinicians and tries to generate a computer program, or proposes a better way of doing it, and tries to develop that method, one comes to grips quite rapidly with the issues that have been alluded to today—the questions of knowledge, the problem-solving process, and all the rest. The immediate effect of the development of such programs is perhaps already here represented by the language that the people who spoke today used so easily when they talked about probabilities, triggering hypotheses, predictive value, and all the rest. That language comes out of mathematics and computer science, and I think is well used by many clinicians. Well before very effective programs evolve, these efforts will have had an impact on clinical medicine.

P. Johnson: I know from the point of view of somebody who tries to construct computer models in order to learn more about the way people work—it's a long and arduous undertaking and it consumes much computer time. I know that one also thinks about using those kinds of things eventually as decision aids. My impression is that currently that is not as practical as we might like it to be.

Question: If we can't distinguish expert and nonexpert clinical problems solvers based on examination, then why do we need to explicate and specifically teach the elements of that process? That is, does explicit knowledge of the process make a difference, and, if so, where?

A. Elstein: One of the things that I think we have learned from these studies is that physician performance is far more variable over situations than we had believed. If we really want to get good assessment of physician competence, we have to assess their performance far more extensively than we believed to be the case before. That would be one reason, I think, that such studies are necessary. I also think part of the reason that we don't find much evidence of growth in these logical reasoning skills among physicians as contrasted with the growth in the knowledge of medical content as a function of experience—we have to look at the educational programs and ask what it is that people are asked to learn. A great deal of what physicians are asked to learn is precisely that which shows superiority over novices. People are not asked to demonstrate systematically that they analyze problems more rationally of more effectively than other people. They are asked repeatedly to demonstrate that they know more than other people. Consequently, it shouldn't surprise us that people who are more experienced demonstrate that they know more than people who are less experienced. They are behaving very adaptively for the environmental demand. I would hope that as we shift the emphasis of assessment toward a greater emphasis on rational analysis of the basic components of the problem, we will see that physicians learn to do that better too. I think it's probably true that medical students and physicians in general will learn to do whatever it is society requires of them. As a group, they are quite bright and learn to do whatever needs to be done. Part of the reason we don't see differences in the formal analysis of problems is that we've not asked that experts show greater sophistication in formal analysis than we've asked novices to show. We've asked neither group to show a great deal of depth of analysis.

E. Stead: We still miss the point. I deal with medical students and basic scientists. The basic scientists never ask the students a thinking question. Anything that has a known answer is a function of memory. It can be a fairly complex function of memory. It may even be aided by a computer machine, but it is always a memory function. All this problem-solving analysis misses that point. When you want to solve something, add to something that isn't known, you ought to build a house that has never been built before. That, by definition, is a function of thinking. But doctors can't carry on their busy practice that way. They've got to deal with things that have known answers. Therefore, it's a memory game. Unfortunately, we haven't set it up with the best memory tools. It's not a question of problem solving. It's a different kind of thing.

A. Gorry: I think everyone who has spoken today with regard to the analysis of clinical decision making would concur with the general notion that the more one studies the way in which people in clinical medicine make decisions, the more one is impressed by how much they actually know. I don't think that is a controversial subject. I would not want it to be thought that the message is that the study of clinical decision making is looking for something that will obviate the problem of knowledge, and make knowledge go away. That's not at all the point. In artificial intelligence, this business is alluded to from time to time. When researchers in artificial intelligence started out, they tried to find knowledge-free theories—cybernetics—where you didn't have to know anything. Now I think it's well recognized by people who work in these areas that people who are experienced know a great deal. So I'm not sure exactly what the wrong point is here, but I certainly would not want to be cast on the side of those who say there is no knowledge involved.

E. Stead: That certainly was not my point. My point merely is that anything with a known answer is an aspect of memory. That is very simple.

J. Murray: While I agree with you in principle, Dr. Stead, I don't think that the exercise has to be quite that way. Let's take a medical student who has learned his physiology—has learned Starling's Law, for example. It's a fact of memory, I agree. But at the bedside, it's a totally different situation. He goes to the bedside. The patient has a heaving chest and you ask him now, what do you see? The chest is heaving. What's the fundamental pathophysiology underlying that? Now very often, the student can't tell you. The student can't apply that knowledge. But the moment you start that train of thought, say this is diastolic overload, diastolic overload makes his heart beat more vigorously, then you are building on that knowledge. Then the student is able to use it. It's not a function of memory anymore—it's really expansion of knowledge based on that fundamental knowledge.

A. Elstein: I don't want to be understood as being in disagreement with Dr. Stead because I am not, fundamentally. I have written, as has Jerry Kassirer and Paul Johnson, about the problems of the organization of medical memory. Purely formal theories of memory of problem solving can never be adequate to account for how a practical task is executed. We're not the first people to discover that. People who have studied the differences between expert and inexpert chess players found twenty years ago that the differences between expert and inexpert chess players are not to be found in how many moves ahead they can see because they can't see any more moves ahead than people who play at the level at which I play (which is very, very bad). The differences between experts and nonexperts in chess are differences to be found in the organization of memory, and the degree to which they recognize positions that they now encounter as familiar positions—ah, I saw one like that once. Those kinds of situations are pervasive in medicine and there is no doubt that the organization of memory plays an important role in medical success. I think the questions that Paul Johnson is trying to get at, the questions that I have been trying to get at in some of my work, and that which Jack Myers and Pople are trying to get at is the following. Suppose that you said that the organization of memory is really important. Now you have said that memory counts for something and that truly formal strategies will never be adequate to account for how this task is organized. What can you tell us about how this memory is organized that would help novices to acquire a useful memory structure? That is the problem that I think we are trying to address.

A. Komaroff: I agree that memory is the issue and that the integration of multiple patterns is the cognitive act that is occurring. I think our problem is that we have been memorizing the wrong thing, or at least not memorizing some of the right things. As Dr. Kassirer pointed out in his closing remarks, what we really need to learn, and then memorize, are the probabilities of the disease, the prevalences of different diseases, and the conditional probabilities or likelihood that given this cluster of findings, the patient has this disease or that disease. It's that type of information that we haven't been seeking in our quest to understand the pathophysiology of illness. Until we have that database, we won't be memorizing all the things that we need to memorize to make the right decisions.

P. Johnson: I just wanted to add a word about the question why we might want to talk about the process of problem solving, if it doesn't serve as a good way of discriminating between people who are good at a task—experts and novices. It seems to me that one of the most important things about learning a process like problem solving in a domain such as medicine is that it itself becomes a tool for gaining further knowledge. One of the things that we've been talking about here really is something called experiential knowledge. It's the knowledge that you gain through the practice of a skill such as diagnosis. The way you learn how to organize knowledge experientially is by applying the problem-solving process that you are taught in medical school. So it becomes a device for acquiring skill once you leave medical school. I think that, to me, is the biggest reason that one might teach that process—not because it's going to serve to tell you who can do and who can't, but it becomes a device for learning.

Question: Aren't we at such an early stage of identifying superior strategies for clinical decision making that we should not promulgate these strategies and try to convince practicing clinicians that one strategy is better than another? Are we perhaps jumping the gun?

A. Komaroff: I think it's very risky to conclude that our analysis has identified a superior strategy. I think it's not impossible that in certain clinical conditions and with regard to certain management problems, we will find that we know enough to be reasonably confident about what is the most expeditious or most cost-effective strategy now, given current technology. More important, though, even when these analyses don't lead to any conclusive evidence that one approach is superior to another, at least major gaps in our knowledge—which we need to fill in order to decide which strategies are superior—are highlighted by the whole analytic process.

A. Gorry: One of the things that gets obscured as we look at the way that clinicians actually do things is that in certain "generic" clinical situations quite a bit is known about how one ought to make decisions. I am speaking broadly of those classes of decisions that lend themselves to such methods as decision analysis. Although it cannot be proved that decision analysis or the use of decision trees or probabilities in a clinical setting will lead to a better decision, I think it certainly can be argued quite strongly for many physicians that the principles of decision analysis, in fact, are ones that the physicians themselves would accept and apply were they introduced to them in a systematic way. Notice I don't say that is true for all physicians. But I think the point is that in some of the complexity of reviewing the present illness and taking histories, we tend to lose sight of the fact that there are some formal methods that could be highly recommended to clinicians in practice.

Question: How satisfied are you with measures of validity in assessing skills in clinical decision making? Are there any studies of the correlation between test results and subsequent performance in practice?

B. Andrew: NO. And I don't think anyone would have let me out of this room if I had said YES.

PANEL TWO

Participants: E. S. Benson (Chair), D. P. Connelly, S. N. Finkelstein, W. A. Gleibe, and D. S. Young

Question: In your opinion, have the various cost containment organizations and practices such as PSRO and health services research groups decreased medical expenditures?

W. Gliebe: There is some difference of opinion about whether PSROs have been effective. Initially, unfavorable reports of their cost effectiveness were published by governmental organizations. Later, more favorable reports followed. There are political implications to interpreting these reports. A favorable or unfavorable view depends on the perspective of the individual making the report. Regarding health services research organizations, such as the National Center for Health Services Research, it is too soon yet to judge their cost effectiveness. This is a relatively new field and it will take time for it to develop a record of accomplishment.

Question: Is there a study of private practice physicians similar to the residency study you cited?

W. Gliebe: Not to my knowledge. There have been very few studies that have actually asked physicians what they think. This, in my mind, is a rather simple idea that may seem too simplistic to some of you. We are trying to gather sufficient data and to make an evaluation over a 20-county area in northwest Ohio. This study would deal with practicing physicians, but we will have to wait at least two years for results.

Question: With your model, how do you get at the test that the physician should have ordered but didn't?

W. Gliebe: I suggest that you could define minimums. You could also ask questions of a physician to see whether he followed some medical protocol. You could use an algorithm as a test of the completeness of a diagnostic study.

Question: I would like to challenge the logic of your administrative solution to the so-called misuse of the laboratory on the basis of malpractice fears. In many instances, the hospital pays the malpractice premium for staff physicians and residents. Do you have hard data that the premium costs are less than costs generated by tests ordered as the result of malpractice fears?

W. Gliebe: That is a good question. With the data that I have, I think that the answer to that question could be computed quite readily. I do have information on the cost of malpractice insurance to the hospital and savings that results from that administrative relationship. Certainly the cost of so-called "defensive" practices can be calculated and compared with the figure of administrative costs of malpractice insurance.

Question: In the long term, would not the fixed costs mostly become variable? That is, would not a 20 percent reduction in tests ordered eventually result in a 20 percent reduction in equipment, overhead, and services? In the long run, therefore, would not the cost savings realized from the reduction in tests be greater than you have calculated?

S. Finkelstein: I remember a quote from Keynes that went something like this: "In the long run, we are all dead." If the assumption is made that fixed costs become variable costs in the long run, annual increments for equipment as a result of depreciation will be gone when the useful life of the equipment is gone. The fallacy here, as I see it, is that the laboratory is going to have to continually update its equipment. Thus, it seems to me, the hospital will continue to have a fixed cost component for use of the equipment.

Question: Why report all 6, 12, or whatever number of tests that are performed by a multichannel continuous flow autoanalyzer when only one is indicated?

D. Young: I think it really depends on your conscience. If you have an abnormal result, presumably it is abnormal for some reason. The laboratory physician would like to feel that this abnormal result should be appropriately addressed by the attendant physician.

Question: Are you recommending either 20-test panels or serum calciums as screening tests?

D. Young: I would not recommend a 20-test panel. The best testing format in my judgment occurs when physicians decide what tests they want to order and then use these specific tests. The evidence from serum calcium would clearly indicate that a large number of patients have benefited from the calcium screen when appropriate follow-up took place.

Question: When you list increases of laboratory tests, do you weight your figures to account for unwanted tests, for example, those in an admission battery?

D. Connelly: In our particular setting, we had a fairly stable set of tests from 1970-1978. After 1978, we introduced a number of multichannel instruments. That is why I chose to terminate my analysis in 1978. Beyond that time, I have no really effective way of determining from the available data what the physicians actually ordered. Over the period of this study, however, from 1970-1978, the test groupings including the admission battery did not change significantly.

Question: Total chemistry tests used rose 128 percent in the 9-year period you studied (between 1970-1978). Considering the rate of inflation and the impact of automation, what change has occurred in real dollar costs (1970 dollars) per patient?

D. Connelly: That is a very good question, one which we did not study. We believe we are doing these tests much more efficiently in 1978 and beyond than we were in 1970.

Question: Have the tests per patient day changed significantly as a whole or for any of the groups?

D. Connelly: Yes, this parameter has changed. We noted an increase in the average number of tests per patient from 30 in 1970 to 40 in 1978. Over the same period, we saw a decrease in the average length of stay from 14 days to 9.3.

Question: The major hospital administration journals deal largely with laundries, lobbies, and kitchens. Many of these costly services in contemporary hospitals are supported in large measure by laboratory income, the so-called "hospital overhead." The problem of the laboratory carrying an undue amount of the cost of these non-profit generating services may be an important one. How does this problem affect your reasoning and your analysis?

S. Finkelstein: This is precisely the reason we went to the laboratory to determine the actual costs of the laboratory as we saw them. The overhead figures that we used to cover the laboratory overhead had two components. These were the "direct overhead" as seen by the laboratory, usually the laboratory director (for example, secretarial costs, etc.), and the "general hospital overhead." The latter was generally allocated on a square foot basis and applied elsewhere throughout the hospital. It is for this reason we did not take laboratory charges as representative of costs. However, you must keep in mind that reimbursement is usually on the basis of costs, except by private insurance carriers who cover a minority of the patients nowadays.

Question: Recently, a young diabetic woman died after treatment for prolonged ketoacidosis. The serum potassium on admission was in the high normal range. She was treated appropriately with fluid and electrolyte therapy, insulin, and glucose. Approximately two hours after the initiation of therapy, she went into cardiac arrest and died. A premortem serum potassium determination gave a concentration of 2.5 milliequivalents per liter. The subsequent litigation has sensitized the emergency room staff so that now most ketotic diabetics have frequent electrolyte determinations made. Plainly, this is an example of defensive laboratory use. This defensive medicine cannot easily be reversed. Would you please comment on this illustrative case?

D. Young: I have a feeling that I would really be on the side of the patient on this point. As you know, it is appropriate to follow the treatment of diabetics in ketoacidosis with frequent serum potassium determinations because, as the glucose returns to the cells, both potassium and phosphate also will return to an intracellular location and the serum potassium will be reduced. It is thus appropriate to monitor serum potassium closely in all ketotic/diabetics under treatment. Of course, some diabetics that are not ketotic do not really have a serious problem of electrolyte imbalance. They might also receive frequent potassium measurements and this might not be as easily defensible.

PANEL THREE

Participants: S. G. Pauker (Chair), E. A. Johnson, J. D. Myers,
R. E. Miller, and H. C. Sox

Question: Please speculate on the likelihood of getting physicians to use algorithms that they have not been involved in formulating? Even if you can get a consensus at the academic level, can you expand their use to the practicing physician?

H. Sox: That's a very hard question to answer, but I think there is enough basis for at least some reasonably informed speculation. As I indicated in my talk, it is unclear how algorithms are used in community practice. We have almost no information. Dr. Komaroff has quizzed some of the people who bought his algorithms. What he found was that by and large they used them not in the form that he had so painfully constructed them, but took pieces out of them that suited the practice, the physician, and the nurse practitioner who were in the practice. It looks to me as if physicians will take pieces of things, essentially ratify them as being appropriate to their practice, and develop a standard of practice that the nurse practitioner, and presumably by inference the physician, is willing to follow in most patients, at least in those patients sufficiently stereotyped to warrant a reasonably stereotyped diagnostic strategy. My own feeling is that physicians are not likely to adopt new strategies unless there is reasonable evidence that those strategies are superior to the ones that are currently used. That is the reason that I and a number of my colleagues have concentrated on trying to look more critically at the diagnostic value of the history and physical examination in relation to diagnosis and test outcome and try to develop strategies that will be demonstrably superior to those that are currently in force.

Question: Will decision analysis ever be applicable to central problems of ambulatory medicine?

S. Pauker: Perhaps, since the problems of ambulatory medicine are so much more common. You don't kill a fly with an atom bomb. Decision analysis is an extremely time-consuming technique and you save it for two kinds of things—a very complex problem that is unusual, or a common problem where guidelines can be used over and over and over again. Dr. Komaroff has been instrumental in applying decision analysis to the development of clinical algorithms. In part, he builds his algorithms and determines the flows by decision analytic approaches. That's a very exciting technique.

Question: Do you think the use of clinical algorithms can reduce the cost of care or maintain a hold if physician assistants or nurse practitioners belonged to a union that demanded M.D. pay for M.D. work?

H. Sox: I think the slides that I showed will answer the point pretty clearly. If physician assistants and nurse practitioners are paid equal to physicians, obviously the cost savings are going to be less and it will take more attention to the content of the algorithm to achieve cost savings. But as indicated by the work of Bob Wood and Paul Rocke from Seattle, it is possible to design algorithms at least for upper respiratory illness and back pain, that can cut the laboratory test costs virtually in half, irrespective of the contribution that the provider's salary makes to the total cost of the encounter.

Question: What is the cost of doing a single case analysis using INTERNIST? How many physician years have been needed to put it into service? What is the cost of acquisition of the computers and operating costs? What will be the role of this in general health care? Can we afford it?

J. Myers: We have estimates regarding the cost of a case analysis by INTERNIST. We are supported totally by the National Institutes of Health at the present time. We are supplied with a telephone network; we are supplied with the computer at Stanford and a backup computer at Rutgers. Our best honest estimate is that the kind of analysis that I showed you will cost about $25, which in the current cost scale of medical care is by no means excessive. The cost might be offset by the selectivity of work-up, by saving time, unnecessary x-ray films, or laboratory tests. We can't prove that, but we have reasons to think that might be possible. The economics of this approach are not at all unreasonable. As one looks ahead a few years there are reasons to expect that the program could be made to operate on self-contained computers that the physician could have in his office. This could be updated with a modern version of the knowledge base periodically—every three to six months. That would not be highly expensive. We see no practical blockade to the use of this kind of system as an aid to the physician.

I have put in approximately four man years in the development of IN-TERNIST and I will be putting in probably three to four more years. We have had a young faculty member who has put in two, a number of fellows and students who have put in some, so I suppose if you add it all up from the medical standpoint, there have been approximately ten man years. From the computer science standpoint, probably the same time has been invested. Now, on the other hand, we have got the greatest part—we estimate about 80 percent—of a "textbook" on internal medicine programmed and checked out. I don't have to apologize for this expenditure of time, nor do I have to apologize to the federal government for using their money. I don't know of any program comparable to this in this country or overseas in its scope or objectives. So if we can swing it, I think we have got a facility that is worth the investment in man hours and dollars both.

Question: Has the decrease in cost associated with reduced tests been compared with the costs of the increased frequency of decision mistakes?

R. Miller: No. I think that is an important question. Are we doing what the operations researchers term "suboptimizing," in other words, making the laboratory most efficient at the cost of making the entire cost of the patient care process less efficient? I think that is a pitfall that we must be very careful to avoid. But there are no hard answers on such commonly posed questions as does accelerated laboratory testing decrease length of stay? What is the magnitude of the false positive problem due to multichannel testing on admission, etc. We must avoid the pitfall of suboptimizing that might result from simply concentrating on decreased laboratory testing.

Question: The chances of aneurysm rupture, the chances of dying from surgery, post MI, are not known for patients with exactly your patient's clinical characteristics. We cannot perform decision analysis with numbers derived without adequate information. What we need first is data on prognosis without intervention that includes all pertinent clinical features of large groups of patient subclasses. The literature contains information about interventions and outcome probabilities. Has there been any attempt to organize or collect such information so as to assist formal decision making?

S. Pauker: First of all, no patients are exactly alike. When you take data from the literature and use that to apply to your individual patient, you are making the tacit assumption that your patient is just like those in the article. That rarely is the case. So you very often need to tune that data using your skill as a physician and a prognostician. Indeed that skill is in part that which you get in your medical training. It would be great if we could collect all the objective data that we need. I expect that given the number of relevant subcategories that will not be happening for a long time.

As we go through the literature looking for data, we often find that the data aren't there in the form that we would like. Until recently medicine and the physician have had no way to deal and use the data that we are now asking for. So there was no reason to put them in the literature. As we are now developing those reasons, authors will begin to report them. I hope that all of you begin to collect and organize the necessary information in a way we can all use it.

J. Myers: I very much agree with your last comments. In certain areas this has begun. For example, Dr. Stead has a wonderful knowledge base on myocardial infarction. They have recorded many parameters regarding myocardial infarction that you won't find anywhere in the literature because nobody in the past has been interested. It is very important that these clinical knowledge bases now be built up. How much I would like to have built our program from these! But if I had relied on individuals to build up each knowledge base, de novo, it would have taken many decades to get where we are instead of 8 years. But that should be forthcoming, and must be encouraged.

S. Pauker: That raises a related issue. I couldn't take our patient with aortic aneurysm and suggest that he be frozen until we could obtain the right data. We needed to make a decision now and in medicine we will always need to do that. We will need to take the best advantage of what we have now, anticipating what may be available later.

H. Sox: There are two ways in which you can use a computer database. One is to feed in the characteristics of your patient and ask for a patient-specific prognosis, in this case, perhaps the risk of death from the surgery. Another approach was used by Lee Goldman, who collected data on a thousand patients about to undergo noncardiac surgery. He observed which patients died and which patients had nonfatal cardiac complications. He was then able to use discriminant analysis to create a rule that identified about eight key factors. The discriminant analysis weighted these factors in a way that optimized the discrimination between patients with and without the bad outcomes of surgery. As a result, now a clinician can obtain this information on a patient and establish where this patient falls into one of four risk categories, very high to very low risk. Thus, it's not necessary to have a computer as the intermediary in this process of using a data base in order to make risk stratification.

Question: How much malpractice insurance does INTERNIST carry?

J. Meyers: This is a question that in one form or another is inevitably asked. We don't carry any because we are still in the experimental and developmental stage. INTERNIST is a consultative program. This program is not in any way intended to replace or substitute for the physician. Information about a case analysis goes only to the physician. I look upon the program as I look upon myself when I am a consultant to a physician. That physician can accept my opinions, he can reject them, or he can take part of them. The same thing will be true of this analysis. Now I know that that is an oversimplified answer, because we are living in an age where a great part of the public unfortunately has more confidence in machines than it has in people. It is a problem to be kept in mind and I am not sure what the eventual answer is.

Question: The evoking strength and frequency values provide approximate conditional probabilities. Do you allow costs of mistakes to weight the choices? The issue being addressed here is that diagnostic errors of different sorts may carry different costs. Missing a treatable disease may be far worse than missing a non-treatable one.

J. Meyers: We are well aware of this concern but at the present time it doesn't fit in. We haven't figured out yet any way that we can give real precedence to a treatable over a nontreatable disease without upsetting the real nature of the analytical program. Right now the diagnoses are based on the best fit method of the model to the information. This concern, I think, would have to be something that the physician should judge. I don't think that it is something that we should turn over to a machine. I remember old Sam Levine, the cardiologist at Brigham, said, "I'm not interested in making a diagnosis of multiple sclerosis, because I can't do anything about that. I want to know whether this patient has a spinal cord tumor which I can remove." So he was perfectly happy to miss the diagnosis of multiple sclerosis all the time, provided he could pick up the spinal cord tumor. I don't want the computer to do that, though. I don't think you would want the computer to do that. If it came down to a differential diagnosis between the two, then I think you are going to have to provide the pragmatism. I don't know how we can get the machine to provide it.

Question: You have shown the applicability of decision analysis to individual clinical problems. In your consulting role, how do you elicit subjective utilities? Could you give examples?

S. Pauker: My major research interest, as is one of the interests of Dr. McNeal is just that issue—the issue of elicitation and use of patient utility values. I really can't go into that in great detail except that in my mind, one of the great strengths of the approach is that is does give a formal way to do that. Some of the consultations that we see are addressed at that specific issue. For example, a 65-year-old man who I saw had peripheral vascular disease. The surgeon had to either perform a bilateral AK amputation or try major salvage procedures. The cardiologist felt that the operative risk of the procedure was going to be 20 or 30 percent. The decision depends on how that patient values his legs relative to his life! I can't answer that question—you can't. We need to go to that patient and some way get that input.

We have done a fair amount with the issue of prenatal diagnosis and amniocenteses. My wife, who is a pediatrician, a genetic counselor, and I have developed a utility model for that situation. We have counseled well over 400 individuals using the model.

Question: Computer programs as described for differential diagnosis, decision analysis, etc., seem to be available to or applicable to the institutions developing them. Can they be more widely disseminated?

J. Myers: The kind of program that we are developing really was not feasible to develop until the last decade. The computer technology that would handle the kind of program represented by INTERNIST has been there only for the last decade. I think we are making good speed and we feel that within two years INTERNIST will be ready for dissemination, after field trial to ascertain its reliability.

E. Johnson: When it is disseminated, each individual institution should accumulate its own experience, its own prevalence rates, and have the opportunity to put their own utility functions in.

S. Pauker: I would suggest not each institution, but each practitioner.

H. Sox: I speak for a group who is trying to develop improved decision strategies that can be written down. The obvious mode of dissemination for these are peer review journals and the obvious rate-limiting step is the referees of these journals.

S. Pauker: Let me make one final comment about that, not that I don't agree with everything that has been said, but let me for the moment—for the sake of argument—come down on a different side. Technology develops and things get published. It doesn't mean that things get read. Technology changes; you can each now own a personal computer. Probably in five years, you can have Jack Myers' PDP-10 to carry around in your pocket, the same way that I carry around a calculator. So over the next few years, technology will not be a limitation. The limitation is the same as it's been in medicine for the last three thousand years. Education. We need to teach each other, teach our students, and teach everyone out there that this is available and can be developed. And we need to attract more people into the field to create the manpower to develop it. And that's you, that's education coming from meetings like this.

PANEL FOUR

Participants: T. F. Ferris (Chair), M. D. Burke, J. M. Eisenberg,
S. E. Goldfinger, P. F. Griner, and L. L. Weed

Question: Since modification of physician behavior appears to be mediated through a change induced in opinion leaders, why should the unit of analysis be the individual physician? Wouldn't a more cost-effective educational strategy be to identify cultural units or teams, for example, a particular medical service or residency program rather than the individual physician?

J. Eisenberg: We do not understand physician behavior well enough at this point to know whether they behave as teams or as autonomous individuals. I suspect they believe their behavior to be autonomous. Nonetheless, the probability is that individual physicians are influenced by other members of their team. I suggest that both team and individual behavior be studied because unless this is done, we may be unable to discover why some physicians respond to behavior modification programs and others do not.

Question: Considering that only two-thirds of the potentially eligible senior medical students at the University of Minnesota take the laboratory medicine elective course, do you have any evidence to indicate that their subsequent behavior in residency and later in practice differs from those who do not take the course?

M. D. Burke: No. It is unfortunate, but we have not had the opportunity to study actual behavior of any students in the postgraduate years. We have studied the behavior of both groups in subsequent senior rotations in clinical medicine and pediatrics. As judged by the clinicians responsible for those rotations, the group who elected the laboratory medicine course performed significantly better than the control group insofar as the appropriateness of their test ordering was concerned. (Ward PCJ, Harris IB, Burke MD, Horwitz CA. Systematic instruction in interpretive aspects of laboratory medicine. J Med Educ 1976;51:648-56.)

Question: How far should we allow the public to indulge themselves in the practice of medicine? Should we establish open diagnostic laboratory facilities analogous to Colonel Sanders' Fried Chicken restaurants?

L. Weed: I think that once computers and medical maps are generally available, the scenario you described will undoubtedly take place. Ninety-nine percent of the practice of medicine on this globe today is self-practice anyway. The important question is the extent or the degree to which the public will become involved. I believe that the boundaries will extend and that lay persons will make use of newly developed tools. I also believe it will be safer because they can inject their own values into the decision-making process. So I would say let it go as far as it will and have the physician work with the patient so that both justify their actions and make their logic explicit.

Question: How do you define excessive laboratory use in the absence of defined indications—in the case of electrolytes, for example?

P. Griner: We do so in two ways. The first involves no more than the application of an intuitive common sense. The second is more explicit and based on retrospective studies.

The first approach is best illustrated by an example: a patient with acute myocardial infarction has an uncomplicated 10-day hospital stay during which he is not receiving any medications of significance, but has electrolytes ordered and duly performed on a daily basis. The house officer then discharges the patient with the order to return to the clinic in two weeks, during which time he has no laboratory determination of any sort performed. What is the logic in requiring 10 straight days of in-hospital monitoring and none once the patient leaves the hospital? That approach is entirely intuitive.

The second more explicit approach is based on the evidence that despite an exponential increase in laboratory testing, for example, an eightfold increase in blood gas determinations over several years—there is no measurable change in reasonably definable outcome measures such as length of hospitalization, complication rate, mortality, etc. In other words, increased use of laboratory data has not shown an improvement in outcome.

Question: How do you propose to implement the changes you advocate in the practice of medicine when you consider the current political and economic environment?

L. Weed: We are working on that right now. The system is now virtually ready to be exported and we are attempting to find a small hospital in which the doctors' offices, pharmacy, etc., would all be electronic. We have some possibilities in mind. The university hospitals are almost out of the question; their fiefdoms are so out of control that they find it difficult to think as a unit. There has been considerable interest from both the British and the Japanese in our system. In fact, representatives from medical institutions in both countries have spent considerable time with us and probably know more about the system than anyone in the United States.

Question: Since hospitals—especially nonprofit community hospitals—hang by a fragile thread financially, and since their major source of income is diagnostic testing of one sort or another, why should such institutions encourage production and test utilization? Would not cost exceed revenue and reimbursement decrease under such circumstances?

P. Griner: The question is an important one. It is true that in most areas of the country reimbursement mechanisms provide no incentive to reduce laboratory or other diagnostic testing. However, in the eastern part of the United States, including Rochester, New York, alternative and more creative mechanisms are already under way. In essence, hospitals are guaranteed an annual income with an adjusted inflation factor based on costs incurred over the previous two years. Here, the incentives are quite different; in effect, they promote efficiency and conservation of resources. Our own experience, after only six months of this type of reimbursement system, is that efficiency is improved and resources are, in fact, conserved.

Question: Will your system make physicians obsolete?

L. Weed: No. But to expand on that a bit, I must explain the system, its participants, and what we mean by physicians. We have a group within the medical system who develop new ideas, build the options, and make the displays—they don't need M.D. degrees. There are others who work out the logic pathways and do the statistical studies—they don't need M.D. degrees either. There is yet another group who actually make the system work by taking this mass of information and applying it in a real and personal sense. Nurses are excellent at this. In my view, we should select from the population at large individuals who love other people, who possess interpersonal skills, who have, for example, a "great pair of hands," and we should train them to apply our information. They should not be taught the basic sciences. But as you well know, no one was ever taught the basic sciences—only the stories of basic science; not the scientific method. Some in the group will require an M.D. degree. However, an M.D. degree in itself should be no guarantee of exceptionally high income. Among the group there will be some who do their job very well and should be paid accordingly. Since "all the graduates of Juilliard are not Rubinsteins" the same does not apply to the remainder.

Question: Because of current reimbursement practices, income derived from office laboratory procedures may be used by primary care physicians to offset other costs. Please comment on this.

J. Eisenberg: There is evidence to show that if a primary care physician in his office practice uses all the diagnostic technology at his disposal, he can triple his income. This, of course, is a function of current reimbursement practices. But it also follows that if the physician decreases his utilization of laboratory and other diagnostic tests, his income will decrease. The magnitude of the problem is a minor one when compared with the potential for reimbursement afforded the non-primary care physician who overuses the more expensive nondiagnostic procedures. The answer to both problems is, of course, altered reimbursement practices.

Question: Since you stated that the problem of inappropriate test ordering may be a lack of knowledge, do you have data to show that improving knowledge leads to more selective laboratory use—particularly in the light of Dr. Goldfinger's comments?

M. D. Burke: Only under the simulated conditions that I discussed in the lecture. To be quite specific, we have evidence that senior medical students use laboratory tests more appropriately under simulated conditions immediately after taking our course than they do beforehand.

Question: It appears that the educational process is best effected by positive role models. If, in fact, that is true—where are these role models to be found?

J. Eisenberg: So far, they have been found on the staffs at university hospitals. I suspect, however, that there is another potentially large pool of positive role models among experienced practicing physicians. We know that older physicians use fewer tests than do the younger group. This may be because we have shown in the case of residents that physicians order fewer tests as they progress or gain in experience. The alternate hypothesis is that the number of tests ordered by physicians does not change with maturity, and the reason older physicians order fewer tests is that they behave as they did 30 or 40 years ago. If, however, the original hypothesis is correct, then it may be that exposing students to the diagnostic strategies of the mature physician would accelerate the maturation process and be a more effective approach to laboratory overuse.

T. Ferris: When I was at Yale, I had such a role model. He happened to be my tutor and his name was Weed. He made great demands upon us in terms of compulsive adherence to therapeutic protocol, for example, in the intensive care of ketoacidosis, and now I'm chagrined to find that what he told us and what we still do doesn't make any sense at all.

L. Weed: It makes sense and it's fabulous—but only for a few patients. It was good for both of us, but irrelevant to society's need.

Question: When an educational strategy fails, what steps do you take to assess the reasons for failure?

S. Goldfinger: I think that is a good question. A better question would be "Do you take any steps at all, or do you just keep doing the same thing?" There is general agreement, of course, that educational enterprises be evaluated. It is very difficult to evaluate continuing education in outcome terms. What is usually done is that the process is evaluated and, in particular, the satisfaction or "happiness index" of the participants is given special attention. This kind of evaluation serves the purpose of the course organizers in that it determines which speakers to reinvite for subsequent courses and so forth. It provides very little information on the effect of a course in any real outcome terms.

Question: How often have you used Bayes' theorem in your last month of ward duty? If so, could you please provide some examples.

P. Griner: The opportunity to adopt a quantitative reasoning approach exists in virtually every case. To answer your question more specifically, perhaps every other morning on attending rounds, a particular problem lends itself to this approach. A common example is the patient who presents with obscure symptoms and signs suggesting the diagnosis of lupus erythematosus. We would first define what we are trying to do. Since the majority of such patients do not have lupus, we would argue that the primary purpose of the test is to exclude the disease. We would assume, based on our own previous experience, that the prior probability of lupus is about 20%. We then discuss the choice of exclusion test. Since we know that serum ANA has a sensitivity of more than 99%, we know that the probability of lupus after obtaining a negative rest result is virtually nil. To be precise, it is approximately two-tenths of one percent. Under these circumstances, I explain to the house staff that given that degreee of assurance they may, if they wish, repeat the test—that approach doesn't worry me as much as if they had failed to interpret the implications of the first negative test result.

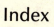

Index

Index

351

Donald P. Connelly is assistant professor and director
of the laboratory data division in the department of
laboratory medicine and pathology at the University
of Minnesota. **Ellis S. Benson** is professor and head of
the same department. **M. Desmond Burke** is professor
of pathology and director of clinical laboratories,
University Hospital, State University of New York
at Stony Brook. **Douglas A. Fenderson** is director
of continuing medical education at the University
of Minnesota.